THE LEADERSHIP TRAJECTORY

DEVELOPING LEGACY *Leaders*-SHIP

THE LEADERSHIP TRAJECTORY

DEVELOPING LEGACY *Leaders*-SHIP

Patricia S. Yoder-Wise, EdD, RN, NEA-BC, ANEF, FAONL, FAAN

Karren Kowalski, PhD, RN, NEA-BC, ANEF, FAAN

Susan Sportsman, PhD, RN, ANEF, FAAN

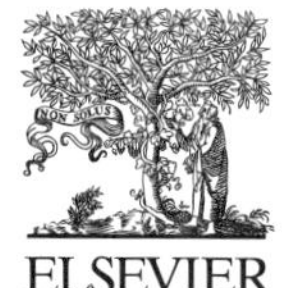

ELSEVIER

Elsevier
3251 Riverport Lane
St. Louis, MO 63043

THE LEADERSHIP TRAJECTORY: DEVELOPING LEGACY *LEADERS*-SHIP ISBN: 978-0-323-59754-8

Library of Congress Control Number: 2020942470

Senior Content Strategist: Yvonne Alexopoulos
Senior Content Development Manager: Luke Held
Senior Content Development Specialist: Jennifer Wade
Publishing Services Manager: Julie Eddy
Project Manager: Andrew Schubert
Designer: Patrick Ferguson

Printed in the United States of America

Last digit is the print number: 9 8 7 6 5 4 3 2 1

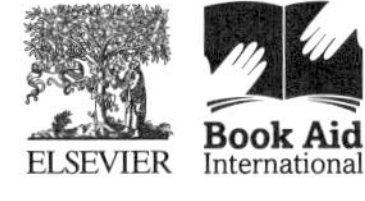

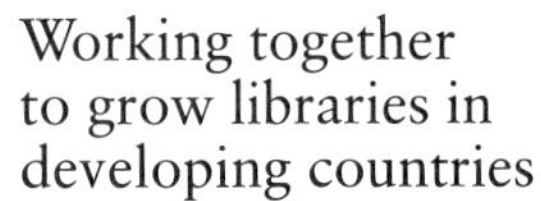

ABOUT THE AUTHORS

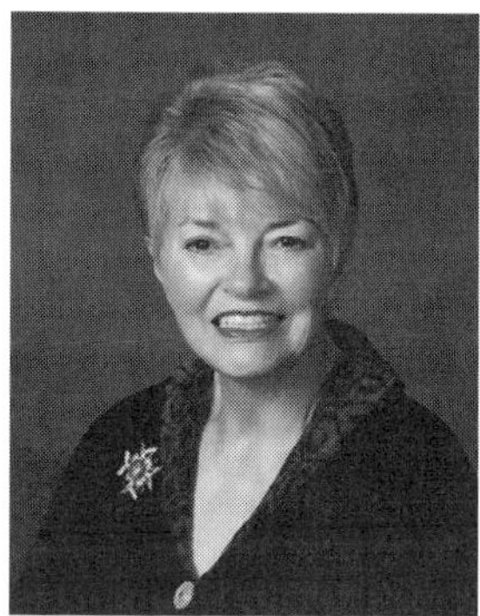

Patricia S. Yoder-Wise, EdD, RN, NEA-BC, ANEF, FAONL, FAAN
Professor and Dean Emerita
Texas Tech University Health Sciences Center School of Nursing;
President, The Wise Group
Lubbock, Texas
Patricia.Yoder-Wise@TTUHSC.EDU
TheLeadershipTrajectory@gmail.com

Pat is the editor (and an author) of *Leading and Managing in Nursing*, a leading text for undergraduate students since 1994. She has held leadership positions in service, education, and professional associations. Pat served as Educational Director for the Ohio Nurses Association before moving to Michigan to serve as an assistant director of nursing and (later) head of a nursing department. After serving as the Director for Continuing Education at the University of Colorado School of Nursing, Pat moved to Texas to help start a school of nursing in a health sciences center in west Texas. In addition to serving as President of the Texas Nurses Association, she also served as President of the American Nurses Credentialing Center, Treasurer of the American Academy of Nursing, President of the Association for Leadership Science in Nursing, and President of the National League for Nursing. She is an Inaugural Fellow of the Academy of Nursing Education and the American Organization for Nursing Leadership and a Fellow of the American Academy of Nursing. Among various awards, including teaching awards at Texas Tech, she has been honored by *Women of Excellence in Medicine*, Young Women's Christian Association, and *100 Transformers in Nursing and Healthcare*, The Ohio State University College of Nursing. She received the *Leaders Legacy Award*, Texas Nurses Association, and serves as Editor-in-Chief for *The Journal of Continuing Education in Nursing* and *Nursing Forum*. The Wise Group provides leadership development and writing consultation. She is also a member of the CNO Academy faculty. Pat is known as a connector and maximizer and is always open to new experiences. She has two favorite sayings: "There are no mistakes in the universe" and "Lead on!" Both help her understand her multiple connections and where we are headed in the profession.

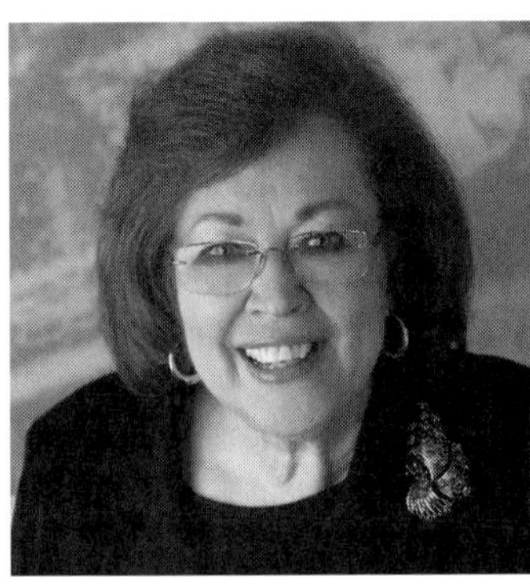

Karren Kowalski, PhD, RN, NEA-BC, ANEF, FAAN
Professor
Texas Tech University Health Sciences Center School of Nursing;
President & CEO, Kowalski & Associates
Larkspur, Colorado
www.KowalskiAndAssociates.com
Karren.kowalski@att.net
TheLeadershipTrajectory@gmail.com

Karren is an educator, speaker, author, Magnet® appraiser, and leadership expert. She has held multiple leadership positions at various hospitals and nursing organizations. Karren is recognized as a dynamic leader in health care and a powerful, engaging speaker. She served as President and CEO for the Colorado Center for Nursing Excellence, the largest nursing workforce center in the country, and was project director for more than 10 major state and federal grants totaling more than $12 million. Currently, she serves as President and CEO of Kowalski and Associates, a consulting group that focuses on education, coaching, problem solving, and leadership development. She has authored numerous articles and co-edited six advanced nursing textbooks. Karren is a Professor at Texas Tech University Health Sciences Center School of Nursing, where she teaches every summer in the DNP program. She also serves as an Associate Editor for the *Journal of Continuing Education in Nursing*, where she is responsible for the monthly column on Teaching Tips, a reflection of her love of teaching and presentations. Karren has served as a Magnet® hospital appraiser since 2008, committing to the program because she believes it has increased the quality of patient care across the country and internationally.

She has held multiple leadership positions, including Assistant Vice President and Administrator, the Women's and Children's Hospital, Rush-Presbyterian-St. Luke's Medical Center, and Chair, Department of Maternal Child Nursing, College of Nursing, Rush University, Chicago.

She volunteers in professional organizations and has served as President of the Colorado Nurses' Association, President of the Association for Leadership Science in Nursing, President of the University of Colorado Nursing Alumni Association, and Secretary of the Nurses on Boards Coalition (NOBC), the national goal of which is to address quality health care by having 10,000 nurses serve on health care and community boards of directors. She has served on boards, such as the American Academy of Nursing; was appointed by the Governor to the Colorado Commission for Veterans Community Living Centers, the long-term care facilities for veterans, which she also chaired; and served on several nursing journal editorial boards.

Karren is the recipient of numerous honors and awards, including being a 2010 Colorado Florence Nightingale recipient, Distinguished Alumnae of the University of Colorado School of Nursing; was selected as one of the Ten Outstanding Young Women of America; and is a charter member of the Colorado Nurses Association Hall of Fame. She was honored as a Fellow in the American Academy of Nursing and a Fellow of the Academy of Nursing Education. In 2015, she was selected from the 30,000 nursing graduates as one of the Top 100 Alumni Legacy Leaders for the 100th Anniversary of the Indiana University School of Nursing.

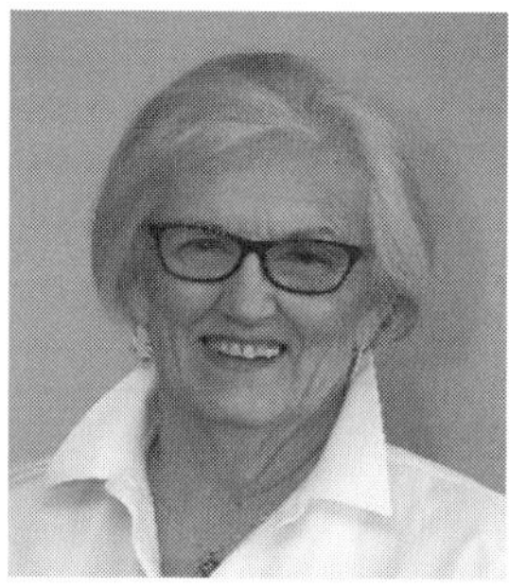

Susan Sportsman, PhD, RN, ANEF, FAAN
Managing Director
Collaborative Momentum Consulting
http://collaborativemomentum.com
TheLeadershipTrajectory@gmail.com

Susy is a Managing Director of Collaborative Momentum Consulting, an independent consulting firm focused on providing nurse educators throughout North American with expert guidance and consultation in the areas of student, faculty, and program performance and leadership development. Her consultation work is informed by her experience as a faculty member, administrator, and leader in both service and education.

Before starting Collaborative Momentum, Susy served as Director of Consulting Services at Elsevier Education Division. Her educational leadership roles included Dean of Health Sciences and Human Services, Midwestern State University, and Associate Dean of Practice at Texas Tech University Health Sciences Center School of Nursing. In service, she was the Vice President of Mental Health Programs at Harris Methodist Health System (now Texas Health Resources) and founding administrator of Tarrant County Psychiatric Center, Tarrant County Mental Health Mental Retardation Center. Susy has published a number of peer-reviewed articles on leadership, simulation, and education and is a contributor to several texts, including *Leading and Managing in Nursing* and *Nursing Now*.

Despite her experience in a wide range of settings, Susy finds common themes threaded throughout her career. She says, "Regardless of the environment in which I was working, there were two opportunities that I found most exciting. The first was the chance to mentor, teach, and collaborate with others. The second was being able to start something new. Whether it was starting a new public psychiatric hospital, establishing a simulation center shared by education and service, or introducing a new program or curriculum (or revising those that were not working), I have always loved finding ways to bring positive change to improve outcomes."

Susy has brought her innovative spirit to a variety of professional organizations, including the American Nurses Association (ANA), National League for Nursing (NLN), and Sigma at the local, state, and national levels, including as President of the Texas Nurses Association. Her contribution to the profession has been recognized as an Outstanding Alumni of the Baylor University Louise Herrington School of Nursing, a Great 100 Nurses of Texas Woman's University College of Nursing, a Fellow in the NLN Academy of Nurse Educators, and a Fellow in the American Academy of Nursing. Her favorite quote from Neale Donald Walsch, which seems appropriate for an innovator, is "Life begins at the end of your comfort zone."

REVIEWERS

Sameeya Ahmed-Winston, CPNP, CPHON, BMTCN
Team Lead
Blood and Marrow Transplantation
Children's National Health System
Washington, DC

Stephanie C. Evans, PhD, APRN, CPNP-PC, CLC
Assistant Professor
Nursing Department
Texas Christian University
Harris College of Nursing and Health Sciences
Fort Worth, Texas

Kami L. Fox, DNP, MS, RN, APRN, CNP-PC
Director
Department of Nursing
Ohio Northern University
Ada, Ohio

Brad Harrell, DNP, APRN, ACNP-BC
Clinical Associate Professor
Director of MSN Programs
Loewenberg College of Nursing
University of Memphis
Memphis, Tennessee

Janine Johnson, RN, MSN
Associate Professor of Nursing
Undergraduate Nursing
Clarkson College
Omaha, Nebraska

Kathleen S. Jordan, DNP, RN, FNP-BC, ENP-C, SANE-P, FAEN
Clinical Associate Professor
Nursing Department
The University Of North Carolina at Charlotte
Charlotte, North Carolina

Francis Nannette Ketcham, PhD (c), MSN, RN, CNE
Clinical Associate Professor
Baylor University
Dallas, Texas

Molly Leer, MS, RN, CNE
LPN-BSN Coordinator
Nursing Department
University of Mary
Bismarck, North Dakota

Dr. Analena Michelle Lunde, DNP, RN, A/P-SANE
Assistant Professor in Nursing
Department of Nursing
Dickinson State University
Dickinson, North Dakota

Barbara Pinekenstein, DNP, RN-BC, CPHIMS, FAAN
Clinical Professor, Richard E. Sinaiko Professor in Health Care Leadership
Nursing Department
University of Wisconsin, Madison
Madison, Wisconsin

Dulce Santacroce DNP, RN, CCM
RN-BSN Coordinator
Nursing Department
Touro University Nevada
Henderson, Nevada

Dr. Crystal R. Sherman, DNP, RN
Associate Professor
Nursing Department
Shawnee State University
Portsmouth, Ohio

Shelly Wells, PhD, MBA, APRN-CNS, CNS-BC, ANEF
Division Chair and Professor
Charles Morton Share Trust Division of Nursing
Northwestern Oklahoma State University
Alva, Oklahoma

CIRCLE OF ADVISORS

Jane Barnsteiner, PhD, RN, FAAN
Professor Emerita
School of Nursing
University of Pennsylvania
Editor
Translational Research and Quality Improvement
American Journal of Nursing
Philadelphia, Pennsylvania

Linda Burnes Bolton, DrPH, RN, FAAN
Senior Vice President and Chief Health Equity Officer
Cedars-Sinai
Los Angeles, California

Karen Cox, PhD, RN, FACHE, FAAN
President and Professor of Nursing
Chamberlain University
Downers Grove, Illinois

Joanne Disch, PhD, RN, FAAN
Professor ad Honorem
University of Minnesota School of Nursing
Minneapolis, Minnesota

Linda Q. Everett, PhD, RN, NEA-BC, FAONL, FAAN
Adjunct Professor
Frances Payne Bolton School of Nursing
Case Western Reserve University
Stow, Ohio

Maureen "Shawn" Kennedy, MA, RN, FAAN
Editor in Chief
American Journal of Nursing
New York, New York

Angela Barron McBride, PhD, RN, FAAN
Distinguished Professor & University Dean Emerita
Indiana University School of Nursing
Lafayette, Indiana

Dedication

As we are proofing this publication, we are doing so from our homes because each of us has been told to stay at home. Yet many of you are going to work each day, often to understaffed and underequipped settings. Out of every tragedy, some bright ray of hope breaks through. We have read numerous stories of nurses stepping up and stepping out to advocate for their peers and their patients, providing care under unbelievable conditions, putting themselves in harm's way to respond to clinical needs, and leading on issues in ways never dreamed of before. The focus of this book is that it takes a group of leaders to create a legacy. Nurses have just demonstrated how they take on the unbelievable and rise to the occasion for the people we serve. Thank you for all you have done and will continue to do. May we never have another test of our leadership like this one!

PREFACE

Welcome to another book on leadership! Rather than providing *the* answers to effective leadership, this book is geared toward helping individuals determine what they need to learn and practice to be highly effective leaders.

Adam Grant suggested that good leadership books do three things. First, they introduce original ideas. Thus, you will find a model for your individual use in developing your leadership abilities at any point in your career.

Second, they support those ideas with evidence and experience. As a result, you will find that the critical elements of the model derive from the literature and our Circle of Advisors, experts who shared their advice about leadership. We incorporated examples of our experiences (and those of others) throughout.

Third, leadership books should be engaging. With this idea in mind, we wrote this book in a style reminiscent of a one-way conversation. For example, we deliberately chose a referencing style designed to keep readers engaged with the message itself. Furthermore, the informal writing style is deliberate—we are talking to *you*! Although you don't have the opportunity to talk with us as you move through the book, you do have opportunities to engage with the content and to contact us directly through email (TheLeadershipTrajectory@gmail.com).

Many nurses who enroll in graduate-level programs arrive with several years of experience in a formal leadership role. In essence, they are already in positions they desire to hold. They have returned to formal education because they seek the knowledge (and the degree) to validate their current practice. Is it easier to learn first and then enter a role? Maybe, but the reality is we all are wherever we are in life. As a result, we find our leadership trajectory is informed by where we've been rather than an imagined version of what leadership might be like.

This book is also designed for all of us who might not be enrolled in an educational program. Many of us are interested in ongoing leadership development. This book is designed to help all of us (both those seeking degrees and those looking to enhance themselves) be better at leading and to develop or refine skills designed to promote leadership at its best.

You will see a model that depicts how you can develop your leadership skills to attain the level of Legacy *Leaders*-Ship, regardless of your position or setting. The content of this book is designed for leading wherever you are in your career and doing so from the power of you versus the title of your position. Each element in the model is addressed separately, and yet each is only of great value when integrated with other elements.

In the big picture, think how an organizational setting influences how you act and what you are supposed to do. The integration of the person with the environment creates multiple dimensions for us. Someone who is undervalued in the employment setting might be seen as a dynamic leader in a state nurse association's board.

In each chapter, we provide at least one reflection to help you recall the leadership talents you already have, determine how you might develop a particular skill or insight, or consider how you can use a skill or insight in your current or future work. To best take advantage of your reflections, we suggest you keep a journal—handwritten or electronic—so you can look back on your thinking later.

Each chapter has an LL Alert (Legacy *Leaders*-Ship Alert), which conveys what not to do in relation to the message of the chapter. We also include an LL Lineup (Legacy *Leaders*-Ship Lineup) to remind you of the big points made in the chapter.

Because we believe that stories make content meaningful and illustrate how you can develop or enhance your own personal story-telling ability, we have integrated stories throughout. Most commonly, these are our (the authors') stories. Although some of you know one or more of us, few if any of us have met Warren Buffet; Martin Luther King, Jr.; Steve Jobs; or any of the other highly influential leaders in the world. We hope the stories of nurses in their ongoing leadership development will provide practical examples to help you develop your own stories.

The chapters are short and pointed. They aren't designed to be comprehensive on a topic but rather to be the catalyst to learning more about the topics each reader identifies as important in terms of his or her personal development. In addition to the usual references (e.g., nursing and business literature), we include a few citations from social media and newspapers. This approach was designed with two thoughts in mind: First, we can learn about leadership from multiple sources. Second, we want to show the prevalence of concern for leadership in our society. If we had sufficient leaders, we wouldn't be writing about what it takes to be a leader or providing pithy comments about being a leader. These examples show how much our society is concerned with leadership. Nurses have the foundation on which to enhance their skills to contribute in even bigger ways than we have in the past. In fact, we are counting on you!

All of these features are designed to help create the best possible level of preparedness. However, all of this, plus all of the other books about leadership, can't make you ready. To quote Tim Cook, CEO of Apple, in his speech to the 2019 graduating class at Stanford, "And when he [Steve Jobs] was gone, truly gone, I learned the real, visceral difference between preparation and readiness.

"It was the loneliest I've ever felt in my life. By an order of magnitude. It was one of those moments where you can be surrounded by people, yet you don't really see, hear or even feel them. But I could sense their expectations.

"When the dust settled, all I knew was that I was going to have to be the best version of myself that I could be."

If someone like Tim Cook couldn't feel ready, we shouldn't add the stress of having such expectations for ourselves. Jobs worked closely with Cook, yet Cook still didn't feel ready. Few of us have the opportunity to learn from masters in their field about what it takes to be the key leader in an organization or division. We do have the opportunity to learn and practice our skills no matter what position we hold or what support systems we have. We have to be as well-prepared as possible to do our best wherever we are and to be ready to take on new challenges when they appear.

Thank you in advance for looking at your leadership potential and being willing to reach new heights. We would love to hear about your journey at TheLeadershipTrajectory@gmail.com and wish you the best!

Lead on!
¡Adelente!

BIBLIOGRAPHY

Cook T. Commencement Address. Stanford University. June 16, 2019. Available at: https://news.stanford.edu/2019/06/16/remarks-tim-cook-2019-stanford-commencement.

Grant A. 2018. Available at: https://twitter.com/AdamMGrant/status/1078275853153374208.

CONTENTS

Strategies Overview

When viewing the model, we see a trajectory from the base, which is composed of our individual purpose, lifelong learning, our values, and the profession—the foundation for the model. The trajectory from the base to the legacy contains strategies that are needed by most developing leaders. These strategies are processes that support leader growth and development. For example, each of us should begin with an assessment of where we are at any given moment in our career and development. Honestly assessing and understanding where we are in relation to our personal growth and evolution as a leader is critical to deciding what the next steps should be in the leadership development process. Self-assessment also involves a process of reflection. Reflecting on where we have been and what was learned from experiences is an excellent strategy, especially when it is focused on how we can do something differently the next time we encounter a similar situation. Reflecting is also a very powerful tool to use in planning for the next event or segment in our career.

Appreciating how we frame information and events brings a deep understanding of what it takes to be successful. For example, do we frame episodes positively or negatively, and how does this perspective, either positive or negative, frame our success? Another aspect of leader strategy is influence. What influences our careers? Experience clearly influences how we advance, such as being selected for the next level of leadership in an organization or not. How does that success or lack of success influence choices or next steps? We also need to consider how each of us exerts influence on those around us. Many of us have been influenced extensively by mentors or other leaders and have clarity about how such influence supports us in learning and growing. Even entry-level leadership allows us to begin to learn how we influence other nurses or not and how nurses influence patients. Nurses have not always been aware of influence or the research establishing varying aspects of influence and what influencing strategies work. Nurses use influence to affect patient care and teamwork, and knowing more about influence has the potential to make us more influential. Nurses as advocates begin with advocating for patients. We learn this is an important role for nurses, as most patients are in a vulnerable or compromised position and might find it difficult to advocate for themselves, particularly in a strange environment. As we practice and become embedded in a team, we begin to think about our peer group and how we advocate for each other to make change in the system. We might want a self-staffing committee or change in a procedure, and we soon discover how to enroll others in our ideas. Eventually, through professional nursing associations, we learn more advanced skills regarding advocating for nursing or for the public (or a special group such as people with physical disabilities), and we learn to advocate for change in the system. Such work may even be at the state or national legislative level. At some point in this process, we learn how to apply advocacy skills for ourselves, our colleagues, and others. We use the principles of advocacy to support other nurses and to advance their roles and responsibilities within the system.

Coaching and mentoring are vital parts of the trajectory because they support the growth of each leader. Coaching focuses on the specific issues and learning required for the present role we occupy, and mentoring focuses on advancement in our careers. Many of us have not had coaches—people who support us to analyze and to think critically about events that have challenged us. They support us to think through what we did that worked and what we did that didn't work and to construct a plan for how we foster growth in both situations. Nurses in early or midcareer can be advantaged to have coaches for a limited period to support growth while on a steep learning curve. At the same time, most of us have had a mentor at some point who has given us advice as to what steps to consider as we advance in our professional careers. Learning about coaching is critical to being able to help others, which is an expectation of leaders.

Leaders create visions about the future and what can be accomplished in the workplace. For example, some nurse leaders create a vision about obtaining Magnet® designation. This requires considerable work and can be a project that has a significant timeline. It requires the ability to sustain enthusiasm over time. A great deal of knowledge and wisdom is required for a nurse leader to balance all the aspects of the Magnet® journey and the smooth running of the organization. Wisdom, for the most part, is gained over a time frame that includes all the aspects discussed previously to gain the skills to be a truly effective leader—one who stands apart and makes a difference for nurses and for patients. Learning how to create a vision and share it in a way that makes it appealing to others is a key leadership task.

Although this trajectory may suggest a linear process, it is not. The strategies are responsive elements to the extent that we could move from wisdom to self-assessment because a new tool is available, or a new insight occurs, or an external event occurs that causes us to seek new information. As we gain additional abilities, we may want to test them for ourselves in some aspect of the trajectory before we assist others with their leadership development.

As you read each of the strategies, you can benefit most by asking yourself if you are using each to its full potential and how each strategy supports the other strategies. The point of this thinking is to create an effective toolbox for your personal development and for your contribution in developing others.

1

Leading to Legacies

Leadership is a rather nebulous thing; Doris Kearns Goodwin said in her book, *Leadership in Turbulent Times* (an apt title for how we describe health care today), that it was the elusive theme of leadership.[1] *Nebulous* and *elusive* are probably two good terms to use in referring to leadership. It doesn't have a set of rules or a formula for success. You can't take two of these and three of those and create leadership. It is highly dependent on the qualities the person known as leader brings to a situation. Yet people can engage in specific activities that help develop one's leadership acumen. What then is leadership? Before we launch into what we think, consider how you would describe what you would say leadership is from your perspective.

> **REFLECTION** How would you describe what leadership means to you?

One more thing to think about in terms of leadership before we really look at what it is: great leaders are what they leave behind. In other words, if we did great things, that is wonderful. Yet we repeatedly hear leaders left positions through retirement or an external position offer only to see something that everyone seemed committed to deteriorate or evaporate. Think how much greater those things could be if we also left behind the commitment and people to continue our great work! A leader's key task is to create a culture where best practices flourish and people grow, or as Claude T. Bissell said, to attain excellence, you must "Risk more than others think is safe. Care more than others think is wise. Dream more than others think is practical. Expect more than others think is possible."[2] *Risk, care, dream,* and *expect* sound like words of commitment to improvement!

A great example of this kind of leadership—one that really makes a difference—was expressed in *The Dallas Morning News* on Sunday, January 6, 2019, in a full-page tribute to the passing of Herb Kelleher—from his employees and retirees.[3] Herb Keleher earned the devotion of thousands of people as a founder of Southwest Airlines (SWA), which is famously known for setting itself apart from other airlines in the way it boards passengers, treats them once on board, and conveys the "rules of flying" in an amusing way. The tribute read, in part, "Thanks for remembering our names. For keeping our airline flying high and our spirits higher. For always being there. For arm wrestling for our slogan. And for turning a Company into a Family." Yes, he wore business suits when necessary, and he also dressed up in ridiculous outfits (like the Easter bunny or Elvis). As an employee, he, too, would jump up to distribute the peanuts (now defunct) to passengers—an expectation for all employees who flew on SWA. He created the culture at SWA using the best data available about how to move people in the quickest and least costly manner. He surrounded himself with people who were as committed to this new approach as he was. He used data AND he used his personal influence to create an airline like no other—one where people wanted to work, where they knew they could be silly at appropriate times (after all the BOSS was!), and where they could participate in what we in health care would call self-governance. The tribute closed by saying: "We will be forever in your debt, and we will aspire to keep your spirit alive." That is leadership of a legacy.

> **REFLECTION** Is your chief executive officer (CEO) a visionary? Does your organization put patients first? Can you think of health care organizations or businesses that convey this same level of commitment to each other? What do formal leaders do to make the organization special?

A legacy leader is someone who isn't the "run of the mill." A leader is someone who goes beyond the basic expectations—no matter what title that person holds. If we believe that anyone committed to others can be a leader, we are probably right. The willingness to influence others, or as Dr. Sylvain Trepanier and others would say—inspire toward a goal—is what leadership is about. And like the social determinants of health, where we live is a factor in who we are. It accounts for some variance in personality and our lives in general, and those factors play into our ability to influence others, according to Berger.[4]

Where to begin in this journey to understand this nebulous, elusive thing known as leadership is a challenge. If you are a fan of Simon Sinek, author of *Start with Why*, you would start with what he says is the most important thing: why.[5] Why consider leadership, and why have another book about leadership? The simplest answer might be what John Maxwell, author and speaker on leadership, says.[6] Our task as leaders is to produce other leaders! And that is what being in a group of leaders is about. Each of us has the responsibility to each other and to those not yet seeing themselves as leaders to engage in a way that makes our commitment to our work overwhelming in the face of obstacles.

When we read the corporate statistics about senior executive leadership (albeit not something every one of us aspires to), we knew we had a major concern to address. Although two-thirds of businesses have programs to help potential leaders advance, only about one-fourth of those programs were seen as successful.[7] And to make a more dramatic statement, about one-third of new CEOs are hired from outside of the organization. Do they come from organizations devoted to leadership development, or is their learning scattered among a variety of opportunities? This is not a positive state of affairs in business, and often health care lags behind what business does! How, then, do we create legacy leaders who can make a difference? The formula these authors provide is quite simple: be clear about the competencies needed for the various roles; assess the five predictors of success—motivation, curiosity, insight, engagement, and determination; map prospective leaders' potential in terms of these competencies; and provide experiences, supported by coaching, that develop strengths in those competencies. While we cannot define competencies for some position that might not even exist today, nor provide specific experiences, we can capitalize on the five predictors of success and through reflection activities, provide some coaching to help you develop those skills. Most organizations have expectations for performance, although not all are stated as competencies, and many organizations rely on external sources to develop talent at higher levels of the organization. Some organizations even ignore an "entry-level" leader's development! If, for example, you served as a charge nurse after an orientation to the role and tasks, you are fortunate. Even at the manager level, we still see organizations that do minimal or no prior development for persons in those roles. We need to do something about this state of affairs!

The reason we must learn about leadership is that health care is too complex to rely on only a handful of people who have official designations as leaders. If we doubt this is true, look at almost any professional association's website and find information about leadership development! Additionally, one of the common stories we hear from leaders who have retired or moved on to another position is that almost as soon as they were gone, so was the key work those people had led. In other words, whatever the work was had not been embedded in the culture or in the people who remained in the organization. Sometimes, that work goes by the wayside because it is too threatening to a new leadership team. More often, however, the key leader didn't have sufficient numbers of leaders committed to the work so that it went on even without the creator of the idea.

While many organizations provide leadership development, at least for a certain portion of the employees, the reality is that leadership is personal. Each of us has a style. For example, some of us tell stories to make a point, others of us ask questions to get to the core of an issue, and still others listen very carefully so we can form a succinct statement about what has just been said in a group meeting. If an organization doesn't select you to be a part of its leadership development work, you can choose to pout, move on to another organization, or take charge of your own development. In fact, taking charge of yourself is probably a good idea even if you are in a leadership development–rich organization. As you will see in the chapter on the *Leaders*-Ship Legacy Trajectory (Legacy *Leaders*-Ship: The Model, LLT), we have a model to help you gain the knowledge and skills you need to be a leader or to strengthen what you are already doing.

Each of us must use personal leadership to develop our leadership talent so that we can be effective in whatever situation we find ourselves. Most of the skills we need to develop are known as *soft skills*. That is, these skills don't have steps to follow or formulas to use such as we might find in analyzing a budget or creating a clinical protocol. The lack of such rules about these soft skills is why one of us always says they are the hard skills to learn, and they are likely to become increasingly valuable, according to Gratton and the World Economic Forum.[8] Surely we want to be prepared for the future!

INTENTIONALITY

Intentionality is critical to leadership—and life. We all have multiple opportunities in life. Some choices we "fall" into for a variety of reasons, and frequently, that is how we learn something. Think of something mundane, but important, such as brushing your teeth. Most of us use the same process, starting at one point and ending back at that point. Some electronic toothbrushes, for example, reinforce this routine by beeping four times as we attend to each quadrant of the mouth. This is a routine, almost mindless, activity.

Other opportunities "call" us. An idea fits with our values or suggests a way to be more effective in what we do. In some ways, we respond almost automatically because we are *called* to action. However, many of those "calls" require an investment of energy. Now we have to deliberately choose to take on the "call" or not. That decision is intentionality. We deliberately do X and not Y. We might even be able to say something such as, "My intent for engaging in the work is because..." We saw this intentionality as nurses, among others, responded during the coronavirus pandemic in 2020.

One way to talk about intentionality is to describe it as purposive. When we have the bigger view of "why am I here," decisions linked to that purpose are done with intentionality. Conversely, when we choose X, in a sense we are rejecting Y. We don't tend to think about the thing we don't do as a rejection, yet it isn't something we choose to do. In those cases where we choose *both* X and Y, we are less effective unless we have close teams who are in harmony with us.

Developing as a leader requires intentionality. Yet some of us are given opportunities we might not even understand at the time. For example, one of us worked for a state nurses association fairly early in her career:

"I met and worked with almost every nurse leader in the state. What I didn't realize at the time is that few nurses have such good fortune. When you affiliate with leaders, it is hard not to follow suit and take on their characteristics and ways of thinking and acting. Most of us, however, have to find ways to create our opportunities—to meet key leaders, to secure exceptional positions, and to love the work we do and our jobs."

Intentionality means that when you decided to read this book, you were intentionally going to take on a new leadership experience. Some of you may be enrolled in an academic course where this book is a required or suggested reading. Others of you may be engaged in an exciting role and you have figured out you could do more if you were more effective as a leader. Still others of you may have picked up the book without the intention of learning about legacies or leadership and then you saw the potential. Whether you were "called" or "falled" to get here, here you are, and now you have the choice to develop your talents as leaders in an intentional manner so that the work you do makes a difference—and that is what it means to leave a legacy. You made a difference.

LEGACIES

The work of four nurse leaders in the 1980s led to reasons why nurses stayed in an organization or left that organization. Margaret (Maggie) McClure, Muriel Poulin, Margaret Sovie, and Mable Wandelt, all members of the American Academy of Nursing, decided to look at what was known as the *leavers* and *stayers*.[9] This work identified several hospitals that later became known as the Reputational Magnet® hospitals and later served as the foundation for the Magnet Recognition Program®, which looks at far more than retention rates and yet remains focused on quality. While these four nurse leaders did not work in the same organization, they came together in a professional organization (the American Academy of Nursing) to maximize their interests in such a way that a legacy was created. This example shows that what we do externally to our work environment also is a place where we can create a legacy. Their legacy is a dramatic one with national prominence.

One other piece about this research work: the research sat idle for years. Then the American Nurses Credentialing Center decided to recognize hospitals that were reflective of the positive findings. Did this work just blossom into a widespread effort? No. Rather, for well over a decade, the recognition of hospitals inched along until the early 2000s, when the idea of a Magnet®-recognized hospital became "the thing." In fact, some CEOs were looking for nurses to fill the nursing leadership position in order to "get one of those!" In our view, that work is the cornerstone of the fourth aim of the quadruple aim—improving the work life of health care providers.[10]

Jean Watson, a professor at the University of Colorado, created the Theory of Human Caring. Her original work involved writing and speaking. What she said spoke to the hearts of many of us, and her work expanded to include the Watson Caring Science Institute. This work has gone beyond the university and beyond a mere theory for nursing; it represents a legacy to the profession—worldwide.[11] Many Magnet® hospitals use at least a part of Watson's theory as the basis of the organizational model for professional practice.

Legacies take time to build and take the commitment of more than one leader. The words from the "World Is Wide Enough" from the Broadway hit *Hamilton* might say it best: "It's planting seeds in a garden you never get to see."[12] The ability to maintain commitment and persist in tending seeds (the people we influence) leads to a legacy.

LEADERS

Leaders are typically thought of as those who hold certain titles. Titles of importance often have the word *president, vice, associate,* or *chief* in them. In health care, people in the C Suite (meaning their title starts with the word *chief* or some word that means official leader) are viewed as leaders. Those titles have little meaning to nurses who work part-time, weekends, or nights. They might know the names of the people in the C Suite, but the leader is whoever is in charge of the unit right now. Dr. Amy Boothe and others put it this way: "In reality, we all move along a leadership-followership continuum based on activities, settings, the presence of others, and our talents."[13] We move from one role in situation 1 to the other role in situation 2. Or we serve as leader until someone else with better expertise, more experience, stronger position title, or maybe even a louder voice assumes the role:

"One of us can even think of an example where the CEO of a hospital deferred to the chief nursing officer (CNO) to handle the organization's response to a major weather disaster. His only statement before going to help transport patients was: Don't let X agency (a rescue organization) take charge! Clearly the CEO realized in such an emergency situation that his highly praised talents were not what were needed, and he stepped out of the way. The CNO, who knew the staff well and was familiar with creating organization out of chaos, rose to the challenge and orchestrated the safe evacuation of patients from the hospital while maintaining attentiveness to the staff."

Another example is when one of us was the associate leader, when the key leader left rather abruptly:

"As the associate leader, I didn't know the politics of the new group I was suddenly thrust into. I vowed that from then on, I was going to do more 'thinking aloud' so that my team knew what they needed to know if I was suddenly absent."

If only one person is seen as "the leader," disaster can ensue if anything happens to that person! Thus, we talk about *Leaders*-Ship development. We mean multiple leaders need to be developed for any organization of any size to be sustainable. As Tagliareni and Brewington say, "...trying to lead as the Lone Ranger is almost always a surefire way to burn out."[14] Being the sole leader in today's world is a foolish approach to leadership because it takes the whole of many people being ready to step in and step up to advance good ideas toward success. Examples of what leaders and followers do are found in Table 1.1. Moving followers toward being leaders is a key goal for people in official leadership positions. And those official leaders need to be ready to follow when that is the appropriate action.

The brief list found in Table 1.1 illustrates how neither group can exist without the other. While some people may have the term *chief* in their title, if it weren't for all those without that word, no chief anything would exist. Rather than thinking of leadership as a hierarchy, as most organizational charts suggest, leadership in action is highly fluid with the hope that the person best able to lead a particular effort is the one who rises to be "in charge." Without this fluidity, official leaders can be stuck in their roles and flounder in their leadership, just as those without titles can be stuck in their roles and abdicate to the official leader. Either way, strong outcomes are less likely. Once again, it is about creating the cadre of leaders so that the leader of the moment can rise to take charge and move things ahead. We saw this occur as the coronarivus spread from one country or community to the next and the person with the best knowledge became the leader.

TABLE 1.1 What Leaders and Followers Do

EXAMPLES	
Leaders	**Followers**
Set the tone	Reinforce the tone
Create the vision	See the practical
Set policy	Provide input/questions
Create trust	Build trust
Create a learning organization	Grow and learn

LL ALERT

- The *Leaders*-Ship Legacy Alert typically represents something about what *not* to do.
- An example of what not to do regarding developing yourself into a legacy leader is to fail to thank people when they offer a compliment for work you have done or ideas you have presented. Take credit without becoming egotistical. Please don't discount someone's input by saying something like: "Oh, it was nothing."[15]

SUMMARY

The goal of this first chapter was to emphasize that having only one person designated as a leader can be disastrous for organizations. That is the "why" of learning leadership. Any one of us may be in a situation where we must act on behalf of others, and we want to be effective when we do so. When we learn the skills of being effective (the how), we have the potential to be influential. When many of us learn the skills, we have the potential to effect lasting change, and lasting change is what creates legacies.

LL LINEUP

- Have a clear picture of the legacy you wish to leave. If you don't have clarity, consider writing your obituary—what would it say?
- Leadership is not about me; it's about we. It takes a team to make a lasting impact.

REFLECTION What would you create as a definition of leadership? If someone called you a leader, what words would you use to describe yourself? What legacy do you plan to leave? Think about what you could do tomorrow to move a group closer to a legacy. What would that look like?

2

Legacy *Leaders*-Ship: The Model

Do you feel as if you are just making it through the day? When someone asks about the legacy you hope to leave, does that seem to be a remote thought? So many of us are overwhelmed by the day-to-day leadership challenges that it is easy to forget that we could leave a legacy, or at least participate actively in establishing or maintaining one, and who among us wouldn't want to do something great rather than something that was just okay?

Recently, we noticed that several leaders who have stepped away from highly visible positions are saddened to know their legacy has fallen apart. (Yes, we know we mentioned this before. It is an important point worth repeating.) Sometimes that seems to be due to a change in executive leadership and the organization moving in another direction. Other times, it seems to be related to the absence of a *team* of leaders to institute, sustain, or grow an endeavor that might be thought of as a legacy. Starting anew with each new leader we might encounter in an organization likely will cause us to spend a lot of time needlessly "spinning our wheels." The Legacy *Leaders*-Ship Trajectory (LLT) model is designed to help us take what we might think of as our ordinary talents and foster them in a way that allows us to engage in creating some incredible and sustainable work that benefits employees and patients. This model allows us to consider how words such as *solid, competent, dedicated,* and *quality* can become *impressive, spectacular, sustainable,* and *legendary*.

When most people hear the word *legacy*, they think that the person who created the legacy is gone. When most people hear the word *leader*, they think of the person in charge. If those views were really the truth, every organization in the world would be in grave trouble. Yes, we ultimately need to have one leader in any organization who is able to say what happens next, and we hope that person has sufficient vision to be in the business of creating a legacy. In the interim, *leaders* (plural) at every level keep organizations healthy and productive, because being a leader is not about a position—it is about a set of behaviors, filtered through values, that is relevant to a given situation. This view applies to all organizations, including health care organizations.

Health care is now the largest part of the economy in the United States. Of the nonagricultural employment data tracked by the US Bureau of Labor Statistics, only professional and business services exceeded the number of people employed in health care and social assistance, and by 2026, the number in health care is projected to exceed all other fields.[1] However, *The Atlantic* magazine reported health care already surpassed other fields in 2018.[2] What makes that such a powerful statement is that health care is less developed than many other businesses in creating leaders. How can the largest part of the US economy not be the best equipped to use the resources it has? We saw or heard about the struggles to use resources wisely during the 2020 pandemic. The purpose of this chapter is to put forth a plan for anyone, probably in any field, to develop leadership skills. That plan consists of a model for thinking about a lifetime of development in leadership, because, as with many other aspects of life, leading is a journey that evolves as we and our environments change. Leading is not a destination, it is a journey; the legacy is the destination and not the final one.

WHY HAVE A MODEL?

Just as Simon Sinek[3] says, we need to begin with answering the question why. People want to know the why of a different way of doing something or a different way of thinking before they want to know the how or what. This is an important consideration because we often start with the "content" and steps before someone is engaged with what we are doing. Because we (the authors) are practical people, we don't offer this model merely for a theoretical perspective. Rather, it serves as a roadmap from getting to wherever you are on your leadership journey to the opportunity of creating and nurturing one or more legacies.

The most pressing reason to have a model to develop leadership is the reality that most of us learned leadership through continuing education, real-life experience, or both. We also had graduate education available to prepare us to lead, but in the full spectrum of leadership, most of us are not prepared at complex levels. Until the last few decades, few of us had a plan we could implement without great challenges, even after we found ourselves in leadership situations. Obviously, a better way is needed if we are going to dramatically change the face of health care in the next decades. That better way is to have a plan. We wouldn't think about driving across the country without a map or Waze, yet few of us have a roadmap for our professional future.

We use models all the time. Models do a variety of things for us. They provide a way of looking at complex issues to see how things interrelate and to serve as a checklist for our thinking. They help us reflect on what was missing or how something came to be, and they can serve as a guide for what we need to do to get where we want to go.

As we wrote this book, we noted that most organizations have undertaken some effort to develop people's leadership skills, at least at the higher levels of the organization. However, the shortage of health care professionals persists, so conceptually, if all of us need to function to the best of our abilities, we all need to develop our leadership skills. Additionally, worldwide, work is seen as having increasing psychosocial risks, some of which derive from restructuring and mergers and acquisitions.[4] Another key factor is balancing the energy you have to devote to the many roles you play at work and away from work. One study showed that people want to increase time in both areas and that is the biggest challenge women workers face.[5] Thus shortages, work organization changes, and the desire to be in two places at once (more at home and more at work) mean that leaders take on new roles of importance in supporting the people within any organization. We need to start with people new to the field of health care or to the organization to gain insight into a new culture. We also need to advance the abilities of those who have remained in the organization. In essence, everyone qualifies for developing greater abilities in leadership. That fact explains the title of the trajectory—Legacy *Leaders*-Ship.

Our approach to care may be based on a model, for example, the illness beliefs model.[6] We may create a model for how we deliver care in a particular organization—we even model what a new patient care room may be like so we can physically test its functionality. Why then would we not want a model that allows us to develop the most needed talent in health care, that of leading others? Simply stated, a model is an example to follow.[7]

WHAT IS THE LEGACY *LEADERS*-SHIP MODEL?

Every model in nursing, and every other discipline, has core elements. Those elements often are broad concepts that are designed to reflect critical components of the whole, and solid models help us understand how we move from concepts to action. Leadership is a great concept, but it is worthless unless actions are associated with it.

The elements in the LLT model (Fig. 2.1) have the potential to change because health care changes, the team changes, new discoveries about care are made, we know more about leadership, we change organizations, or we redirect our energies to take on some aspect of leading we never engaged in before. Sometimes that change is small—for example, as intelligence evolved to include emotional and visual in addition to intellectual. Some parts remain untouched—for example, the idea of a trajectory and the need to consider both personal and environmental factors. Other elements can make dramatic changes—for example, what we need to know in the two triangles of the model. As an example, a few decades ago, we wouldn't have included mindfulness; now it is a critical element associated with effectiveness.

Each part is important and has value in its own right. However, the synergy among the elements is what provides an exponential effect. Further, because this model is designed for anyone and is derived from the view that "it takes a village" to be effective in creating sustainable legacies, the model is intended to be used by all the leaders in any group. That means the model for leadership has to be dynamic and individualized. As a result of that thinking, the LLT model has five component parts built on the foundation that we already have from our clinical and functional performance:

1. Values—these represent the driving forces behind why we do certain things and not others.
2. Lifelong learning—this represents how we stay relevant throughout our careers.
3. The trajectory—this represents how we continue to develop our competencies as a leader.
4. Personal elements—these are the elements we need to continue to hone to be effective as individuals.
5. Environmental elements—these are the elements we encounter in various leadership situations.

Each of us may use a model differently—after all, we are not replicas of each other. Testing out what works for each of us is important, and we all need to have some idea of what things we should be testing to be effective leaders. That is what the LLT model does.

As we said earlier, *Leaders*-Ship is not a typographical error. Rather, it is a deliberate tactic to remind us all that if we wish to leave a legacy, we cannot do so by ourselves. As Simon Sinek says: All of us is better than one of us![3] In those rare instances where one person does achieve a legacy status, that legacy sometimes fades shortly after the leader departs. However, when a team of leaders is committed to making a difference, the legacy has the potential to be sustainable. For those

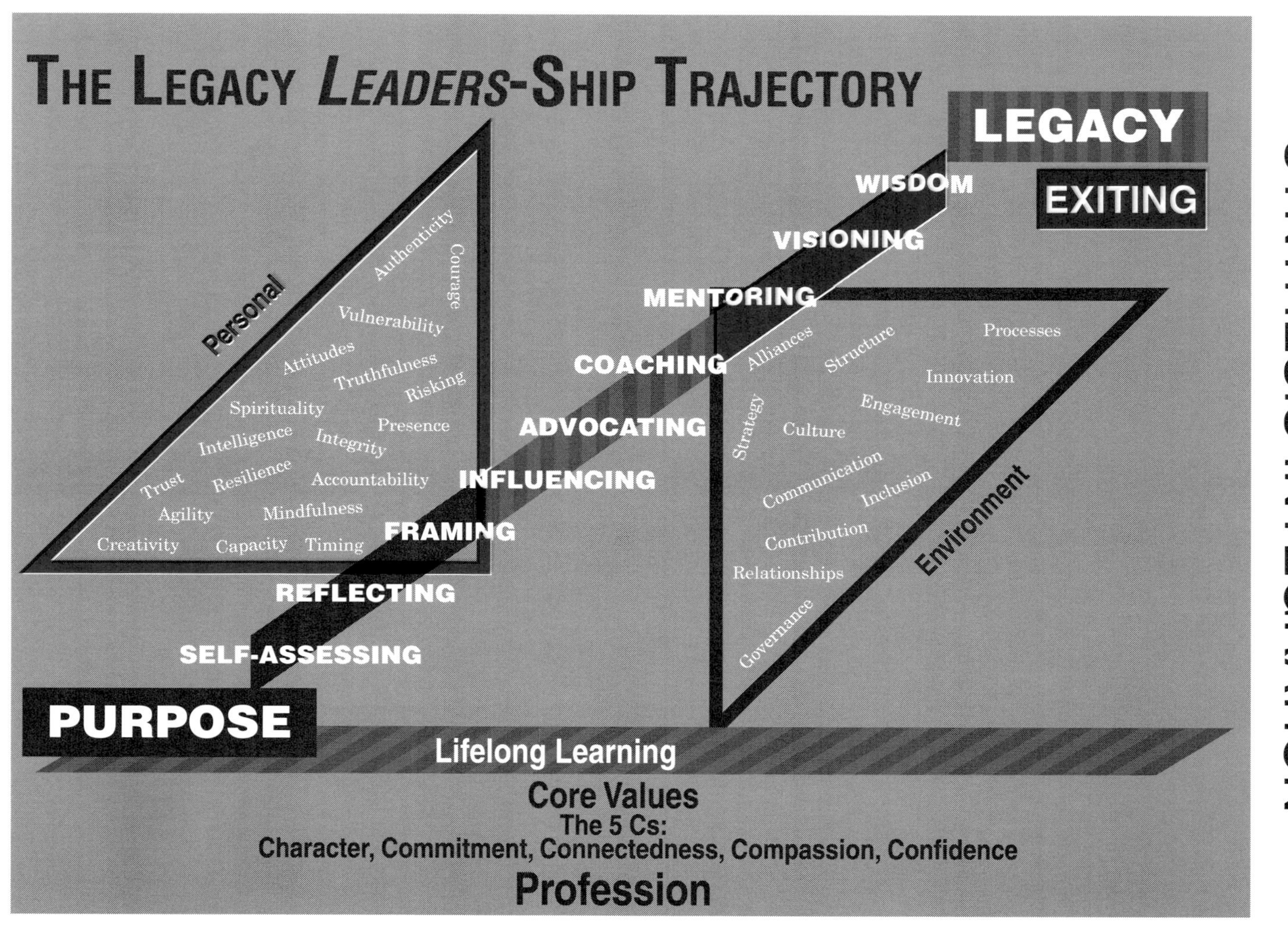
SYNTHESIS INTEGRATION
SYNTHESIS INTEGRATION
SYNTHESIS INTEGRATION
SYNTHESIS INTEGRATION
THE LEGACY LEADERS-SHIP TRAJECTORY
LEGACY
EXITING
WISDOM
VISIONING
MENTORING
COACHING
ADVOCATING
INFLUENCING
FRAMING
REFLECTING
SELF-ASSESSING
PURPOSE
Personal
Authenticity
Courage
Vulnerability
Attitudes
Truthfulness
Risking
Spirituality
Presence
Intelligence
Integrity
Trust
Resilience
Accountability
Agility
Mindfulness
Creativity
Capacity
Timing
Alliances
Structure
Processes
Innovation
Strategy
Engagement
Culture
Communication
Inclusion
Contribution
Relationships
Governance
Environment
Lifelong Learning
Core Values
The 5 Cs:
Character, Commitment, Connectedness, Compassion, Confidence
Profession

Fig. 2.1 The Legacy ***Leaders*****-Ship Trajectory.** This model is designed to help leaders at any point on their journey develop skills that lead toward creating a legacy. The model is surrounded by the words *synthesis* and *integration* because simply accumulating knowledge and demonstrating some skills are insufficient to be established leaders in any role. Those skills and knowledge must be synthesized and integrated into the way we perform our roles on a regular basis.

The *background* of the model is gray—similar to how leadership is often described. Leadership is not a series of steps or an algorithm. Rather, it requires operating in the gray zones of knowledge and relationships and actively synthesizing and integrating the cues we gather about our skills and the environment. The gray background represents the idea that leaders often must operate without precedents, complete facts, or clarity of a situation.

The *bottom* of the model reflects that leader skills are built on a professional foundation. Nursing, as an example, has specific expectations for what constitutes professional and ethical practice. Those expectations are incorporated with core values, such as the 5Cs in this model.

Lifelong learning extends across the model elements because we change and so does the environment—even if we aren't changing roles or our environment. To remain contemporary in practice, ongoing learning has to occur. We may carry forward long-established practices if they best fit a given situation, or we may determine we need to employ new approaches.

The *trajectory*, really the core of the model, begins with the word *purpose* and ends with the word *legacy*. Without a clear purpose, leaders might respond to any opportunity. If, however, leaders are clear about their purpose, they use each of the words in the trajectory to enhance their leadership skills. Although the sequence of some of those words is not fixed, if our purpose isn't clear, getting to a legacy may be a challenge. Typically, we need to be clear about the first three words (*self-assessing, reflecting,* and *framing*) if our purpose is to be successful. Likely, as we move through our professional lives, we take on the knowledge and skills of influencing, advocating, and coaching, which appear on a different-colored background. They often are exhibited once we feel confident in our work. We then employ all of the prior strategies to be effective in mentoring, visioning, and sharing wisdom.

The *two triangles* cross through the trajectory rather than merely abutting the trajectory. *Personal* is lower on the trajectory to indicate that understanding the self must precede understanding the environment. This placement conveys that both personal and environmental factors may influence our trajectory and alter what we do in any given situation because the assessment of our abilities or the environment in which we find ourselves may alter our trajectory. Thus, if an environment demands something with which we are unfamiliar, we may need to return to self-assessing and reflecting before moving ahead again.

Finally, the word *exiting* is placed below and abutting the word *legacy*. Not everyone exits a position or organization once a legacy potential is established and it's clear others can carry on the legacy. However, the goal of creating *Leaders*-Ship is to enhance the potential that good work lives on beyond the time an individual influenced that work.

---

of us who love Apple products, the death of Steve Jobs created anxiety. Would Apple ever be the same? Although it probably is different today than when Jobs was leading the organization, Apple didn't disintegrate or create bad products—the culture was engrained in the team! That is the goal we all have in our work. We don't want to do something just for today, although we expend a lot of energy focused on the things that are "in our faces." Rather, we want to make a difference for the people with whom we work and for the patients and clients we encounter in our organizations. Remember the lines mentioned in the first chapter from "The World Was Wide Enough": "It's [think the word legacy] planting seeds in a garden you will never get to see."[8] This doesn't mean that leaders won't see some wonderful outcome from their efforts. What it does mean is that the full impact of what we do today, if sustained, will produce something that may not even have been imagined as possible.

In a sense, the LLT model is a personal model. It builds on the talents we have developed in our primary professional work (as a nurse, as a critical care nurse, as a neonatal nurse, and so forth). It provides for the core inputs (the personal and environmental aspects), the activities that contribute to personal development (the trajectory), and eventually what the impact will be (legacy). How each of us gets from where we are to where we can be may vary; however, all of the aspects of the model are core elements to reach the pinnacle of creating a legacy.

If you choose to do so, you can use the model outline in Fig. 2.2 and create a personalized LLT model. What creating your own LLT model could do for you is to create your

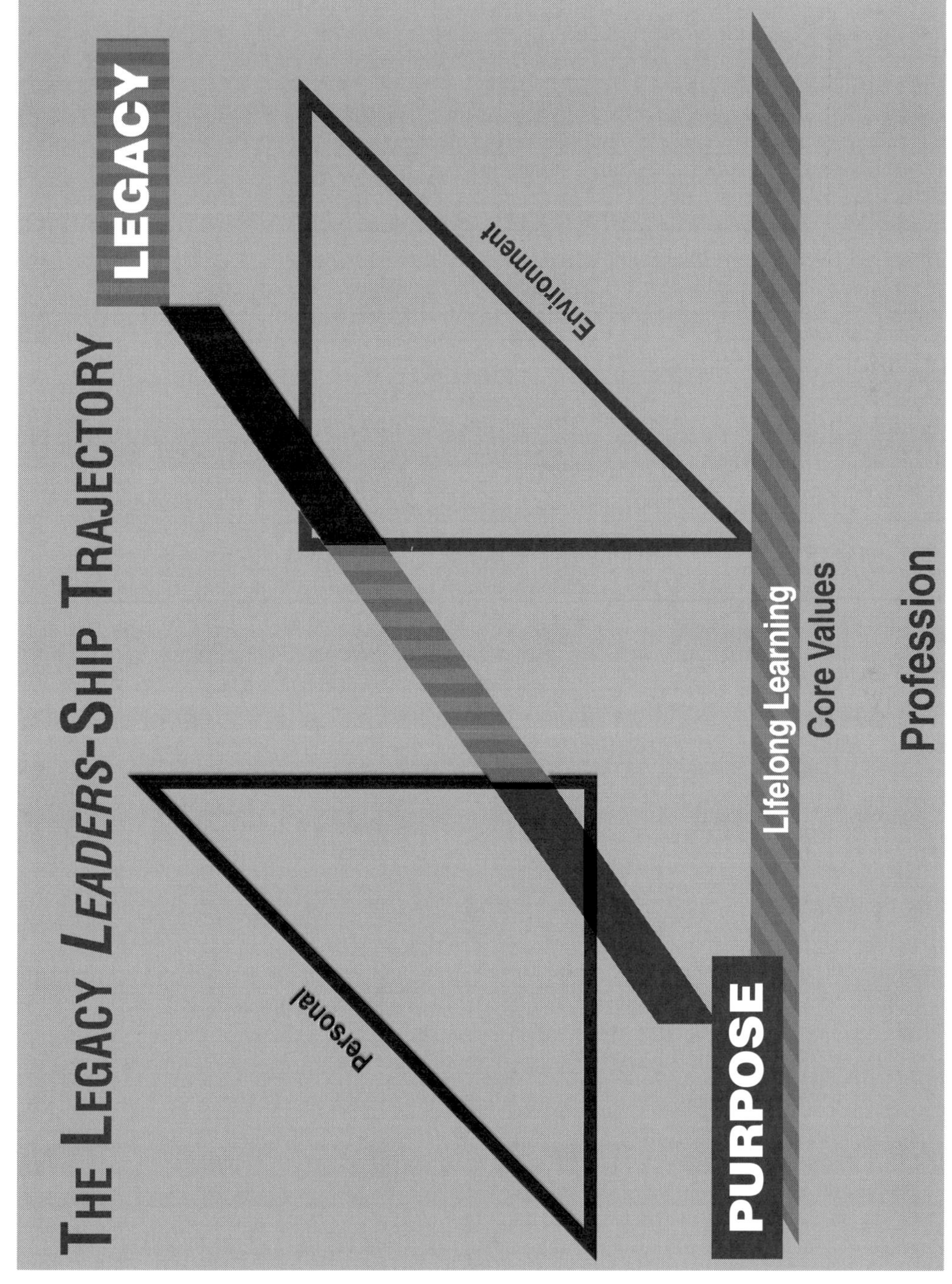

Fig. 2.2 The Legacy *Leaders*-Ship Trajectory Model Outline. Use this blank model to fill in the words that exemplify your own leadership journey.

own meaningful words, to emphasize those elements that you need to attend to, to identify what your current talents are, and to translate that plan into a timeline.

HOW WAS THE LLT MODEL DEVISED?

The model you find in this chapter is derived from several sources (see Fig. 2.1). First, this model represents our thinking about leadership from having served in numerous roles within health care organizations and associations over several decades. Second, it is grounded in the leadership literature—some of which is apparent in the health care literature and some of which is found primarily in the business literature. Third, this model reflects what other resources, such as authoritative websites, general publications, and video presentations, say about leadership. And finally, this model represents the thinking of individual leaders in nursing who served as our Circle of Advisors.[9] During this process, we asked individuals to respond to the overall model and to offer any suggestions they had for key concepts that needed to be included. Throughout the whole process, our goal was to be lumpers instead of splitters—that is, to use a broad term that could encompass several ideas rather than detail the hundreds of words that have been associated with the concept of leading. This conscious decision was based on our desire to keep the number of words that stimulate thoughts for others to a lesser rather than greater number. Thus, if you do not find your favorite words related to leadership, they probably are embedded in one of the words that does appear.

If you look at the literature related to leadership, you might find almost any word that conveys something good and desirable. Dr. Linda Cain and others,[10] as one example, undertook a project to identify key behaviors and attributes to distinguish high-performing nurses from others so that those individuals would be sought for employment, development activities, and promotional opportunities. A content analysis of eight focus groups, comprising 65 participants from various positions including patients, families, administrators, physicians, and nurses, produced seven themes: teamwork, patient advocacy, communication with patients and families, caring, approach to care, work attitude, and personal attributes. These themes are focused on, as the title of their article suggests, high-performing nurses. Why then did we not adopt these categories as a way of thinking about leadership? The answer is simple: we are building the idea of leadership development on the expectation that all of the attributes about nurses would be in place through the initial and ongoing professional education and experiences that nurses use to become successful as nurses. What we need to develop in order to be successful as leaders is the focus of the LLT.

When Dr. Vickie Hughes looked at the literature to determine what made a leader a standout leader, she found many descriptors.[11] Her findings from a 10-year review created a four-category view: personal traits, behaviors, clinical expertise, and context. The LLT model does not address clinical expertise because we viewed the LLT model as an addition to one's clinical (and functional) expertise. The characteristics, as you will see, are reflected in the LLT model as personal. Those five characteristics identified by Hughes (integrity, approachable, motivational, emotional capacity, and social intelligence) are ones we expect of key leaders. That means they are characteristics we should begin developing early in our intent to have a leadership career. The context in Hughes's work is seen as environment in the LLT. The environment, or context, conceptually dictates the behaviors we exhibit. The behaviors of mentoring, role modeling, and communicating effectively are either viewed as part of the environment or are the elements found on the trajectory line. Examples of what Hughes found in the literature are shown in Table 2.1.

LL ALERT

Remember, no formula exists for creating effective leaders. If one existed, someone would have bottled it and retired a wealthy person!

REFLECTION If you haven't already looked at the model, think about words that you would use to describe a leader you admire. Think also about the context where that person exhibits the characteristics you believe to be of value. And, finally, think about what activities you would have to undertake to become skillful in your workplace at exhibiting those characteristics. If you have looked at the model, consider whether the words are words you would use and view as important.

The above is the FIRST reflection related to the model. Through years of research, Kouzes and Posner concluded that the way to learn leadership is through reflection.[12] And the best way to do it is to take 10 to 15 minutes in a dimly lit room without any distractions. (This would include no cell phones, computer, paper and pencil, and so forth, except what you need to record what you think.) What you are doing is really consolidating information—in this case, from your experience. This deliberative process of thinking about leadership and individual performance adds a dimension to the way we learned leadership before. We aren't merely gaining experience—we are thinking about our performance and how situations and people differ, and we are creating our own list of lessons learned.

TABLE 2.1 Examples of Words Describing a Standout Leader as Identified From Hughes's Review

Characteristics	Behaviors	Clinical Expertise	Context
Five major categories	Three major categories	No categorization	No categorization
Integrity	Mentor	Competence	Situational factors
Honesty	Reflective practice	Adaptability	Capital
Moral code	Role model	Rapid thinking	Influence
Approachable	Sets example		
Open	Effective communicator		
Motivational	Good listener		
Warm	Open		
Emotional capacity			
Caring			
Emotional intelligence			
Social intelligence			
Ability to influence			

Based on Hughes V. Standout nurse leaders...what's in the research? *Nurs Manag.* 2017;48:16-24.

THE LEGACY *LEADERS*-SHIP TRAJECTORY MODEL

If you participated in the first reflection, you already know that the words we have chosen to portray the model are not etched in stone. They are derived, as we said earlier, from a variety of sources, and yet you may call something by a different name or see a particular word as a subset of another characteristic. In one sense, the model is like a jigsaw puzzle. You have to put all the pieces together to create the whole. In a difference sense, the model is more like a spider web, with each creation being distinctive based on placement (environment) and talents (personal). And pulling on one piece affects the other pieces in the web.

First, the model is surrounded by the words *synthesis* and *integration* to symbolize that nothing happens by itself and the synthesis of ideas and skills is what makes us distinct as leaders, especially when we integrate them in varying environments. The presence of those two words is designed to convey that the model is dynamic, even though we may have tendencies to see things in a particular way or rely on our favorite skills. If it weren't for this dynamic state, we likely could create a formula for leadership that would reflect which elements were the primary drivers in various situations and a checklist for when to use one formula versus another.

The foundation of the model is your professional self. That element reflects your clinical expertise and your functional skills and abilities. Many of us have similar elements in those areas, for example, being a geriatric nurse specialist and being able to lead a team.

The LLT model begins at the bottom with values—in this case, the 5 Cs. These words are based on prior work two of us did related to leadership.[13]

Each of us has some core values. Without core values, we might learn about leadership and yet be rudderless, going from one view to the next without thinking about the impact on those who are following. As Chef Jeff Henderson says: values are what divide people in this country.[14] His point was made clearer when he said that he grew up without values and only learned those when he was in prison. Most of us don't have to go to that extreme; in fact, many of us probably were raised with parents or a significant other who helped instill values in us. If we weren't that fortunate, we learned from someone—a teacher, a religious leader, or a friend—that we needed to be grounded in something. Watching and listening to others help us form values. What others say and do reinforces our views of what a value means, and we become frustrated when someone says one thing and does another—that is when actions conflict with stated values.

Immediately above the core values is the idea of lifelong learning. In addition to our years of work in continuing education and the importance of continual learning (as identified, for example, in the Institute of Medicine—now the National Academy of Medicine—report on *The Future of Nursing*),[15] we know that in today's world, if you aren't learning, you aren't standing still. You are falling behind.

Thus learning throughout a lifetime about specific work and what it means to be a leader is critical.

Next, the trajectory moves from purpose (why are we here?) to legacy (how did I help make something great?). The words along the trajectory convey how to develop so that we, too, can be a part of leaving a legacy.

To the left of the trajectory is a triangle impinging on the trajectory line. It represents the personal characteristics and skills we need to possess (or develop). To the right of the trajectory is another triangle impinging on the trajectory line. It represents the environment and the factors that influence us to behave and think in certain ways in a specific culture. Each of those triangles contains words that are designed, again, to build on what we already are as nurses. Yet some words are ones we would find in undergraduate education. What is the difference between undergraduate education and personal leadership experience? The difference lies in the intricate nature of what a leader is expected to be versus someone who is learning nursing. An example might be communication. We probably all are no longer surprised when one of the "causes" of anything (good or bad) is attributed to communication. Yet communication at high levels of leadership is very different from everyday communication we might hear in a patient care area. Think about Dr. Margretta Madden Styles creating a watch word for her presidential service at both the American Nurses Association and the International Council of Nurses. Her famous watch word was "march." Her view was the word "march" was a call to action. In other words, conceptualizing, planning, and so forth were insufficient; we had to take action if we were to be effective.

REFLECTION What might your watch word be?

Each of those elements of the model is described in subsequent chapters to convey the important ideas behind the words. Conceptually, we could start anywhere in the book because the only sequencing in the model is having values in place, increasing skills as we move along the trajectory, and starting with self rather than environment.

SUCCESS TIPS

What you get out of the model depends on the effort you put into using it—just like any other endeavor. You have options: you can read the words and check off having read the book (in case you were ever asked); you can put some effort into reading the text and pausing to think about the questions; or you can focus on developing your leadership talents and consider what is stated here and then think what meaning that has for you. Then you can answer the reflection questions and devote 10 to 15 minutes of uninterrupted, undistracted pondering (as suggested by Kouzes and Posner) about what you have learned and how you can use that knowledge to be a better leader.

You can use the blank model and fill in the words that have meaning for you to create your own version of being a leader. Those words, however, should have some connection with the current (or in some cases historical) literature. They also should make sense to others.

Finally, you can use the model as a measurement of your leadership abilities. By routinely comparing what you think you are doing (and how you are doing whatever you are doing) with the model, you can at least have some perspective of what elements are missing, or need further development, in your leadership toolbox.

LL ALERT

- Don't ignore the model and how it can be used, and don't avoid reflecting—it's how we really learn.

SUMMARY

We all need a plan. To take on that plan, having a model to force us to think about important elements makes us more productive. Health care is still in the era where not all leaders have been formally prepared at the graduate level or have been fortunate enough to have enrolled in a leadership intensive experience designed to quickly develop critical leadership skills. Therefore, we must make a commitment to developing the talents we have and enhancing those we don't have. The LLT model is designed to engage us in thinking about values, lifelong learning, a leadership trajectory, and personal and environmental elements that can produce legacies. The ultimate goal is to create positive outcomes for the people for whom we care so they can care for the people who come to our organizations for care and development.

LL LINEUP

- Choose your words carefully—they guide your development.
- Use a model to take an in-depth look at where you are and what you need to do.

REFLECTION What happened today? Did you seek out people with whom you don't normally interact? Where would you place yourself on the trajectory? Which talents are already personal strengths? And to use Joe Tye and Bob Dent's question: "What would you do if every job paid the same and had the same social status?"[16]

3

The Profession and Values

Every effort toward leadership builds on something. In the Legacy *Leaders*-Ship Trajectory (LLT) model, we build leadership development on two critical elements: the profession and values. Each is related to the other, and together they form the basis for what each of us develops to be better leaders.

THE PROFESSION

The bottom of almost every model represents one of two things: the underpinning or the goal/outcome. In the LLT model, the "bottom line" is the underpinning of the model. Think about all of the words and abilities you might attribute to the word *nursing*. All of those are subsumed in that element and are what we learned in our initial academic preparation. They were reinforced in our experiences, and they form the basis for the nature of our leadership. We assume that we practice in legal and ethical ways, that we maintain the competencies we need for the area of practice on which we focus, and that we serve as role models for being good citizens of the world. We enact what Vincent Van Gough said: "Your profession is not what brings home your weekly paycheck, your profession is what you're put here on earth to do, with such passion and such intensity that it becomes spiritual in calling."[1] While we may assume that some people in our profession are seeking leadership development because it can lead to more money and status, that is not the intent of building on the foundation of nursing. We suggest that the profession is the launchpad from which we can develop enhanced leadership skills because much is already expected of us.

Those attributes of practicing in legal and ethical ways, of being competent, and of serving as role models probably contribute to nurses being recognized as the most trusted profession.[2] Our selflessness is not unique to nursing, yet it seems to be a word commonly associated with us. The DAISY Foundation, for instance, has capitalized on all of the best about the profession and found a way to recognize the outstanding exemplars of what nursing is about.[3] The foundation says it honors nurses for their compassionate and extraordinary care no matter where they practice. The Daisy Award provides the opportunity to celebrate nurses who give of themselves to provide extraordinary care for patients or learning experiences for students.

The term *profession* represents several fields, each of which has associated values. For example, nurses are associated with caring. On the other hand, we don't think of truth as a value of someone whose life is focused on crime. We associate truth with certain professions, such as those related to religion, health care, or the judicial system. In fact, in the judicial system, truth is part of the mantra of "seeking truth and justice."

VALUES

Most organizations today have values statements. Sometimes they are emblazoned on a wall near an entrance or etched on glass or prominently displayed on various documents. The key is this: Are they emblazoned and etched in the hearts of the members of the organization and prominently displayed in actions, both large and small? Simply put: values are just words if they aren't exhibited by everyone in an organization because they believe in those values.

Have you ever seen a statement of values where a dozen or more words are listed? While we may have multiple values, when we cannot prioritize those values into a succinct few, we may be too unfocused—or at least not helpful to the people in an organization. Being able to state an organization's values is an important expectation for all employees. If values are simply cute acronyms for key words and are not embedded in the organization, they are not serving the members of the community well.

Recently, we (the authors) saw an organization's list of values. They numbered more than 10! That means if you remember words by counting them off on your fingers, you have to enlist your toes. It isn't that any of the words were inappropriate. The wide-ranging set of words simply didn't allow the organization to be clear about what its bottom-line values were. This example is unlike a couple of nursing organizations we know. Both the American Organization for Nursing Leadership (AONL, formerly the American Organization of Nurse Executives [AONE]) and the National League for Nursing (NLN) are succinct in their values. One of us had a first in-depth exposure to AONE's values while serving on the strategic planning committee. The values were succinct, and the whole strategic plan fit on one piece of paper! When anyone read that document, they knew what AONE valued and where it was headed. Similarly, when NLN moved its offices to Washington, DC, its core values were etched on the glass surrounding the main conference room. It is not possible to enter the headquarters without seeing the four words (caring, integrity, diversity, and excellence) boldly displayed. Many nurse educators agree that NLN always adheres to its values. Those two examples are representations of clear organizational values.

Being able to state personal values is equally important. Steven Hayes, a professor at the University of Nevada, says, "Values are what bring distinction to your life."[4] In other words, they set each of us apart from others and let us find kindred souls who have our same (or similar) values. He goes on to say that values are inexhaustible and only embraceable and demonstrable. In other words, if our values are real, they don't wear out or apply only in certain situations, and we cannot help but exhibit them to others—they are us!

Even more important to the individual is being able to see where the statements of values fit with organizational values and where conflict occurs or is likely to occur. If we really paid attention to an organization's values before we decided to engage with an organization, we might experience less moral distress. A great question to ask a prospective leader during an interview is: "How do you see yourself living the values of our organization?" If the person provides simplistic answers or the answer sounds scripted, those values are at the "emblazoned-on-the-wall" stage for that person! Similarly, a person being interviewed for a position within an organization should ask for an example of how the values of the organization were implemented in practice *in the last week.* (Note the inclusion of a specific time. Every organization has "The Story" everyone uses as the example of values. The real question, however, is whether that was a one-time occurrence or if it is a lived reality!)

All human beings have a set of values—whether they know it or not. Those values can direct some people to behave poorly because one of their values might relate to seeking attention at any cost. Personal values can also direct others to behave well because they care about their fellow human beings. Personal values ignite action without a "thinking through" what values we have, which apply in a given situation, what the benefits and liabilities of action are, and so forth. Personal values simply ignite us to action.

TABLE 3.1 Leadership Development Model by Miles and Scott (2019) Linked to Gardner's Tasks of Leadership

Miles and Scott	Gardner
Individual	Envisioning goals; renewing; affirming values
Group	Managing; explaining; achieving a workable level of unity; motivating
Society	Serving as symbol; representing the group externally

From Miles JM, Scott ES. A new leadership development model for nursing education. *J Prof Nurs.* 2019;35:5-11; and Gardner JW. On leadership. New York, NY: Free Press; 1990.

The leadership development model presented by Miles and Scott identifies three areas in which we must address values.[5] They are individual, group, and society. These three areas have grouped the work of Gardner's tasks of leadership into the most relevant areas.[6] Table 3.1 shows the relationship of the three areas of values with the corresponding tasks of leadership.

REFLECTION What are your key values? How few can you name? Those are really your core values.

THE 5 Cs

When Karren and Pat wrote "The 5 Cs of Leadership" in 2003, we considered the most prominent words beginning with the letter C that appeared in nursing's literature (see Table 3.2).[7] We could have chosen T—trust and truthfulness come to mind instantly. Or we could have chosen V—and the idea of vulnerability rises to the top. Patrick Lencioni would advocate for T because so much of his work centers around building trust.[8] Similarly,

TABLE 3.2 The Five Cs of Leadership

Compassion
Confidence
Commitment
Connectedness
Character

From Kowalski K, Yoder-Wise PS. The five "Cs" of leadership. *Nurse Leader.* 2003;1:26-31.

Brene Brown would advocate for vulnerability, based on her years of work on this topic.[9]

Meanwhile, you may wonder why we chose the letter C rather than some other letter. The answer relates to the word most commonly associated with nursing's best attribute and the word most commonly associated with the root of most issues. Both words start with C: *compassion* (or caring) and *commitment*. For example, we don't hesitate to respond to crises when they arise, as was demonstrated with nurses volunteering to go to the coronavirus "hot spots"; we often seek unusual solutions for unusual requests. Nurses are the ones who slog through extreme weather to come to the aid of colleagues and to serve their patients. Additionally, nurses have been described as the glue in many health care settings. That is because we are well *connected*. We value our relationships with patients and their families, and we often think of the people we work with as our families. *Confidence*, another C word, reflects the profession's continued growth in competence and skills in caring for the broad spectra of health care issues in a wide array of places. And finally, we know that the core of successful people, defined here as making major contributions to the profession, is what may be the most important C—*character*.

Each word alone has great implications for exhibiting leadership in nursing. Together, however, these five words suggest that we have the potential to make a huge impact on health care leadership, similar to the influence we have had on patient care.

Although health care has changed dramatically over the intervening years, those five words still hold great relevance. And while you might find those words sporadically throughout course syllabi or position descriptions, deliberative development plans to build these skills are almost nonexistent. The main exception could be viewed as building confidence. Simulation, as a key example, fosters the development of confidence. Yet these five words provide a solid foundation for the development of leadership. Without these elements in place, we may evolve in headship (position titles indicating a formal leadership position) but not in leadership (the skills of leading irrespective of position).

Many other C words come to mind that could describe the foundation for being Legacy Leaders. Additionally, other letters could be used to create a list of words to describe the essence of nurse leaders. However, rather than creating more words that could become overwhelming, we want to use these five still-relevant words as the cornerstones of how to build leaders for the future.

Fig. 3.1 reflects a view of these cornerstones. The word *cornerstones* may seem a strange analogy—after all, most cornerstone analogies are based on four: the number of corners in a square building. What makes sense to us—and hopefully to you—is that character is the central foundation, as shown in Fig. 3.1.

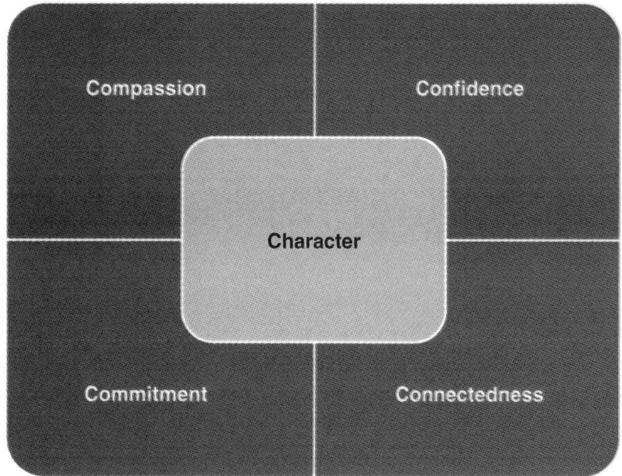

Fig. 3.1 The 5 Cs of leaders as the cornerstones.

Compassion (Caring)

Compassion is described as an openness to feelings. The term *caring* is synonymous with the profession, and if a leader wants to be effective in that profession, caring must be evident. However, this caring goes beyond the concern for patients an organization might encounter. This C relates to how leaders must truly care for the people within the organization. This caring, or compassion, can't be expressed as one races down a hall. It can't be scheduled, as in a monthly meeting, and it definitely can't be scripted to convey the almost identical message for each person. It must be spontaneous and genuinely linked to a specific person. Think, for example, if you have been really sick and you finally return to work to be greeted with a "glad you're back" message and then everyone goes about their business as if you simply had a day off. Think how differently you would feel if your immediate supervisor came to you—even if you had been at work for a few hours or a few days—and asked how you were in terms of the specific issue for your absence and if you needed anything special. When that kind of communication occurs, we feel as if that person truly cares about us and our welfare, whereas the "glad you're back" message may make us feel as if we were needed to fill a slot.

When one of us worked at a small organization in Michigan, one of the nurses was absent one day because her dog was quite sick:

"When she returned, several people questioned her thinking: Why were you at home with a sick dog? For some people, a dog is just a dog. For others, it is another member of the family (as was true in this case). I began my conversation with this nurse by acknowledging how much more welcoming a

dog is on a typical day than any member of the family. No one else rushes out to the garage expressing great delight that YOU are home like a dog does! In this case, that conversation starter allowed us to talk about numerous issues."

Finally, in a study by Groysberg and his team, caring (compassion) was ranked first or second by 68% of the respondents.[10] It was viewed as creating improved teamwork and engagement, among other positive outcomes. The only culture style that exceeded that response was results (89% chose that as their first or second response), which is about achievements and the ability to do the best and most that you can. Caring is the connection that people seek in preferring one employment opportunity over another or working with a particular group of people rather than a different group. Although it is intangible, it is highly influential.

Confidence

Basically, confidence is the view you have of yourself as able to achieve whatever you set your mind to. Self-assurance is an attribute necessary for leadership—and for nursing. Patients don't want to hear that you might be able to take care of them, and people with whom you work don't want to hear that maybe you could pull something off if really forced to do so. Patients and the people you work with want to know you are confident in your personal and professional abilities and that you understand yourself sufficiently not to be foolish in your expectations. As we said in 2003, you have to know what you don't know in order to grow, and if you aren't growing, you aren't simply stagnant—you are falling behind. The intensity of health care (and the world) today demands that we have a clear perspective of who we are and what our abilities are so that when we say we can do something, everyone can rely on that something being done. One of the tools we will discuss later that really helps us think about the contributions we bring to any group is the StrengthsFinder assessment.[11] Basically this tool helps people understand what their natural tendencies are so that they can build on those abilities. What does that have to do with confidence? Well, if you operate as much as possible from a position of strength, you feel more confident, and if you feel that way, you actually become that way. Or as Amy Cuddy, former Harvard professor and author of *Presence: Bringing Your Boldest Self to Your Biggest Challenges*, would say, you really can fake it till you are it because you act your way into what you want to achieve.[12]

What prevents us from being self-assured, or confident, is fear. Karren uses the letters of that word to convey a different message: False Evidence Appearing Real.[13] We may tend to give ourselves negative messages (I can't balance my checkbook; I'm so dumb!) or we assume the worst possible scenario when confronted with something new (What if I say the wrong thing? Will I be dressed the right way?). In a sense, when confronted with something challenging, many of us do the prom night routine. If you went to your high school prom, you tried to second-guess various details of the event to the point it was almost difficult to have fun, and having fun was the purpose of the prom!

Commitment

Most of us have heard older relatives lament the world today, especially in terms of commitment. A common phrase they use is "a man is only as good as his word." (We choose to think that phrase was the use of man in the same sense as the "all men are created equal" meaning, today, humankind.) Commitment basically means if we say we will do something, we do. No one wants to follow a leader who waffles and says one thing and does another or who commits to a goal or a deadline and can't keep that commitment. We see this inconsistency played out on a frequent basis when we look at organizational statements of values. When those words aren't committed to, employees talk about them as words on the wall or lip service, and they have difficulty feeling compelled to adopt those words as their own. A way to think about commitment is to think of whatever you say you commit to is a promise.

Short-term commitments are fairly easy to live up to. They last a few hours or days. Long-term commitments, however, are more challenging, primarily because of all the intervening variables that occur as we move through months and years. People who have sustainability toward a goal are critical to a group's effort in long-term situations. They are the ones who remind others of why the group is doing something and what value it brings to the organization or people.

John Maxwell, in his video series, says that nothing happens until we make a commitment.[14] Although we may be part of a group, we aren't really engaged with the work until we commit, either publicly or privately. A strategy we (the authors) use in group work is to go around the room and provide the opportunity for people to state their commitment or to raise questions before we move ahead as a group. Maxwell also points out that an external commitment tends to make people happy. We see we are here for a bigger purpose than just ourselves. Yes, we select positions for a variety of personal reasons, but that doesn't mean we will stay or be engaged with the work if we don't see it as something more than "just about me."

Connectedness

If you look back to the model in the prior chapter, you will find the word *relationships* in the environment triangle.

The basis of that as an important factor derives from this C, the desire to be connected to other people and to meaningful work. We often start out with a small trusted circle of colleagues and friends. Some people never really expand that circle much and, by doing so, limit their influence and resources. Meeting and knowing others provide you the opportunity to have a wider range of influence. That influence might be within the organization or external to it. Equally important is that you have more resources available to you. Being able to reach out to someone across the country or the world to talk about an issue you might be experiencing can assure you whatever the issue is, it is not unique to you and you have an external opinion available to you.

The key work of leadership is influence or inspiration, and it is impossible to influence others if we aren't connected to them. We can feel a part of something, such as a concert, because we are all in the same space, listening to the same music. To be connected, however, means that we have to reach out to others and find mutual understanding and feelings to have a true connection. It is the basis for creating relationships with others so that we have the opportunity to influence them and to be influenced by them.

Character

At the core of Fig. 3.1 is character, and it is centered there for a very specific reason. How we interact in society derives from our character. Character dictates how we behave even, or should we say especially, if others aren't watching. In a tweet on May 15, 2019, Adam Grant, Harvard professor, stated that the ends never justify the means because they are the measures of your character. Character dictates whether we are honest, trustworthy, accountable, caring, and so forth. Think of this: your leader is a good, honest person who makes a mistake. What do you do? People tend to gather round and be supportive. Now think of the leader who is self-centered, takes credit for everything, and makes a mistake. What do you do? This time, people often let the leader struggle through without help or support from the team unless the leader has directed others to do certain things.

Our character derives from a variety of influences. Family, faith, and friends are three common sources. Character is what causes us to experience moral distress when something happens that doesn't fit with our values. Because so many ethical dilemmas occur in a typical health care setting, we would benefit from thinking very deliberately about how we developed our character, what our limits are, and how we handle conflicts with values. Character is the core of who we are, and when we stop being us, we are no longer successful.

Is character important to leadership development? Well, the US Air Force Academy must think so. The Center for Character and Leadership Development publishes the *Journal of Character and Leadership Development.* Most leadership development efforts in health care settings do not address character. Yet the Air Force does so on a regular basis. Chad Hennings, writing in one of the issues, says people who strive for excellence are the force of character, people who always do their best.[15] He further points out that "we don't talk about topics like character and virtue enough."[15] That applies to health care! John Maxwell puts it another way—your success stops where your character stops.[16]

> **REFLECTION** How could you initiate a conversation about character and virtue in your organization? Would you feel secure enough to do so? Who likely would be your allies?

THE INTEGRATION/INTERCONNECTEDNESS OF THE 5 Cs

As with any other set of characteristics, each element has value on its own and leads toward quality. The integration of the elements, however, produces something even more powerful. To be effective leaders, we need to have compassion (or caring). To learn about others and express our caring, we have to be connected. Both of these require some degree of confidence to reach out to others and take a risk in telling them what we think. Most of our work, sometimes even in our personal lives, requires a commitment to something bigger than we are, and at the core of everything is who we are as people—our character.

CREATING A VALUE MODEL IN TOUGH DECISION SITUATIONS

Steven Johnson, author of *Farsighted: How We Make Decisions That Matter the Most,* suggests a strategy for consciously using our values in making decisions.[17] We likely always have our values influencing our decisions, but we may not have consciously considered them in an effort to get to a decision. We don't recommend using this approach for most decisions, yet sometimes we really get stuck and can't decide which avenue to take.

Identify values you hold in relation to the decision to be made. Assign a score of 0 to 1, with 1 representing a highly rated value for you. These values might include equity, security, caring, integrity, or any other value you hold dear. Place these on a vertical axis. On a horizontal axis, list all the options you might consider related to the decision to be made. Those might entail doing nothing,

TABLE 3.3 Generic Example of the Values Model

		OPTIONS		
Values	**Weight**	**Alter the Offer**	**Refuse New Assignment**	**Leave**
Honesty	0.9	90 = 81	90 = 81	90 = 81
Caring	0.7	90 = 63	50 = 35	50 = 35
Balance	0.5	50 = 25	90 = 45	50 = 25
Excellence	0.8	95 = 76	50 = 40	50 = 40
Totals		245	201	181

In this example, the best option is to alter the offer.

speaking up, negotiating with the person in charge, and so forth.

For the intersection of each value with each option, assign a score from 1 (low) to 100 (high). This score is based on how a particular action fits with the intersected value. As an example, doing nothing might score a 10 when compared with caring and a 90 when compared with security. Multiply the weight of the value times the score of the option. For each option, add these new numbers to form a final score. The option with the highest score indicates what best fits with the values you identified as important.

Table 3.3 poses a generic example of how the model might look once each of the values and options has been identified and weighted or scored. You might be asked to assume a new role that conflicts with an ongoing family obligation. Your options for action might be alter the offer, refuse the new assignment or leave. If you choose to use this model, please do so only for those decisions where you are waffling among choices. Note that this model allows you to consider multiple options by extending the horizontal axis. It isn't a mere listing of pros and cons for each. It requires you to return to what values you hold most important and use them as a driving force for the options you identified.

REFLECTION Consider what words have the greatest meaning to you in your professional life. Write those down. Does a theme emerge (for example, a specific letter), or is an acronym possible to help convey core values? The NLN's is DICE (diversity, integrity, caring, excellence).

LL ALERT

- Don't take the easy way out in avoiding an issue because every position in health care has some leadership potential.
- Don't avoid exercising that potential because avoidance limits what we can contribute to making a person, a group, or a system better.

SUMMARY

We come to leadership development with a rich foundation in nursing. We think we have been well prepared to focus some of our energies on developing more specifically in the role of leader. We all have values. Some of us simply aren't aware of what they are. Leaders know what their values are and if they are in alignment with those of an organization. Our (the authors') values remain in the 5 Cs. That doesn't mean we don't have other values. What it does mean is we have boiled our words down to a manageable, recallable set of words that have real meaning to us in serving as leaders.

LL LINEUP

- Use the talents you gained through the education and experience of nursing as the base for developing your leadership abilities.
- If the 5 Cs don't resonate for you, create a list of values (keep that list to five or fewer).

REFLECTION Consider what you value in life and nursing. How have those values shaped choices you made related to your career?

4

Lifelong Learning

If you are at work, think of what you are doing right now. Did you learn that in your first nursing education program? (Did your role or work even exist then?) When you graduated from your school of nursing, did you know everything you needed to know to meet the performance expectations of your first position? Have you specialized? How did you do that? Do you remember your first phone? Is the phone you have now capable of more functions at faster speeds? How did you learn to use the new phone? Obviously, the point of these questions is that continuing to learn is critical for our personal survival and even more important in terms of patient care.

The Institute of Medicine (IOM; now the National Academy of Medicine) released *The Future of Nursing* report in 2010. Among the eight recommendations, several related directly to education, either by using that word or a related one. These educational recommendations were (1) achieving higher levels of *education* and training through seamless academic progress, (2) doubling the number of nurses with *doctoral degrees*, (3) increasing the numbers of nurses with a *baccalaureate degree* so that 80% of registered nurses working with patients/clents hold that degree, (4) creating *nurse residency* programs, and (5) ensuring nurses participate in *lifelong learning*.[1] Over the intervening years, all of us (the authors) have been actively engaged at the state level working to implement these recommendations.

Most states know where they are with the first four recommendations on the list. They are all related to more formalized preparation and outcomes. The latter ones, however, are fairly unknown. How many groups and organizations have created a program they call a residency program? We know some have, but surely those that are known don't represent the whole of the efforts. Many have created an accredited residency program through the Practice Transition Accreditation Program (PTAP), with the American Nurses Credentialing Center (ANCC). Some facilities have created programs that are not accredited, causing some confusion about the name "new graduate residency program." In addition, how many nurses participate in continuing education beyond that required of an employer or what is needed for licensure? While most certification programs require nurses to participate in continuing education, not all nurses are certified. No "roster" of offerings across the spectrum of nursing exists so that any individual could see where to build depth and where to find breadth in learning. Additionally, support for learning across various health care organizations ranges from someone who provides some learning opportunities on a part-time basis to a complex department of many specialists.

What we really don't know is how many nurses participate in lifelong learning. In part, this is because of what lifelong learning really is.

WHAT LIFELONG LEARNING IS

Michael Bleich calls lifelong learning "intentional learning" because it must be deliberate and specific to us as individuals.[2] Lifelong learning is a long-range focus on the individual who uses a variety of resources to meet needs or interests in an attempt to remain relevant and informed. It begins at some point in life, frequently after the completion of a person's initial education. The resources may include formal degree programs; formal, organized, continuing education courses; print matter (such as journals); software (such as videos and simulations); and serendipity (finding something from an unrelated newspaper article or television show, an overheard conversation, or a tweet that causes the person to seek further information). Because lifelong learning has such a broad definition, it is difficult even for the individual to document where or how something was learned. We can count the number of academic credits earned and the number of formal continuing education participation hours. We can even count some reading we do because a journal or professional organization has determined it would take someone a specified number of hours to read the article. The other "spur-of-the-moment" and unexpected learning situations typically do not have any way to be documented as learning. Finally, during the early stages of the pandemic, we engaged in what one of us calls "real-time" learning, meaning we learned as we were doing.

If you are an admirer of Theodore Roosevelt, you might appreciate that Roosevelt was a "lifetime learner."[3] John Coleman, author of *Make Learning a Lifelong Habit*, argues that learning can't just be fun and we can't just engage in it sporadically. Rather we must form a habit, such as what Roosevelt did. One specific strategy he suggests to meet learning goals is to develop a learning community. Our most likely examples in nursing are journal/book clubs. He also suggests considering massive open online courses (MOOCs), audiobooks, podcasts, iTunes U courses, and learning apps. Technology can enhance the idea of creating the habit of learning, and it leads to the idea of a lifelong learner.

Dealing only with new learning is insufficient. For example, learning to "unlearn" is also a critical approach to improving. If we couldn't unlearn, we would probably still be dealing with barber shops providing illness care! If we unlearn nothing else, we should attend to processing negative experiences. Because they typically have intense emotions associated with them, negative experiences become the driving forces in our perceptions of many situations. Career coach J.T. O'Donnell suggests that we write a story about our career because it often includes the intense emotions we have experienced throughout that career. Her intent is that we learn to drop the emotion and move ahead. She calls this the Experience + Learn = Grow model. In short, when we examine those intense experiences we see as creating our career, we can isolate the negative so that we can move on![4]

One set of authors suggests we need to consider seven key practices to be successful in lifelong learning. Those seven practices appear in Table 4.1. Using van Dam's model, Jaqueline Brassey, Nick van Dam, and Katie Coates elaborated on these practices. Each of the practices makes sense on its own, and combining them can potentiate lifelong learning.[5] We just looked at why we would want to do some unlearning to lead to growth, but think of the vast opportunities in nursing to expand the way we consider new information, innovations in practice, and new opportunities to lead. Keeping ourselves mentally stimulated throughout life allows us to make connections in thinking that we wouldn't be able to do if we didn't continue to learn. As Bradley Staats says, "To succeed in this new environment requires continual learning—how to do existing tasks better and how to do entirely new things. If we fail to learn, we risk becoming irrelevant."[6]

The idea of stretching our learning is the same concept as a stretch goal in performance. A stretch goal is designed to maximize a person's contributions. The idea of stretching our learning suggests that we connect unlikely facts and concepts and consider what that new thinking might mean for what we do. This practice leads to another practice of great importance for each of us: building a personal brand. We all have a cadre of people we know to call upon if we have a certain type of problem. We have "branded" that person as good at X task. If we brand ourselves, others will think of us when they need help with an issue we have mastered. And that idea ties in with the idea of doing what we love. For example, if we love to learn and we love the idea of leadership, teaching others about leadership is a great way to take what we learn and help others be better prepared.

If lifelong learning occurs throughout one's career and not all of it can be measured in some standard unit, how do we know if this large part of continuing learning has value? In part, we may think of the value John Maxwell alludes to when he says we shouldn't focus on what people do, but who they are.[7] Learning enriches who we are even though a lot of learning may relate to what we do. As an example, learning opportunities can reinforce our character.

A key to the future is a zest for learning.[8] Although many jobs in society will never be replaced by artificial intelligence (AI), it will affect how those jobs are performed. Without lifelong learning, people could lag behind what the new work requires. Problem-led leaders are those driven by challenges rather than a set of descriptors attributed to a role. When combining a zest for learning with the approach of problem-led leadership, we realize we must continue to learn.[9] We might even consider the idea of metacognition: thinking about thinking. How we learn to think better and more effectively is one strategy that helps us be more effective as leaders. One of us had the opportunity to develop a psychiatric hospital on behalf of a community mental health organization:

"I thought I was hired to tackle this development work because I was an expert in psychiatric nursing. Such was not the case! I was hired because I had an entrepreneurial spirit and had shown that spirit previously on several projects about which the hiring managers were aware. My zest to learn and my ability to be a problem-led leader made me the ideal candidate for the position."

The idea of lifelong learning also can be seen from an economic perspective. In *The Third Education Revolution,* Jeffrey Selingo says that our current view of education will not sustain the 21st-century economy, which will require "continual training" to keep current and to gain new skills.[10] We love the term VUCA (volatility, uncertainty, complexity, and ambiguity) because it describes today's health care world. Just when we think we have a good grip on something, we find a new process, medication, expectation, etc., that sometimes makes us think we know less and

TABLE 4.1 Seven Key Practices for Lifelong Learning

1. *Focus on growth.* People either have a view of being fixed or as having the potential for growth. To be effective in life, having the idea that you can continue to learn and that IQ is not a fixed state—nor is the brain's capacity—will allow you to learn what you need to know to succeed.
2. *Become a serial master.* Traditionally, we had broad, general knowledge of an area, such as nursing, and one area of expertise (say, hospice care). To be effective in the future, or actually today, we need to have multiple areas of depth. So, we may need to be expert in hospice care, and leadership and family nursing, and....
3. *Stretch.* If all we did every day was the same thing, we likely would be bored. Yet in an era of VUCA (volatility, uncertainty, complexity and ambiguity), we have to work in areas where we are uncomfortable because our work is evolutionary. But that newness becomes comfortable after a while because we have gained confidence. Taking on learning something new involves deliberative learning.
4. *Build a personal brand.* Whether deliberative or not, we all have a personal brand. That brand reveals our character and commitments. And unless we are becoming irrelevant, our brand is evolving because we are constantly learning to stay relevant.
5. *Own your development.* If we look at turnover statistics, we quickly see the need for this element. We cannot rely on an employer to provide us with everything we need to know. We are accountable for ourselves, including defining and then fulfilling what it is we need to learn and master.
6. *Do what you love.* Why would we spend our lives doing something we didn't love? Yes, we may have had jobs we hated and yet we went to work every day. If we really hated what we did, we would have to have some overriding benefit to compensate. For example, if we were paid $1 million dollars a year to do something that wasn't illegal or immoral and we hated it, we might last that year, and we might be willing to do whatever that work was because we could see the financial benefit of such income. In the end, however, what we try to do is choose to do something we love because we have a greater sense of accomplishment.
7. *Stay vital.* Think how much more effective we are when we are rested and well nourished and loved. This state of well-being allows us to learn—sometimes even for the sake of enjoyment. We remain relevant to our lives and the life of the organization.

Based on Brassey J, van Dam N, Coates K. Seven essential elements of a lifelong learning mind-set. 2019. Available at: https://www.mckinsey.com/business-functions/organization/our-insights/seven-essential-elements-of-a-lifelong-learning-mind-set?cid=other-eml-alt-mip-mck&hlkid=6f43374516d344afb1465e60d533e628&hctky=2599421&hdpid=4a586936-e25d-452d-83b4-969eb0daa091.

less. While that feeling is anxiety-producing, it is really a good thing. If we weren't connected to what was going on, we wouldn't feel that way! Selingo refers to education of the future as short spurts. This short-spurt approach cannot replace our need as a profession to continue formal education to be sure we are educated to meet the evolving expectations of the profession. It does suggest, though, that we can't simply rely on our organizations to offer some learning opportunities or that we occasionally attend a national conference. Rather, it suggests that we get focused on what we need to know and immerse ourselves. Further, nurse managers may have many people directly reporting to them. If a manager has 53 people reporting directly, how is it possible for that manager to know what *your* specific learning needs are or to meet them? The answer, of course, is it is not possible, and therefore, we have to be in charge of ourselves.

From an economic perspective, consider what organizations' priorities might be. Likely they are going to be focused on the highly skilled to make them even more productive. That is good news for us. Even though many processes in nursing have been automated, the result hasn't been reduction of the number of nurses to provide quality care. We evolve to do different things and to change our sole focus from one patient to populations until we are needed to focus on one person at a time. Our ability to be flexible in the way we provide care makes us highly valuable to any organization.

One more thought about lifelong learning: the emerging generations in the workforce may have the view of work as the gig economy, one where nurses are freelancers or have short-term contracts as opposed to permanent jobs. Clearly, they will need to be self-reliant about learning in order to stay marketable. Rather than spending their time making certain the various requirements for employment are met, they can focus on learning. Will they need learning coaches? Will continuing education courses need to be online with videos and podcasts? How will we reach those who have solo practices or practice in small, rural settings? The implications are great to assure that the recipients of care have access to competent providers. Leaders have an accountability to help others to learn, and they also have accountability for their own learning. Taking advantage of what an organization provides as ongoing learning opportunities is smart—but it is insufficient. Each of us can figure out what the emerging innovations in health care are, what we see as our role in those innovations, and what we want and need to learn. That is one example of why we have experienced a growth in learning about leadership in health care. We need leaders to carry us from the present to the future!

> **REFLECTION** Think what your current work might be like if you could automate those things capable of being automated. What will you do with the time opened up by this support?

LEARNING IN AN ORGANIZATION

We would argue that if learning hasn't occurred over a period of time, the individual is not only stagnant but falling behind. If we think about Rogers's theory of diffusion of innovations, we know that laggards comprise a small yet critical part of the people in any organization.[11] Laggards are a risk to patient safety, and we quickly see that not only are they reluctant to take on the new, but also they may be an actual danger to safety. Unlike a few decades ago, new graduates come into the profession with the knowledge that they are expected to continue their education. They understand why laggards are potentially dangerous to an organization. They know if they want to be their best, they have to continue to learn. Why then don't organizations support this learning in a more proactive way? Francesca Gino and Bradley Staats say that our traditional obsessions may be the cause of failing to improve continuously.[12] When addressing the bias toward action, they suggest the organization support the idea of building in breaks, allowing for thinking times, and using reflection. These make total sense, and yet when we think about the intensity of work in any setting where nurses function, we know breaks are infrequent and short. Even chief nursing officers find thinking time a challenge to schedule and keep.

Many new graduates know the practice of reflection, and James Kouzes and Barry Posner, probably the leading researchers about leadership, say that is how you learn leadership.[13] Sometimes, however, those who understand reflection and its purpose slip into the practice of "rehashing" as opposed to deep thinking about what went well, what didn't, and what to change and how. Using a structured process to reflect can be highly valuable, with the intent that deep thinking about what we learned becomes our focus. The intent, of course, is to be better the next time.

Francesca Gino and Bradley Staats also talk about the tendency of people wanting to fit in.[12] They suggest that we focus on helping people develop their strengths, becoming engaged, creating new kinds of experience, and then using that experience. Some organizations can get so focused on filling slots that the thought of developing people is lessened. Even organizations with solid, well-staffed professional development programs cannot address the needs of all learners. So learners need to learn to give voice to their needs, especially when they seem unrelated to their current role. Quality doesn't improve itself; it takes well-informed, motivated individuals to move an organization's effort toward quality. That requires ongoing learning!

If people are fortunate, they have the opportunity to work with someone who understands how important professional development is. As an example, Sydney Finkelstein says that great managers spend time with the people for whom they are responsible, and the focus of that time is, in effect, tutoring.[14] Further, through his research, he found that the foci of these intensive interactions were professionalism, points of craft (the how-to of the work), and life lessons. These great managers used the "teachable moment" to share information to make learning more effective. If those moments didn't occur, the subjects in his study manufactured them! They were expert at customizing to the individual what that person needed to know, they asked questions, and they modeled the behaviors expected. This is how we should learn and how we should help others learn.

> **REFLECTION** Using the work of Finkelstein (discussed earlier), consider how you can reflect on or consider those strategies for yourself in your organization.

INNOVATION IN LIFELONG LEARNING

We must acknowledge that educational institutions and organizational departments of learning have a vested interest in education—that is their business. Despite that, many colleges and universities have focused solely on degree-granting efforts. That is laudable, especially in cases where a shortage of educators exists. However, we need to consider how to be more effective about leadership development and lifelong learning in general. The idea of a personal learning cloud, a comprehensive online resource for learning, has the potential to be much more in-time learning focused.[15] In-time learning is personalized, socialized, and contextualized, and learning outcomes can be tracked, which is a common concern with continuing education participation!

REFLECTION What issue are you grappling with that is really challenging? Could you map what type of learning you need? Who could be a learning consultant? What outcomes are possible if you are effective in addressing this issue?

Georgia Tech created a new vision of its contribution to society. Susie Ivy reported on a new commission's report that basically reshapes how Georgia Tech views learning.[16] This report suggests that the institution should redirect its view by 2040 so that it isn't viewed as a physical campus and that it is the hub of learning, not just a place to earn degrees. To achieve this, educators will need to become learning advisors and to facilitate learners accessing the learning opportunities they need or want. Note first that Georgia Tech does not have a nursing program. However, if other educational institutions embrace this new view, we will eventually see that we have great support for lifelong learning. In the meantime, lifelong learning is primarily the responsibility of the individual. Embracing opportunities to learn not only keeps us relevant to what we need to do now but also lays the foundation for what our future contributions may be.

No matter how we go about committing to lifelong learning, we must be our own integrators/synthesizers of what we are learning. Have you ever gone to a meeting with a colleague and later discussed what you learned only to come away confused? How could your colleague possibly have heard what he heard when you heard something totally different? How could your colleague point out something was a great takeaway point and you don't even recall the point being made? In addition to people learning in different ways, we tend to seek (and thus hear and see) specific things that resonate for us. This kind of experience happened to one of us early in her career:

"A colleague and I went to a national meeting. My colleague came home and reported on the meeting by basically saying the sky was falling. On the other hand, I saw the outcome of the meeting as setting directions for the future. Who was right? We both were because we were coming from different perspectives. That response apparently happened to multiple others who attended the meeting because action on the topic took decades to become significant."

A colleague of ours attended the famous 1965 House of Delegates meeting of the American Nurses Association where the "Position Paper on Nursing Education" was presented. This was the first effort calling for nurses to be educated at the baccalaureate level. Our colleague was a diploma graduate at the time, took to heart what she heard, promptly secured the bachelor's degree (and subsequent degrees as well), and had an illustrious career. The idea of hearing a controversial issue and deciding what you will do is an example of an individualized learning outcome.

Grabbing knowledge, thinking about its meaning, reinforcing it with experience, informing others, and then acting on what we know and can do is what continues to push the profession forward. Two key events in nursing have really moved the profession forward. One, mentioned earlier, is the report, *The Future of Nursing*, with a commitment to follow through on the recommendations. The second is the Magnet Recognition Program®, researched by the American Academy of Nursing and implemented by the American Nurses Credentialing Center. Magnet® has evolved its standards to continue to move the profession ahead, stated an expectation for 80% of nurses to be prepared at the bachelor's level by 2020. and required evidence of how learning occurs in the organization and how that learning changes practice. So even though learning is an individual responsibility, our commitment to such activity is enhanced through external expectations that allow us to justify to others what we are doing to improve ourselves. The real key is the subtitle of Bradley Staats's book, *Never Stop Learning*.[17] The subtitle directs what we can do: *Stay Relevant, Reinvent Yourself, and Thrive*.

LEARNING BY FAILURE

Have you ever been unsuccessful at something? If not, we think you haven't pushed yourself much. Failure is a part of life. Merriam-Webster gives us a delightful way to cloak a word we tend to avoid in something that doesn't sound so bad. Failure is the omission of occurrence or performance.[18] Now we don't have to say we failed—we can say we had an omission of performance! Actually, we would like for all of us to say: Wow! I had a growth opportunity fall into my lap! Failure is permanent if you don't do anything about it. Bradley Staats puts it this way: "You can begin by understanding that despite fear of failing, people actually overestimate their future suffering."[17] One of us had such an experience when she was downsized from a large health care system:

"My initial response was 'the sky is falling,' which was followed by 'I'll never work again!' However, as I would say later,

'This downsizing was one of the best things that ever happened professionally.' It set the trajectory for the next component of my career."

So, part of our unwillingness to try something new stems from our fear of failure. To make the situation worse, we think the worst possible outcome is the likely result of the failure. Despite all of the optimism we (the authors) have presented here about failure having good qualities, we recognize that many of us still work in environments where people look for what we call a "designated blamee." In other words, rather than figuring out the whole of the situation and how to correct it for the future, some organizations busy themselves with looking for someone to be the culprit—even when the situation is clearly riddled with potential suspects and the system itself doesn't work. In those situations, we advise caution in taking on risks beyond what we normally do in our regular work. The organization can't tolerate the discussion that should ensue to identify issues and their resolution.

Think about this: if you learn from some mishap and reflect on what led to the outcome, you have answers to consider for the next time. In essence, failures are major learning experiences (MLEs). We don't advise going about creating failures to increase your learning, but when you do fail, have the "right" attitude about it and take the learning you gain to do your best next time.

LL ALERT

- Don't become so involved in learning that you forget to live.
- Don't risk being irrelevant because you didn't test and adopt or adapt that learning.

SUMMARY

In order to develop anything, and especially leadership abilities, lifelong learning is essential. Without the attitude that we are never "finished as nurses," as Nightingale[19] said, we are doomed. We may hate learning some part of a job, and yet if that knowledge is integral to being successful, why would we not commit to learn? If we want to move along a continuum to be better leaders, why would we not commit to a lifetime of learning?

LL LINEUP

- Have a plan that includes formal (degree and continuing education) and informal (learning from others in unstructured ways) learning.
- Determine what to learn next on a regular basis.

REFLECTION If you have been out of a formal academic learning program for more than 3 months, consider what you have done that would provide evidence of being a lifelong learner. How have you spent your learning time? What have you done in a traditional continuing education credit approach? What have you done in a serendipitous manner? How have you integrated that learning into what you do? Have you met or exceeded any externally imposed expectations such as continuing education requirements for licensure or certification? If you are in a formal academic learning program, consider how what you are learning makes you more relevant to your current work. How does it better prepare you for the future?

5

Purpose

Why do we do what we do? Why do we exist? What difference will we make for others? These are the kinds of questions we ask when thinking about the term *purpose*. Purpose gives us direction. In our personal lives, it directs how we relate with family and friends. In our professional lives, it structures what we do, and if we are fortunate enough to have a big-picture view, we know that purpose is bigger than any of us and it directs an organization to a greater outcome.

WHAT IS PURPOSE

Another word for purpose is *intent*. Every health care service says something about making people's lives better in terms of their health. Yet we look at multiple organizations and see very different ways of being. That must mean organizations have more than one purpose. For example, some organizations must make money because they have financial shareholders. Others serve their purpose through a religious venue and limit some services (such as abortions) and support others (such as an active chaplaincy). Yet all of these have the purpose of providing some type of service that is designed to support people. Understanding the full purpose (or multiple purposes) is critical to being satisfied in an organization. But what about purpose at the individual level?

Each of us has some purpose driving us (or pulling us) toward some goal or goals. For example, Tim Cook, CEO of Apple, shared that he left a successful position at Compaq to join Steve Jobs at a fledging business on the verge of bankruptcy because the values at Apple aligned with Cook's values. He saw he could live his view of his purpose. When our purpose isn't clear or we have multiple purposes, our effort in serving and achieving each is diffuse. A purpose is really the why behind the what. Others see the what and sometimes make assumptions about the why. Therefore if you think your why is important, you shouldn't rely on others guessing correctly what that is. In a sense a purpose is like a vision. You know where you want to go, yet only when the information is actually shared do others understand where you are headed and why. Sinek and others say, "Your vision is only actionable if you say it out loud. If you keep it to yourself, it will remain a figment of your imagination."[1]

We all have work we do. We often can teach someone else how to do at least some aspects of our work. The real question is why do we do what we do? What gets us out of bed every day?

> **REFLECTION** If you aren't clear about your purpose in the world, stop reading and ponder that question. Create a succinct statement you can share with others. For example, although each of us (the authors) has a different purpose statement, we can all agree that a big part of our "why" statement is about developing others to be solid leaders. What is your purpose?

Purpose, as the Legacy *Leaders*-Ship Trajectory shows, is built on people's professional backgrounds and their values. It is supported or evolves through lifelong learning. If you yourself haven't said this, we are confident you have heard the phrase "I found myself" (or my niche or my passion). These words mean that the person has been floundering or deliberately testing thoughts, careers, lifestyles, and so forth. No matter if our purpose was evident since childhood or it became clear yesterday, the point is that all of us have a purpose, even if we aren't yet clear what it is. People without homes who are struggling to survive may have the purpose of survival; others who have great wealth may have the purpose of making more money, or they may have the determination to donate generously to a specific cause or multiple causes. Even people who seem to wander through life may have a purpose even if they cannot espouse it. Some people are still in the floundering stage and have difficulty engaging in some activity that might be relevant to them. From all of that, we can say this: most people have a purpose, and once they are clear about it, they are guided by it, just as they are guided by their values.

In Boris Groysberg and colleagues' study, purpose garnered only 9% of the respondents' choices for first or second place about what was important.[2] The first two choices were results (89%) and caring (63%). In a way, this makes sense because if an organization isn't producing results, it is likely to become extinct. If it isn't caring, turnover occurs more frequently than in organizations where caring is evident. Purpose is about idealism and something beyond ourselves, and in today's fast-paced world, we sometimes have difficulty seeing the bigger picture because so much is right in our faces. Purpose, however, is what can take us to new ways of being because it allows us to see the world in a different light.

A 2019 report focused on looking at purpose and various life factors suggested that having a higher purpose is positively connected to a longer life and negatively connected to cause-specific mortality.[3] This study suggested, in essence, that when people see a bigger reason for being other than the obvious, they live longer and have fewer instances of heart, circulatory, and blood conditions. As a result, we might think of purpose as being a critical component of our health status.

GETTING TO PURPOSE

Most of us do work that we love—except for the parts we hate. For example, all three of us (the authors), if "forced" become detail oriented. For a big-picture perspective, however, we are looking for the sense of what is happening and what that means in our respective worlds. Yet all of us can figure out whether we are focusing on the right things. Steven Hayes, a professor of psychology in Nevada, offered 10 signs indicating you know what matters.[4] Table 5.1 cites those signs and provides examples for us to consider in our personal and professional lives.

The beauty of being clear about purpose is that it allows us to sift through the numerous opportunities that present themselves (or we make for ourselves) and select those that are most rewarding in terms of our purpose. We typically don't do one set of totally unrelated things for our personal life and another unrelated set of things for our professional life. We integrate our efforts in our wholeness and choose among the options to more closely approximate our end goal in life—to achieve our purpose of being.

The Sense of Enough

We all know the feeling of having eaten a particularly good meal, and we may even say something about the possibility of eating more. But we don't. We are sated. Think of an emotional sating, when whatever you are doing or who you are in the moment is enough. That is what the sense of enough is about. It doesn't mean that, just like eating, you won't repeat tomorrow the processes you used today. You are doing what you are doing (or being how you are) because you feel fulfilled. That fulfillment often relates to work reflecting your vision of your purpose.

Readily Naming Heroes

Hayes suggested that part of how we know what matters is because we can identify the people who helped us get to where we are.[4] We suggest you carefully think about making this list public because in naming some, you have omitted others. If, however, you clearly had one or two people who stand out in your life, by all means acknowledge them. Whereas some of us may describe how these people helped shape us and our thinking, we may not feel the same about certain people or leaders. Why offend them when we are seldom asked to list our heroes? If you are asked to do so, you might try honoring the "hero of the day," meaning you have many and today you are recognizing one person and why that person is your hero. If you are effective, people will ask for the next day's hero too. Rather than list people, consider this: it is sufficient for you to know who they are and then to thank each person personally.

Singling Out Life's Sweet Moments

Why would we single out specific moments? We have some ideas that might be useful to you. First, those sweet moments tend to make us smile (we are engaged emotionally). Second, they provide us with the opportunity to look at those moments and consider what message we can take away in terms of what we value. What specifically made the moment "sweet" or memorable? Can we link our sweet moments to our purpose? If not, do we need to consider what our perception of our purpose is?

Identifying Our Greatest Pains

Some of these pains may tell us what to avoid. Others may tell us those pains point out conflicts with our purpose. Think for a moment about the troublemaker in an organization, one who may be the bully. That person derives pleasure in causing angst for others, and generally the rest of us experience that angst because whatever is the focus of the bullying doesn't fit with our values or contribute to our purpose. Think if you have heard someone say, "It pains me to tell you this…." That person may be saying he or she hates giving bad news or that the expectations of being honest or cooperative were violated. Often, painful moments or events are in opposition to the sweet times and to our stated purpose and values. Our pains provide a window to what we value, including our purpose in life.

The Next Life-chapter Theme

People without purpose "go with the flow." They often can't describe what tomorrow may be like, let alone the next life-chapter theme. Those of us with purpose may not be accurate

TABLE 5.1 Understanding Purpose and How It Relates to Both Personal and Professional Perspectives

Sign	Personal	Professional
You feel *a sense of enough*, rather than a need to measure whether you have more or less than others.	Most of us have heard the phrase "keeping up with the Joneses," meaning the feeling to buy or do something just because a neighbor or friend has or does something. When we have enough, we are pleased for others and don't necessarily transfer it into our lives.	Being certified is a good thing so long as it is based on the desire to validate your knowledge and skills rather than accumulating one more credential.
You can *readily name* your heroes.	We often name our parents as such. They definitely had some influence. But who else has made a dramatic impact on our lives?	Some of us might name someone like Florence Nightingale or Lillian Wald. But, again, can we think of someone in our day-to-day lives who has influenced us a lot? What about a DAISY nurse?
You can *single out the sweetest moments* of your life.	We can probably recall some wedding vows that caused us to think how two people had found each other and were now so committed to each other they would let nothing stand in their way. Or maybe we think of the birth of a long-awaited child. Or the opportunity to hear a veteran tell about his or her passion for fulfilling the mission.	Lucky us! We often get to experience these because so many people are grateful to nurses during an illness. Those moments make us glad to be nurses and renew our commitment to the next person we care for or care about.
You can *identify your greatest pain*.	Hayes says "we hurt where we care" (p. 56). If we didn't care, we would ignore a snub, or if we were in pain, we would consider what we could do to avoid or minimize that pain.	As professionals, we experience various pressures in a typical day. When we consider that caring is a word always associated with us, we understand why we feel betrayed when we are unable to provide the best care possible to patients or when we know what we have to do is not supportive of the people who deliver that care.
You don't know the content, but you can *identify the theme of the next chapter of your life narrative.* [PLEASE read this one again. This to us is a clear-cut view of whether or not you are purpose driven.]	You can see the potential for love and loss. You get that these are part of the life cycle and you can have the potential to make the best of whatever evolves. You may have a goal of having a family vacation, building a home, or starting a community group.	Unless you have already mapped out a professional plan and know what you need to learn more about and with whom you need to connect and where you can find the support you need, you need to start such a plan right now. (We say this because when we postpone such critical action, we might end up like Scarlett O'Hara and worry about that tomorrow. Remember the movie *Gone with the Wind* ended without our knowing whether she took on all of the issues she needed to address. No better time to start a plan than right now!)

Continued

TABLE 5.1 Understanding Purpose and How It Relates to Both Personal and Professional Perspectives—cont'd

Sign	Personal	Professional
It's *what you would do if nobody were looking.*	Think of some people you know who belong to certain community groups because they can be seen. If others weren't watching, would those people still want to do whatever those community groups do?	Nurses have been called the unsung heroes in health care. Few of us do something so that others see what we do. We do what we do because we are committed to a group or a project or a belief. So, even if no one notices, we don't typically stop doing what we believe in.
Your decisions *make you feel like getting up in the morning.*	If you are a parent, you may go to bed "dead tired" and emotionally drained, and yet the next morning you are delighted to see your children.	Many quotes appear in the literature about how nurses feel about their jobs. One of our favorite quotes suggests that we LOVE our work and hate our job. That is why we are ready to get up and get back to work the next day.
You can, in only a few minutes, *write about what matters.* [And you should.]	Think about how people introduce themselves. They often say wife (husband), father (mother), daughter (son), nurse. The sequence of what we say may be more meaningful than we intend.	A common statement nurses make relates to keeping patients safe—no matter what role we play in the profession. We want to see others grow, have the resources they need, get obstacles out of the way, and allow anyone who needs care to receive the best possible care.
You have a *strong desire to communicate your interests* to others.	People who take on leadership positions in the community are able to say how what they do relates to how they see their purpose in life.	Nurses who take on leadership opportunities in health care are able to say how what they do relates to how they see their purpose in their profession.
You *use your mind as a tool to humanize* rather than objectify yourself.	Consider why we choose certain community involvement over other opportunities. Is our choice made because this was a convenient choice—close to home, good hours, not too intense? Yes, at some points in our lives we choose those options, and then we find that the experiences aren't necessarily satisfying or we learn something about the experiences that allows us to connect one or more of them to our values, and we see how these experiences become expressions of how we see our purpose.	[Now read that second column again and substitute *nursing* for *community*. Can we not say the same thing for our professional lives?]

Column 1 represents work found in Hayes S. 10 signs you know what matters. *Psychol Today*. 2018:53-9, 90.

in what the next chapter is, but we know where we are headed and what we anticipate. Intervening variables (e.g., some personal tragedy) may derail us for a short or long while, but in the end, we know where we are headed.

When No One is Looking

This statement characterizes the concept of character. It suggests how we really determine to live our lives. It also tells us what our real purpose is. We have probably all told a fib (often described as a small lie). Those tend to be about inconsequential things, such as what you think of someone's clothes or a statement that did not harm others. However, would we get in front of a room full of people and give them false information, a situation that frontline nurses described when confronted with the rapidly changing information in the first months of the coronavirus outbreak? Not speaking the truth does not reflect our character for most of us. Yet we can probably name some people who do this routinely.

> **REFLECTION** What people are on your list of heroes? What people are on the list of what causes you pain?

Wanting to Get Up in the Morning

If we don't look forward to going to work (or having lunch with a friend, etc.), we are probably doing the wrong thing. Wanting to get up in the morning suggests an eagerness about what we do and who we are that makes work and interactions a pleasure! Admiral William McRaven, in his book, *Make Your Bed: Little Things that Can Change Your Life...and Maybe the World*, suggested that small routines, such as making your bed, make a difference in how we approach our work and lives. Consider what small changes you could make that will lead you to having a great impact on others![5]

What Matters

In one sense, being able to state what matters is a shorthand way to convey our purpose. For example, many people say family comes first. That brief sentence conveys messages such as work comes later, don't call me for overtime, don't ask me to take on the chair of a committee, and so forth. What matters conveys where our true interests lie and what we value in relation to how we spend our time. An example is that the macro level of behavior conveys what matters.[6] We all know what micro-behaviors are, even if we haven't called them that. They are our gestures, our manners, and so forth. The macro-behaviors, however, are more subtle. An example is if our schedule matches what we say matters. When it does, we are in harmony. When it does not, we aren't. A good way to check where we are with macro-behaviors is to think about how what we say matters and then review our schedule to see whether it reflects those values (what matters). For example, a leader in a formal role who says he is totally focused on people in his service area but hasn't personally seen anyone individually in months is in disharmony. Someone who says he values maintaining positive interprofessional relationships can show multiple meetings where at least one other discipline was present—and probably even can show one-on-one meetings with people from a different discipline.

Communicating Your Interests to Others

This isn't intended to be effusive statements about the latest thing you have learned. This communication could be repeated daily or annually because it is at the core of who you are. When you communicate your interests to others, you allow them to help you, and you are declaring your view of what is important in your world. It also has the potential to encourage others to share their interests.

Humanizing

The final sign relates to humanizing. Brene Brown, for example, suggests we allow ourselves to be vulnerable as a way to connect with others.[7] Obviously, this strategy has to be exhibited only in healthy workplaces; otherwise, you might be attacked for being weak or inadequate or wrong. The idea, though, is to help others see you as a person, not as a role or a position. Understanding the needs of others and offering support is a demonstration of humaneness and vulnerability. A simple example is when someone sends another person home because that person's parent or child is ill and needs not only health care but also family support. We become human when we put the person above the work that person is expected to produce.

ANOTHER LOOK AT PURPOSE

Another way to look at purpose is to consider how passion becomes a purpose by knowing something matters. Being clear about our passion and how to sustain it to be a passion is what allows us to take on some work for a lifetime.[8] The purpose of "a purpose" is to inspire others, and inspiration is a key obligation of being a leader. As Simon Sinek says, our obligation is to make other leaders.[1] Additionally, passion links with performance in one of four ways.[9] When passion is low and performance is low, little energy is expended. In essence, we are close to being bored. An example of this might be cleaning a room when we don't really like cleaning. When passion is low and performance is high, we likely do not enjoy what we are doing but we are fairly intense because expectations for performance are high. For someone who doesn't like driving a car, this task would be unenjoyable. The person has to pay attention because performance expectations (such as not hitting another car) are high. When passion is high and performance is low, we are enthusiastic and yet not really doing anything such as producing outcomes. When many people sing in the shower, they know they are doing it not because they are great singers, but because they love to sing and they hope no one else hears them. When both passion and performance are high, we are engaged in our calling and putting forth our best efforts. When people love to cook and are really good at it, they have both high passion and performance. When we reach that point, we are, as Csikszentmihalyi says, "in flow"—that magical point where our boredom and anxiety balance each other to keep us actively engaged.[10]

REFLECTION Think back to the last time at work when you felt absolutely elated. What were you doing? Why were you doing whatever it was? How does that activity relate to your passion and performance?

In a study about the characteristics of nursing directors that influence nurse satisfaction, one of the themes was Nurse Director Passion and Vision Foster the Quest for Excellence.[11] This means nurse leaders must have a vision or purpose that others understand. Further, using a purpose to create a *career* legacy map can ensure that you have meaningful work in nursing.[12] Who among us doesn't want to do meaningful work in our profession, especially in the things beyond our job? When we are clear about our purpose, we select the things beyond our paid employment in a deliberative way.

In our work, we have the opportunity to create an organization, department, or unit vision. That statement has to encompass what we do and why we do it. In nursing, our work isn't just about accomplishing a certain number of tasks in a given period. Our work is about creating healthier communities. Saying words that connect the head to the message is insufficient. We can mouth many messages. To be believable, we have to include our hearts![13] If we can move others to tears or to beaming pride, we have a clear organizational purpose. When we say our purpose, we are believable only if our passion is connected to the words.

REFLECTION When you think about your purpose and why you want to take on leadership abilities more intensely, are you beaming or moved to tears? If not, you may not have perfected your view of your purpose yet.

The clearer we are about our purpose, the more likely others will understand and value what we want to achieve. Daniel Pink, in his book *Drive*, says that we have to feel something. When only the head is involved, we seldom get to feeling something. "Autonomous people working toward mastery perform at very high levels. But those who do so in the service of some greater objective can achieve even more."[14] He goes on to describe how former US Secretary of Labor Robert Reich assesses an organization. Reich calls it the "pronoun test." He listens carefully to determine whether an organization is a "we" or a "they" type of organization. When we are "we," a true connection of us and the purpose exists. When we are "they," we can move on to another place because where we are is not compelling.

REFLECTION Consider how you talk about your organization. Do you refer to the people you might supervise as "they"? Are the people above you in an organization "they" also? Or are all of you "we"? Words matter.

If we take the work of Robert Quinn and Anjan Thakor and apply it to individuals versus the organization, we might find a plan for ourselves that will work. Table 5.2 makes that comparison for our consideration. Whether at

TABLE 5.2 How to Build a Purpose-Driven Organization/Person

The Framework	The Leader's Help to Others	The Leader's Personal Development
1. Envision an inspired workforce.	Expose others to positive examples of an inspired workforce.	Seek out situations where people are engaged and speak of their work in glowing terms.
2. Discover the purpose.	Seek others' opinions of their work and its impact on the organization and community.	Analyze what you love to do and why you want to do it. Actually write a personal statement of purpose. Why are you here?
3. Recognize the need for authenticity.	Use the purpose to drive decisions and actions.	Use your purpose to drive decisions and actions.

TABLE 5.2 **How to Build a Purpose-Driven Organization/Person—cont'd**

The Framework	The Leader's Help to Others	The Leader's Personal Development
4. Turn the authentic message into a constant message.	Repeat the message again and again. Ask of any activity or decision: How does this contribute to our purpose? If the answer is unclear, consider if the activity or decision is the best fit for the organization.	Consider creating a personal mantra that relates to or evokes your statement of purpose. Post it where you see it every day. Carry it in your phone—and in your head and your heart.
5. Stimulate individual learning.	Capitalize on the desire of employees to want to learn and grow.	Capitalize on your own desire to learn and grow. Make a leadership development plan.
6. Turn midlevel managers into purpose-driven leaders.	First, unless all leaders are connected to the purpose, the purpose stands little chance of being embedded. Second, because most employees relate with their direct leader, if all aren't engaged in the purpose, staff miss out on the full potential of a purpose.	Although our statements of purpose are our own, if we share them with others, we have the potential for others to buy into our intent in life. If we do not share our statements of purpose, at best, any support would be happenstance.
7. Connect the people to the purpose.	Now the key is to help everyone see how what they do on a regular basis ties in to the purpose. This becomes transformative.	We are already connected to our purpose—after all, we made our personal statement of purpose. Yet we likely haven't looked at what we do on a daily basis to see how what we do connects (or not) with our intended purpose. When we become more purpose driven, we eliminate the "noise" in our work and contribute more clearly to what the purpose of our being engaged in something is.
8. Unleash the positive energizers.	We frequently refer to these people as the champions—they have specific expectations to "spread the word" and model how it is to be engaged with a purpose.	Although we could unleash those around us who know our purpose and believe in us, we can be even more fundamental than that. We can identify those things that stimulate us, that connect to our purpose, and that make us more interested in doing better or more. Those incentives derive from within us.

Column 1 represents work found in Quinn RE, Thakor AV. Creating a purpose-driven organization. *Harv Bus Rev.* 2018:78-85.

the organizational level or the individual level, without a purpose larger than ourselves, we are as rudderless as a ship tossed about in the sea.

LL ALERT

- Don't forget that being too purpose driven means we miss a lot.
- Don't be "difficult" to work with because you see only your purpose in life, as if no other purposes mattered.

SUMMARY

Assuming we have a clear purpose statement about developing our leadership—we know where we are headed and some key steps to get there—we now have the opportunity to expand our purpose. That might be helping someone who hasn't clearly defined a purpose, or it might be taking what we have learned and making certain others have access to that same knowledge. Think about that statement this way: if we really are judged by the company we keep, we want to be sure we are in the best company. So from a leadership perspective, the more leaders we have where we spend our greatest time (which typically is work!), the more connected we can be, the more goal directed we can be, and the better outcomes we can produce. We are maximizing our leadership potential—and everyone else's.

LL LINEUP

- If you don't have a statement of purpose, make one.
- If you have one, measure everything you consider doing against it.
- Practice using your purpose as a context for others to understand why you do as you do.

REFLECTION Think about how ineffective or effective you are when multitasking. After a period of such activity, do you feel relaxed, tense, successful, unsure, or something else? Finally, ask yourself why you were multitasking. Was it to meet a deadline? Was one of the tasks boring? Were you trying to feel superior because you could do two things at once? Now consider if you have multiple purposes. Which ones have greatest value? Are you ever in conflict about the purposes you are serving? Can you be clearer about what the true purpose is?

6

Self-Assessing

Just as Kouzes and Posner would say you learn leadership through reflection,[1] we would say you cannot learn leadership if you haven't conducted your own self-assessment. For example, how would you feel if you were taking swimming lessons from someone who said they never went into the water because they didn't really know how to swim? One of us recalls someone she knew who would always say, "I read in a book once…." Reading about something, including swimming, doesn't mean we can actually do it! We would instantly think we made a bad investment. Why, then, would we accept someone telling us how important it is to know yourself but had really never participated in such activities? We might feel we were the guinea pigs in an experiment or at least, like the example noted, we were being asked to do something that the person who was doing the asking didn't believe in because he or she had never done what was being asked!

WHY DO SELF-ASSESSMENTS?

Most of us wish to live our lives in a fairly autonomous manner. We don't want others telling us what to do, how to do it, or, more importantly, who to be. We can be rebellious and function in an autonomous manner, which, of course, is not advisable because no one would want to work with us: the Trouble Maker. Rather, we can increase our understanding of ourselves (yes, even if our employers don't expect us to do that) and have that insight about who we are as we think about what we want to do with our lives. In essence, it's about the drive to have autonomy in working toward what we see as our purpose for being here and doing what we do.[2] When we have a growing understanding of who we are, we are better at understanding why we do certain things and we are better at helping others see why learning about self is important. The concept of "leading yourself" remains one of the fundamentals of leadership[3] and thus is a logical place to begin or strengthen the pursuit of a legacy.

THE TOOLS

If one perfect tool existed, we would all use it! Fortunately, many tools exist that contribute to our understanding of the elements that comprise leadership. Our task is to find and use those tools for greater insight about who we are so that we are more effective in whatever role we are in or are pursuing. This list of tools can be quite lengthy, so we are focusing on some of the more readily accessible, less costly tools in an attempt to make self-assessment a relatively easy process. What is important, though, is to remain aware of emerging tools to capitalize on the information they provide.

Rather than discuss all known tools in a general manner or a handful of tools in depth, we have chosen to provide basic information about several tools that tend to be readily available. A summary of this information can be found in Table 6.1. Note, however, that we encourage you to follow up with any tool that has been determined to be reliable and valid and sometimes involves fees for use or interpretation. The point is: the more you know about yourself, the more effective you can be in any position you might hold.

OTHER STRATEGIES

Having knowledge from assessments is insufficient. They are great starting places, yet they don't complete the full picture of who we are and what we do. Some further assessment can derive from two other major sources: others and yourself.

Others

Others can provide feedback to you about many aspects of your behavior. For example, you may want to break a habit of saying *I* or *me* instead of *we* or *us*. You can ask a trusted (and confidential) colleague to note each time you say *I* or *me* when you really mean *we* or *us*. And attaching a penalty (some denomination of money, for example) each time

TABLE 6.1 Sample Self-Assessment Tools Contributing to an Understanding of Self

Tool/Source	What It Measures	Why It Might Be Useful
The Leadership Framework Self-Assessment https://www.leadershipacademy.nhs.uk/wp-content/uploads/2012/11/NHSLeadership-Framework-LeadershipFrameworkSelfAssessmentTool.pdf	Composed of seven individual tools to measure the elements in the model.	A straightforward tool to determine our insight into the seven areas of the framework.
Zero to Three Leadership Self-Assessment https://www.zerotothree.org/resources/413-leadership-self-assessment-tool	Based on reflective leadership. Focused on formal leadership positions.	May be helpful in strengthening our ability to reflect.
How Good Are Your Leadership Skills? https://www.mindtools.com/pages/article/newLDR_50.htm	Questionnaire is to be completed after watching a video, which has embedded information about the five traits of leadership covered in the questionnaire.	Can be used as a refresher or an orientation. Video and subsequent tool focus on key information.
Collaborative Leadership Self-Assessment Tools https://northwoodscoalition.org/wp-content/uploads/2016/10/Chapter-7-Collaborative-Leadership-Self-Assessment-Tools.pdf	Six assessment categories from the Robert Wood Johnson Foundation's work.	Highly appropriate for nurses because of the nature of collaborative work.
StrengthsFinder 2.0 http://strengths.gallup.com/110440/About-StrengthsFinder-20.aspx	Talents that reflect our "go-to" responses.	Widely tested in various cultures with millions of responses in a database.
Grit Scale https://www.nytimes.com/interactive/2016/03/01/us/01grit-quiz.html	Based on Angela Duckworth's work. Interactive site.	Helps us determine how "gritty" we are (which is a characteristic of successful people).
Emotional Intelligence 2.0 http://www.talentsmart.com/products/emotional-intelligence-2.0/	Based on Bradberry and Greaves's work. The leading emotional intelligence (EI) test.	Assesses our current state of EI, which the literature says is critical to successful leadership.
Give and Take Assessment https://www.adamgrant.net/	Based on research by Grant.	Helps us know which one of three types best describes us.
Originals Quiz https://www.adamgrant.net/	Based on research by Grant.	Helps us see how we relate to others in terms of being original.
Authentic Leadership Self-Assessment Questionnaire http://people.uncw.edu/nottinghamj/documents/slides6/northouse6e%20ch11%20authentic%20survey.pdf	Assesses four components of authentic leadership.	Helps determine our degree of authenticity.
How Mindful Are You? https://hbr.org/2017/03/assessment-how-mindful-are-you	Based on a strategy to be effective.	Assesses how we see ourselves in exhibiting mindfulness.

TABLE 6.1 Sample Self-Assessment Tools Contributing to an Understanding of Self—cont'd

Tool/Source	What It Measures	Why It Might Be Useful
Clance Imposter Phenomenon Scale http://www.paulineroseclance.com/pdf/IPTestand-scoring.pdf	The tendency for individuals to see themselves as imposters.	Recognition of feeling like an imposter can free up energy.
DiSC https://www.discprofile.com/what-is-disc/overview/	A valid and reliable tool designed to portray an individual's behavioral differences.	Helps us to see why others act differently than we do and why they are equally valuable in the big picture.
Myers-Briggs https://www.mbtionline.com/	One of the oldest assessments; designed to help us understand our personality type.	Helps us understand people are different in specific ways.
Keirsey Temperament Assessment https://www.keirsey.com/	Designed to categorize individuals into one of four types.	Helps us understand people are different in specific ways.
Insights Discovery https://www.insights.com/us/products/insights-discovery/	Based on work of Carl Jung. Four-color model.	Understand style, strengths, and values we bring to a team.
Leadership Influence Self-Assessment Instrument Shillam CH, Adams JM, Bryant DC, Deupree JP, Miyamoto S, Gregas M. Development of the Leadership Influence Self-Assessment (LISA©) instrument. *Nurs Outlook*. 2017;66:130-13.	Preliminary validity and reliability established. Based on Adams Influence Model.	Assesses the distinctive ability leaders need: influence.

this occurs provides a greater incentive to change behavior. That is a simplistic example, and one we all can probably relate to.

One concern with asking others, however, is our tendency to ask a trusted colleague we like and who likes us and also who may not be able to say what we really need to hear. So we need to consider having at least two trusted colleagues. One of those needs to be more direct in conveying messages and able to deliver the messages we really need to hear.

Think for a moment of the jokes about how clothing makes us look. One of us asks: Does this look good on me? (First, note the hint of the direction the response should take: yes, it looks good on you.) Really good colleagues will tell you that the tie does not go with the jacket you have on, the color makes you look too pale, the pattern seems too informal, or something similar. But many of us don't want to create controversy and just say something to convey that the person looks fine. If we can't take on the potential for controversy over a piece of clothing, will we be able to challenge someone's thinking or vision?

REFLECTION Consider the "bigger" habits and what you might want to change. For example, do you jump in when someone else is struggling and provide a solution? In emergencies, that is probably good; otherwise, it thwarts that person's self-development and may convey that you have in mind one right way to do something and you just provided that answer. What habit do you want to change that will help you relate well with others? How can someone else help you make that change?

Self

The next source is self, and the key strategy is reflection. When we participate in reflection, we have the opportunity to consider any aspect of a situation. We can consider if we were dressed appropriately, or if we had prepared adequately for the group we were going to work with, or if we said inappropriate things (or used inappropriate words), or if we failed to interact with others, and so on. The point

TABLE 6.2 Unappealing Behaviors of Leaders

- Taking more than an equal share of something
- Eating with mouth open, lips smacking, and crumbs falling
- Interrupting coworkers
- Multitasking during meetings
- Raising one's voice
- Saying insulting things
- Taking sole credit for a team's work
- Forgetting colleagues' names
- Spending more money than in the past
- Taking unusual physical risks

From Keltner D. Managing yourself: don't let power corrupt you. *Harv Bus Rev.* 2016:112-5.

is we get the opportunity to figure out what went well and what could go better next time.

Realistically, we likely will never have the opportunity to replay whatever the situation was we just experienced. But if we think about the nature of the situation rather than the specifics, we likely can see we will encounter it again. As the saying attributed to many, including Lee Iacocca and John Gardner, goes: we will again encounter the opportunity, brilliantly disguised as a problem. Our task is to think about the big-picture view of what a situation is like so that we can use it as a resource for the future. In other words, rather than focus on specifics, if we see the "themes" in situations, they can be applied in other situations. For example, if we learned how to chair a meeting on a clinical unit, can we not take what works well there and apply that learning to a different setting once we have assessed what that other place is like?

One of the elements to consider in a self-evaluation is your response to growing leadership capabilities. The caution is that as people rise in organizations and seem "more important" in life, they may take on undesirable characteristics. Dachter Keltner identified several negative, sometimes disgusting behaviors the leaders in a group took on.[4] Table 6.2 summarizes some of those key points.

> **REFLECTION** Look at Table 6.2 and tally the number of habits you exhibit. If you have none, don't adopt any in that list! If you identified some, consider how to become aware of when and where you exhibit these behaviors and how you will change them.

Keltner also offers three thoughts for practicing graciousness, an exhibition of good power: empathy, gratitude, and generosity. Being gracious conveys to others concern for them, not for yourself or your position. In addition to boosting others' perspectives of your use of good power, they tend to see you as deserving of respect and influence. Examples of showing empathy include asking questions and paraphrasing important points, as well as being an active listener and signaling concern when appropriate. To show gratitude, leaders can say (and write) thank you, publicly acknowledge the value each person has made toward an effort, and use touch appropriately. Finally, to exhibit generosity, consider how to spend one-on-one time with people for whom you have responsibility, delegate high-profile responsibilities so others can "shine," and share the credit.

> **REFLECTION** Consider a recent situation where you thought you learned a lot. What "takeaways" did you gain from that? What was the name (yes, actually name it) of the situation (for example, conflict, praise, money, relationship) of the situation? How will you use it in the future? Please list at least two practical examples.

USING SELF-ASSESSMENT TOOLS

One final overall thought: when we seek self-assessment information, we sometimes are skeptical of it. Why do we do that? We may feel humbled by the information we receive (through tools or others), yet we may be uncomfortable hearing or reading words that suggest we really are special in some way. People look at others for comparison and think, "I'm not in any way as capable or as good as they are." This phenomenon has a name: the imposter syndrome.[5] The Clance IP Scale is used to determine whether we have imposter characteristics.[6] Higher scores on the imposter assessment tool suggest that this phenomenon might actually be interfering with our lives. On the other hand, are we really stretching ourselves if we have a low score? People with low ability on this assessment tend to see themselves as better than others, whereas people with high ability tend to assume that whatever the behavior is, it must be really easy because "I get it and of course everyone else thinks it was even easier." That thinking is reflective of the imposter syndrome.[7]

The imposter syndrome occurs more frequently in women than in men. It is present when we are unable to internalize accomplishments, and practicing mindfulness can be helpful. When we move from one position to another, we often experience this feeling because we are dealing with a new setting, or new people, or new expectations. We shouldn't be incapacitated by those changes.

LL ALERT

- Don't overindulge in using tools to assess yourself.
- Don't think a different tool will necessarily provide a different answer.

SUMMARY

Many tools exist to help us better understand ourselves in terms of developing leadership abilities. Our task is to be selective and make a plan for using the assessments we find helpful. Being deliberative in seeking feedback from others can help us understand how we appear in real time.

LL LINEUP

- Select at least one assessment to complete now.
- Select an assessment (from Table 6.1 or elsewhere) to complete on an annual basis.

REFLECTION Consider that several assessments have associated action plans. Which assessments did you use? Did they have an action plan? If not, are you able to make one? Were some more valuable than others? How will you use this information? Make a plan to use what you learned about yourself and track that for a week.

7

Reflecting

Reflective practice is the capacity to think about action and events and to enter into a process of continuous learning.[1] This is a method to study our leadership experiences and to improve our functioning. It's a process of learning from our experiences while analyzing what worked well and what we might like to do differently. Remember, Kouzes and Posner[2] said the way to learn leadership is through reflection. As an example, one of us often thought the cause of waking up at 2 a.m. was about menopause and estrogen:

"I quickly realized that it was actually driven by any difficult personal or work situation from the previous day. Learning to write down my personal thoughts on paper before bedtime caused the 2 a.m. wakeup with negative thoughts and recriminations to stop."

This technique may not work for everyone; some people are able to process verbally by talking with a friend or colleague or even thinking through a structured process—these two techniques are also reflective practices. Some of us work best by writing our thoughts and processing our experiences, learnings, and plans on paper before going to sleep. This work doesn't have to be done at 2 a.m.! Although this doesn't work for everyone, the reflective process is critical as a thought process, and the subsequent writing about events and accompanying deeper analysis facilitate growth as a leader.

Deepak Chopra works with leaders across the globe. He supports them to reflect on important questions, such as "Why do I want to be a leader?," "What brings me joy?," "What will my legacy be?," and "Who are my heroes?" Chopra teaches how to relinquish resentments, hostility, fear, and shame and go to a deeper level of awareness. Many of these leaders believe they were "just lucky" or that they were in the right place at the right time. Chopra believes that success is opportunity and preparedness merging, which is an outcome of awareness.[3]

THE EVOLUTION OF REFLECTIVE PRACTICE

The classic work of Chris Argyris and Edgar Schön[4] advanced a theory that advocated two types of reflective practice. Reflection-*on*-action involves reflection on an experience or an action already taken and consideration of the positives from the action, as well as what could have been done differently. Reflection-*in*-action (or reflecting on action in real time) is the second type. Considering best practices for communication and relationship building, we have found that successful leaders refrain from quick, sarcastic responses or "put-downs." Effective practice does not focus on the smart or cutting comments that many of us think we should have said if only we had thought of it in the moment. This is about thinking more clearly and asking questions; it is about being curious about other human beings and what they are thinking or feeling. What has created the upset? The goal is to understand other people's emotions and thinking, rather than to attempt to practice "one-upmanship."

Later, Shoen identified a third perspective: the idea of reflection-*before*-action, which focuses on thinking through a particular situation in advance. In other words, preplanning an interaction and reflecting on the best possible outcome, the worst possible, and whatever is most likely. This approach can help in dealing with surprises or being completely "blindsided" in stressful situations. As an example, one of us practiced this strategy every time she had to provide legislative testimony. Thinking in advance about the questions that could be raised allowed her to represent nursing in a more positive way than if she had to respond to questions that should have been anticipated but hadn't been thought about.

The focus on reflective practice in health care was refined by a professor of nursing, Christopher Johns, of the United Kingdom. His work over the last three decades has emphasized reflecting on clinical practice for nurses. For leaders, our practice is leadership, and most of his work is easily transferred to the practice of leadership. He encourages each of us to begin with our own thoughts about an ideal practice (in our case, leadership) or the practice observed in a nurse leader.[5] We can then reflect on the incident or experience and examine the gap between the actual occurrence and our ideal approach. He calls this the contradiction between real and ideal behavior to the same situation (reflection-on-action).

This reflection helps identify what we might do differently or reinforce what we did very well.

In this country (the United States), these ideas were taken up by critical care nurses late in the last century.[6] Nurses, along with other health care professionals, have incorporated reflection into practice settings and found both advantages and challenges to the practice. One benefit of reflective practice is increased learning, which is obtained by examining both the positive and negative aspects of the learning experience. This reflection could include not only the clinical aspects of patient care but also the very real problems with communication breakdown that occur between nurses and other health care providers. Learning often comes from what didn't work as expected. Close examination of the experience can promote deep learning, and the emotion of the experience is sealed in the practitioner's memory. We can always recall crisis situations. How often have you said, "I'll never do that again?" When the reflection is done in a rational manner, both personal and professional strengths can be identified, as well as areas for improvement. Reflecting on events supports leaders to pay attention to interactions with others and to envision our ideal practice as a lived reality. The act of reflection can also increase our resiliency.[7] It can support us in being more proactive, rather than reactive, and provides the opportunity to think through what we would do differently. Imagine the reflections of the nurses who served as frontline leaders in providing care for COVID-19 patients, tracking contacts, and testing concerned people.

Reflective practice allows leaders to continue to grow and improve our leadership practice through being mindful of situations and interactions. Being mindful translates into leaders becoming aware of patterns of intention, resulting in feelings and actions without distorting them with defensiveness, habit, resistance, and ignorance.[5]

Educational needs may also be identified. We may say: "I really need to learn more about X," which can lead to new knowledge and even a new skill set. When deep self-assessment occurs, a deeper appreciation of beliefs and values can evolve in a way that may actually change your attitudes and behavior. Such deeper understanding can lead to an improvement in personal and leadership confidence.

WHAT MAKES LEADERS REJECT REFLECTION

Jennifer Porter believes reflection is about nuanced, careful thought.[8] Effective reflection involves conscious consideration and careful analysis of beliefs and actions for the purpose of learning and growth. Limitations to reflective practice exist due to a lack of understanding of the reflective process by some practitioners. Some nurse leaders are uncomfortable evaluating or challenging what they see about themselves and in focusing on the analysis of beliefs and actions for the purpose of learning from the process. Some leaders become defensive about the weaknesses identified through reflection and, naturally, discard the positive aspects of the reflection—the behaviors that were effective. Reflection requires that we pause amidst the chaos, sort the observations and various aspects of experience and behaviors, and consider multiple perspectives and interpretations. From this approach, we create meaning while refraining from "beating ourselves up for what we did or didn't do." The more objectivity, the better! Reflection can seem very time consuming to some leaders who are primarily action oriented, and these people resist devoting the time needed to be highly thoughtful. Some leaders are focused solely on the return on the "bottom line." Because the reflective process requires time and dedication to observe an outcome from the practice, we can become impatient. Even though we know some processes take time, we want immediate results. For a combination of these reasons, some of us refuse to consider using this tool. Reflective practice is not easy, but it can be incredibly rewarding.

JOURNALING

Many leaders use journaling to facilitate their reflective practice. Journaling is the depiction of ideas or events in a person's life either in an electronic format or handwritten in a notebook. The value of recording events and experiences promotes open-mindedness, observation, self-awareness, critical analysis, problem solving, evaluation, and synthesis of learning.[9] A reflective journal needs to be useful to the leader. It's a cue that stimulates memory and must be honestly written. A journal is for the author, not for anyone else.

Journaling can be used to describe and evaluate key events or interactions. It is an effective process to identify and process recurring themes. Because it is written, it is easy for us to refer to previous similar events. This reflection can assess and reveal habits in behavior, enabling us to act on nonproductive behavior.

The most difficult aspect of journaling is getting started.[9] Begin by setting aside writing time (this works best by entering this task in your calendar). Before beginning to write, think about events objectively, including any ideas you have about the events. Don't be concerned about writing style or how it looks. Some leaders journal in bullet points or phrases, and some write in a narrative style. The purpose is to reflect on the event and what happened, what you thought and felt, and any associated motivations. Think about what evidence supports your thinking and analysis.

TABLE 7.1 Questions to Define Ideal Leadership Behaviors

- How do you see your role as a health care leader?
- What is your purpose?
- What made you choose leadership?
- How effective do you think and believe you are as a leader?
- What leadership values can you identify?
- How do you demonstrate your professional values and code of conduct?
- What is your vision?

You might begin by asking yourself a series of questions that could help you define your ideal leadership behaviors. This ideal can provide a model to compare with the actions in the event being analyzed. Table 7.1 illustrates some questions to consider.

This thought process can help you create professional ideals for both practice and learning. If you have not formed a habit of systematic reflection, now is the time to begin.

REFLECTION Using the questions in Table 7.1, create a view of your ideal leadership behaviors. Is that how you wish to be seen?

After creating ideal leadership behaviors, choose a form of reflection that can work for you. In addition to journaling, you could choose from a list of questions identified by Harry Kramer[10] that appear in Table 7.2, put them in your computer or handwritten journal and use them to stimulate your thought process when considering an episode or event where you know learning occurred. The questions can serve as a systematic process to analyze the occurrence. Or you could also talk to a colleague or a coach, who can ask similar questions to support the analysis. Focus on what is to be learned and relinquish berating yourself for those things you believe you mishandled or "should" have done differently.

As you progress along the trajectory (your career) and you expand the ability to reflect, you will notice a deepening level of thinking about and understanding your behavior and motivation. One of the most important aspects of reflecting is the deep, thoughtful consideration of noticeable patterns, both those that work and those that are problematic. As a result, it becomes easier to choose responses, even in stressful situations.[11]

Rose Sherman believes that following a line of self-questioning can establish a pattern for reflective practice, and after several reflective practice journal entries, a pattern that works for you will develop.[12]

TABLE 7.2 Questions for Reflecting on Your Leadership Practice

- What precisely did you do? Describe in detail.
- What was your intention for the interaction?
- What made you choose specific behaviors?
- What was the goal of those choices?
- What were you attempting to achieve?
- What is the chronology of events?
- How successful were your choices?
- What were the criteria you used for analyzing the event?
- What were some options you might have used?
- Could you have dealt with the event in a better way?
- How would you act differently in future similar events?
- How do you feel about the entire event?
- What knowledge or skills were demonstrated in the event?
- How do you believe the other person felt about the interaction?
- How did you analyze the event compared with past experiences?
- What would you do differently in future interactions?

TABLE 7.3 The Three-Step Approach to the Reflection-on-Action Process

1. The event/experience
2. Your reaction
3. Lessons learned

AN ADDITIONAL APPROACH TO REFLECTION

The Center for Creative Leadership[13] developed a straightforward three-step approach to a reflection-on-action process. As a thought process, you might take 10 minutes and think through this process. Or you might take 15 minutes and "journal." Table 7.3 identifies those three steps.

When looking at the event/experience, consider its relevance. As objectively as possible, think through as many aspects of the event as you can remember (do this reflection as soon after an incident as possible—the same day works best). Describe the interaction, including where it happened and who else was involved.

Next, think about your reaction. What behaviors did you display? What were you thinking at the time? What were you feeling? Describe how you reacted to the situation. What did you want for yourself in the situation?

Could you see possibilities? If you were upset, could you ask for a timeout to consider more aspects of the event?

The last step is to look at lessons learned. This is the most important step because it is preparation for the future. What did you learn from this interaction? What did you learn from your reaction to the situation? Did you notice any patterns? Could you identify any "triggers" that stimulated your reaction (perhaps certain words or gestures or a history with the person)?

Thinking about and responding to these questions can facilitate analysis of events or issues that can produce growth as a leader.[14] This shorter process can evolve as you gain experience with the reflective process.

LL ALERT

- Don't activate the critical voice in your head that tells you how stupid you are and how you should not have done or said the things you did.
- Don't detract from learning by making yourself wrong.

SUMMARY

Leaders may not have associates or close friends who can provide effective feedback. Reflective practice and journaling are excellent tools whereby you can assess, analyze, and act on a much clearer outlook regarding specific events or actions taken. Thoughtful reflection can support you in evaluating behaviors in events and interactions and in learning and adjusting for future events and interactions. This is a process of continual learning and growing.

LL LINEUP

Effective legacy leaders are continuously growing based on experiences:

- Focus on continual growth.
- Practice reflection three times a week for 30 days.
- Describe any change in your behavior or processes at the end of the 30 days.

REFLECTION Think about the last time you were involved in a difficult situation, one in which you felt blindsided or inadequately informed and you felt your performance wasn't the best. You may have been speechless or felt like a "deer in the headlights." Think through the chronology of events and begin writing. Use the questions in Tables 7.1 and 7.2. Think about what your ideal leader would have said or done in this situation. Look for gaps between the ideal and the actual. Use this information as the basis for how you might change the behavior the next time a similar event occurs.

8

Framing

One of the skills leaders need to learn and use often is the art of framing. Framing basically means the process of deliberately presenting or receiving a message in a certain light. As senders, leaders know which words are inflammatory and which ones convey the same intent without distressing everyone. We all likely understand the framing related to political issues. Framing often is designed to find the "common ground" even when people don't think they have anything in common with "the other side." It also can be used to create greater divides, if that is the intent.

A colleague of ours was the state nurses' association president and mastered the craft of framing. During a legislative year in Texas, nursing needed money. To the Democrats serving in the House, we spoke about the services this money would provide. To the Republicans serving in the House, we spoke of the money saved by doing what was proposed. Either view was valid and produced the same outcome. Had we used only one perspective, we likely would have been defeated in our request for funding.

A frame can be in the foreground (as the example just illustrated) or it can be in the background—for example, when we provide a description about the setting or the background that brought us to a particular place. Even specific words make a difference! Many of those words are in the form of adjectives that begin to paint a picture to portray one view or another. Framing is designed to influence our attitude toward something to create a positive or negative light. First described in 1974, framing is a deliberative process we use mainly to influence others.[1] However, we can frame things for ourselves so that we have a context in which to interpret information. For example, if someone fired us, we could see this as the end of our career. Or we could deliberately choose to reframe this event as the release from the current position so we can move to the future. That kind of reframing allows us to continue to move forward.

One of us was downsized from an administrative position as part of a system-wide reorganization (in part due to economic factors):

"I had the presumption that every situation had one 'truth.' What I thought in this downsizing was that I hadn't performed well and was being fired. Although that might have been dramatic, it was what I thought. I then realized multiple perspectives comprised my situation, and some of the factors had little, if anything, to do with my performance. The economic situation, as a glaring example, was totally beyond my control. This reframing helped me make downsizing more palatable and allowed me to reflect more deeply on the situation from a realistic perspective. That perspective, plus many people in the state seeking my services, turned my thinking around to what could be versus what was."

As an example, using the Legacy *Leaders*-Ship Trajectory model, and assuming we have taken to heart the preceding information in the book, we are clear about our values and our purpose. We have reflected on our self-assessment, and we now have a way to frame ourselves as *leader*. We may choose to lead in a very specific, localized project or in a widespread, national endeavor. Those choices may help frame how we see leadership enacted. In the first, we may be much more focused on providing feedback; in the second, we may be more focused on influencing. Both require our conscious effort at framing. Another example of framing has to do with titles. We create a frame when we hear or see certain titles. For example, the word *chief* in front of almost any word creates the frame of importance. Yet in certain circumstances, we don't care what someone's title is—we care what that someone can do.

THE HANDWASHING STUDY

One of the most famous framing examples occurred in health care. Adam Grant and David Hofmann created two messages regarding handwashing, and one of them was more powerful.[2] The two messages were as follows: (1) hand hygiene prevents you from catching diseases, and (2) hand hygiene prevents patients from catching diseases. Thus the first message was about the provider, and the second was about patients. Two ways of evaluating the effects were used. The first involved the amount of soap used, and the second was direct observation. Pre- and post-measures were taken. In the first approach, the message about patients produced an increase in the use of soap by 17%; the message about you basically remained flat. The second approach involved direct observation. Again, the message about you basically remained flat from pre- to post-measures, whereas the message about patients increased the numbers of positive observations by almost 9%. In short—simply changing the word *you* to the word *patients* increased a desirable behavior. That one-word change reframed the message. If we now translate this to the messages we give ourselves, we can see the value of framing.

THE POWER OF YET

In a President's message published in *Nursing Education Perspectives*, one of us shared the story of Michael Oher, a famous football player, as depicted in the movie *The Blind Side*.[3] To make a long story very short, he had to be tutored by Miss Sue to improve his grade point average so he could get into college and receive a football scholarship. Michael was given a math problem and basically said he didn't understand it. (How often have we thrown our hands in the air and said that we just don't get it?) Miss Sue corrected him by saying, "Yet. You don't understand it yet." The word *yet* suggests that no matter where we are in life, we can be different in the future. It is reframing!

REFLECTION The importance of the word *yet* cannot be overstated. Have you converted any of the negative messages you might give yourself to a more positive message simply by adding the word *yet*? If not, consider why you have not. If it is because you never give yourself negative messages, good for you. Otherwise, help yourself by using framing.

THE ART OF PERSUASION

Robert Cialdini, professor emeritus from Arizona State University and the founder of Influence at Work, is one of the better-known authors who discuss persuasion.[4] If we think about persuasion, we are, in a sense, creating frames for others to hear. Through research, Cialdini identified six elements related to human behavior. Those six principles appear in Table 8.1. Those words have meaning to us. Although we will see these words again in the chapter on influence, they are here because using the principles helps us frame messages so that others hear the messages in our desired context. To be effective, however, we have to know the person or people with whom we are talking. For example, one of us, while visiting with members of the US House of Representatives from her home state to advocate for nursing funding, mentioned that her husband was a veteran. What does he have to do with Title VIII funding (an ongoing issue of appropriations and authorization that provides federal funding devoted to nursing)? Probably nothing, but Texas congressmen tend to be very patriotic. They heard what she said differently after they knew she was the wife of a veteran.

TABLE 8.1 The Six Principles of Persuasion

Reciprocity	Consistency
Scarcity	Liking
Authority	Consensus

REFLECTION Look at Table 8.1 and consider how these principles can be used by leaders and whether they feel genuine. Please consider these words before you read more about them.

The principles of persuasion are inherent in many situations. Although the examples Cialdini provides are derived from research, we can make analogies in terms of health care. Think, for example, of how reciprocity works on a clinical unit. If one of us is always helping the other out without receiving help in return, the exchange is missing, and the volunteer often stops the helpful behavior. On the other hand, if I help you today and you help me the next time we work together, we begin an ingrained habit crucial to a team's functioning—working as a group to accomplish the work. An example of framing using this principle is to tell yourself that the last-minute work you are doing for someone else can be reciprocated. What is critical, however, is to frame the message to the other person who needed this work. When that person thanks you, don't say something such as "It was nothing." No, it really was something, and you pulled it off! Instead say, "Thank you, and I know if the situation were reversed, you would do the same for me." That is advice from Robert Cialdini in a business application, but it works in health care, too! That is a perfect example of framing.

We probably use the principle of scarcity every time we have a promotional opportunity. Manager and director positions are fewer than those in direct care positions but greater than the number of chief nursing officers. The "up" side of scarcity could be the feeling we experience if we are chosen for one of those positions. Another example of scarcity can be seen in any transition-to-practice program where only a select number of new graduates can be supported. Thinking again about how we use framing in health care, we could consider an aspect such as recruitment practices (we are the only hospital within 100 miles with an accredited transition-to-practice program). Individually, we can frame messages about who we are to convey that we should be considered for a particular role or opportunity.

Our authority not only derives from our legal status (registered nurse) and our position (the title we hold) but also from factors such as the credentials we hold. These credentials most commonly relate to clinical or functional certification and formal education. Additionally, our competence in our role can determine whether we are a trusted member of the team. We see this influence play out when we have to call someone in the middle of the night to make a remote decision about care. Framing allows us to shut down arguments (or maybe even prevent them). If the president of a group such as the American Association of Critical-Care Nurses told us something about a new critical care procedure and how it is within the purview of nursing, we would listen with great anticipation because this new procedure has just been framed as part of nursing practice by someone with authority.

Consistency can be demonstrated in how most of us become engaged with committee work. We start with something that isn't a critical committee and continue to be involved with other committees and positions until we are chairing the Shared Governance Committee or a Clinical Unit Facilities Development Project. The point is we took a first step, and if we fulfilled our commitment, we were seen as a "keeper" and so were asked to serve on other groups. A clinical example of this consistency is seen in a colleague of ours (the authors). She is skilled at being what we would call professionally bilingual—translating that complicated medical terminology into everyday language that patients get right away. She has framed something scary in such a way that people always hear her as if she were a friend telling them about something new. That consistency in approach to framing the message helps people work effectively with a new diagnosis or treatment.

The next principle relates to liking. This is played out every day when we take breaks with our colleagues. If, in the earlier example, we saw you produce good work consistently, we would be more likely to respect/like you because you have the same work ethic we do. As a result, we would ask you to do things that relate to goals we want to accomplish. Now think of this in another way: If we have two physicians to consider for an organizational committee and one functions in a holistic manner, respects other members of the team, and communicates in a professional manner, we select that person. We don't knowingly appoint a disruptive, surly member to the team. And when a friend asks us to do something, even taking a position on an issue, we are less likely to shut them off or turn them down. The "like" helped frame the message we received.

Finally, we see the principle of consensus plays out whenever we have any kind of fund drive. The reason we have something like a thermometer showing the amount of money or number of staff who participate in something is to convey the message that others endorse the effort and the more who do, the more each of us should. The "frame" is that we are almost at what we need to be, if only you would help a little. Consensus can also be played out with negative consequences by such strategies as asking the most powerful person in the room to speak for or against something first or by downplaying the minority opinion in a discussion of options.

One of us worked with a group where she could predict that the most important item on the agenda was always the next-to-last item. The chair would announce we were almost out of time and needed to adopt whatever the agenda item was. We all felt pressured to adopt the item and knew that we would not be seen as team players if we had questions. That didn't prevent our asking questions, but we were very careful what questions we asked because we knew they had to be powerful ones. Incidentally, the last item on the agenda was one the chair didn't want to deal with—"Oh, we are out of time. I'll place this on the agenda for next time." After a couple of those movements of the same item, one of us would suggest we start with that item at the next meeting! When we did this, we typically reframed the issue so it seemed less threatening.

One of our favorite examples, illustrated in a Stanford Executive Series video of Dr. Cialdini, includes understanding how we tend to agree to buy something.[5] We are much more likely to buy something that is related to preventing a bad thing (such as insurance for a roof replacement) than we are to support a good thing (such as something that might make the environment better). We don't normally like to "scare" our patients or each other, yet the research in marketing suggests prevention of a bad thing (fear) is a far more effective approach to bringing about desired change than is conveying positive messages. An example of this principle might be the fear of having a heart attack versus the desire to be healthier.

THE MOST EFFECTIVE CONVERSION IN FRAMING

Probably many avenues exist to reframe something. One of the most effective strategies we have found to force ourselves to reframe is to begin a statement or thought with the phrase "on the other hand." This phrase forces us to create a different message from the one we are using or receiving. This is especially effective when the topic is controversial. The phrase "some people would say" has the same effect of helping others see a different view (or frame).

LL ALERT

- Don't jump to consensus, especially if doing so is just to go along with the group.
- Don't negate the power of framing.

SUMMARY

How we hear a message and how we translate messages to ourselves and others can determine our response. The glass can be half full or half empty depending on the viewer's perspective. Our opportunity is to help the receiver of any message to hear it in a way that is reflective of that person's values.

LL LINEUP

- Use the phrase "on the other hand" whenever you think a group is getting to a conclusion too quickly or is ignoring the input of a minority opinion.
- Practice reframing messages, such as those you read in a paper or on social media or see on television, so that you are better at reframing when you must.

REFLECTION Consider some message you received recently that was hurtful or made you angry. Now convert that message to a new frame!

9

Influencing

One of the top talents a leader can have is influencing. Let us repeat that: one of the top talents a leader can have is influencing. Influencing is how we pull any of our other abilities together to affect those beyond ourselves. We obviously cannot do all of the work, whatever it is, ourselves. So we have to be influential to have others work with us to accomplish work.

Influence is defined as "the power or capacity of causing an effect in indirect or intangible ways."[1] Unlike many sources of power, which tend to be more overt, influence is subtle. That subtleness is what makes influence so appealing. People typically come away from being influenced without feeling controlled. Influence is the soft glove of guidance as opposed to the iron glove of control. Most of us prefer to have our opinions and actions shaped rather than controlled.

The ability to unite people in a common effort is a core expectation of a leader. That ability is powerful in both informal and formal leaders, and that is why we (the authors) believe we cannot rely on having only a handful of leaders in an organization. We all have to be able to exert our influence, and hopefully it is aligned with the organization.

If we don't take on the task of influencing others, our leadership is all about self-leadership, and although that is a good thing to have, it is insufficient. We all must be able to influence others because we may be in a situation where the person with the least authoritative title is the one with the best knowledge and is needed to override those with titles that may sound more knowledgeable. As we emphasize more interprofessional work, we become more acutely aware of the importance of influence, because no profession wants to cede to another the control of their profession (nursing). Over the history of nursing, we have had periods, some more intense than others, where other professions wanted to dictate what the profession of nursing should and could do. The idea that one profession would control another limits the full utilization of talent available to the healthcare industry. Being able to influence can be more powerful than being able to control.

Many leaders in healthcare and other endeavors prefer to think of influencing as inspiration. Inspiration is defined as the action or power of moving the intellect or emotions.[2] Actually, the first (preferred) definition refers to inspiration as divine and has to do with the sacred. In other words, inspiration speaks to our emotions and causes us to want to do something rather than merely "buying in" to an idea.

This concept of divine makes perfect sense to us (the authors) in many situations. We influence people all day long, and we also want to inspire some people in some situations to take on challenges they might not normally assume because we see the potential in these people. When they sense they can take on a challenge, we have succeeded in inspiring them to see themselves as we see them. Our task then is to inspire them to see how the challenge relates to their values and their purpose in life (not just in nursing). That inspiration, in our view, is analogous to thinking of influence on steroids. Inspiration is a form of influencing, and its intensity and relationship to values and purpose make it even more powerful. When we hear someone say, "I'd follow him or her to the ends of the earth," that person is not talking about influence. That is inspiration.

WHAT IS INFLUENCING?

First, let's look back at the chapter on framing, where Table 8.1 presented the principles of persuasion (or influence). Robert Cialdini's principles of persuasion don't merely allow us to reframe our thinking about something—they are the basis for influencing others.[3] Influence can be seen as the capability of using indirect processes to create an effect. These indirect processes have been described in various ways to the general public: presence, charisma, and aura. Note that they are all somewhat ethereal words. This is not by mistake. A formal position provides an expectation of influence, but we probably have all known someone with a great title and limited ability to sway others to a particular point

TABLE 9.1 The Science of Influencing

Element	Meaning and Example
Reciprocity	We feel obligated to repay in kind what another person has provided us. (Favors and trades)
Scarcity	Opportunities seem more valuable to us when their availability is limited. (Fear of loss)
Authority	We have a strong sense of duty to authority within us; because obedience to authority is most rewarding, it is easy to comply automatically with that authority. (Expert knowledge and competence)
Commitment and consistency	Once we have made a commitment, we will encounter personal and interpersonal pressures to behave consistently with that commitment. (Small-step action)
Liking	We mostly prefer to say yes to the requests of someone we know and like. (Similarity and respect)
Social proof/ consensus	One means we use to determine what is correct is to find out what other people think is correct. (Snowball effect)

Elements derived from Cialdini R. Influence: the psychology of persuasion. New York, NY: William Morrow Co.; 2006.

of view or action. We also can likely think of someone without the accoutrements of position who called us to action.

Cialdini's six principles of persuasion (reciprocity, scarcity, authority, consistency, liking, and consensus) help us influence others (see Table 9.1). Although every professional exchange we have does not include all of these principles, they are powerful when used together. Alone, each principle has the potential to make us more influential. For example, our ability to help others, especially if we are an expert in some aspect of our profession, creates great influence. Hypothesize that we are in a meeting and the nurse who works in infection control suggests a specific protocol for working with a patient. We are far more likely to align with that person's thinking than we are if someone with limited experience with infections suggests something—even if both individuals suggest the same approach. In this situation, another influence principle is likely at play, and that is scarcity. In addition to having relatively few people employed in infection control, they, theoretically, are the ones who are most familiar with the current evidence related to infections. Most of us who are not faced with solving the problem of infections on a daily basis aren't as familiar with the literature about infections. So in addition to having authority, the person from the infection control services has scarce information. It is the authority of the person working in infection control and the scarcity of the information for the larger group that help influence the group in deciding what to do.

We all likely have had experience with someone whose consistency is "flipping." In other words, if asked what to do in a particular type of situation, on day one the answer is one thing, and the next day, it is something different. Those who experience that inconsistency do one of several things: stop asking, seek a second (or third) opinion, avoid interactions with the person, or seek a higher authority. As one of us is fond of saying, "You can be predictably good or predictably bad. What leaders cannot be is unpredictable." On the other hand, being so totally consistent that people can predict what might be said may not be a good thing either. If a goal of an organization, for example, is to innovate, always getting the same response may limit creativity.

REFLECTION Consider if you work with someone who is totally predictable. Do you seek that person's input, or do you simply keep that person informed? Do you work with someone who isn't predictable? How do you feel when you need a response from that person?

Another way of looking at influence is found in Jeff Adams's model. The Adams Influence Model, created in 2016, provides a way of thinking about the wholeness of influence, which is the basis for one of the self-assessments, LISA.[4] Fig. 9.1 illustrates the model. The model has three levels of influence, the social, the interpersonal, and the personal, and it consists of the agent of influence and the target of influence. Both major elements (agent and target) have subelements that influence any interaction: knowledge-based competence, authority, status, communication traits, and time and timing. All of those elements interact to explain how influence occurs. Knowledge-based competence, authority, and status might be similar to Cialdini's view of

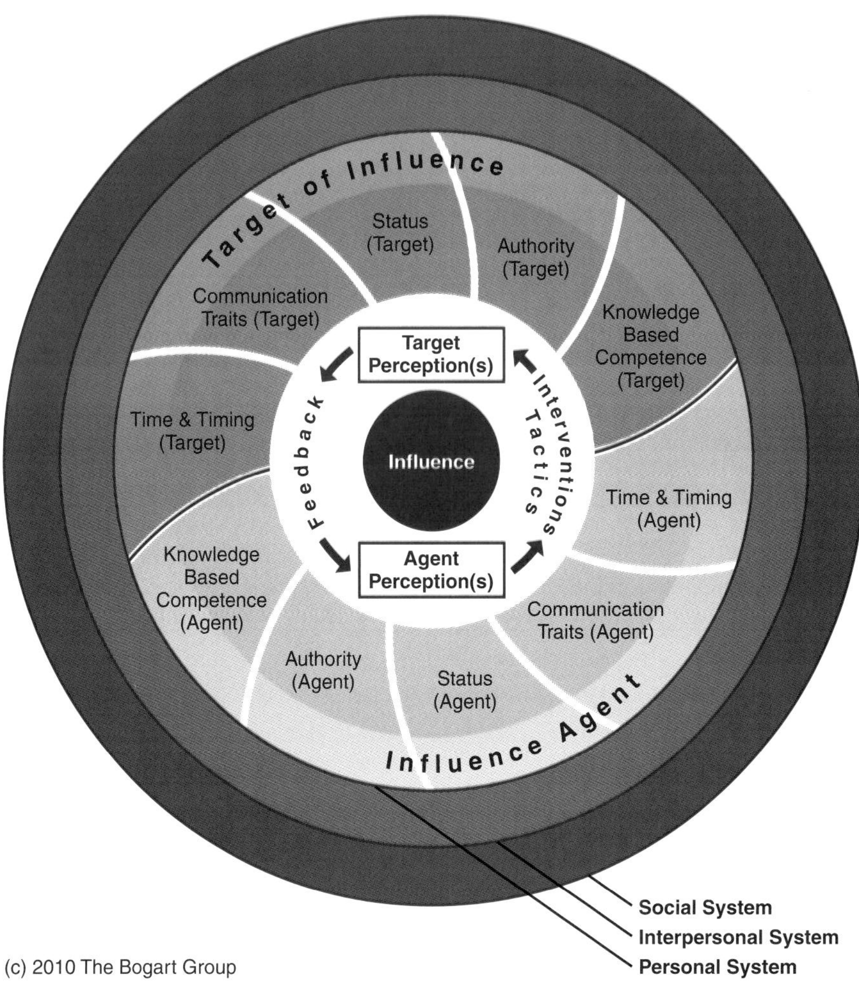

Fig. 9.1 The Adams Influence Model. © Jeff Adams, LLC. Adams JM, Natarajan S. Understanding nursing influence: development of the Adams Influence Model using practice, research, and theory. *ANS Adv Nurs Sci.* 2016;39:E40-56.

authority. Communication traits and time and timing seem to be different aspects from what Cialdini discusses. Our ability to communicate in various ways is critical to our ability to influence others. Because individuals are influenced through multiple electronic communication means, communication is even more challenging.

An important consideration in influencing someone else has to do with timing. Time and timing should be thought of as a resource. People with more time to create relationships with others can be more influential because they are deliberately connected to others. If they have the perspective of timing, they know when to broach a subject and when to just wait. Think how many arguments start on Thanksgiving Day because someone is blocking the television or talking during "the" game (the reason the television was on)! The timing was off, and now everyone just wants that person to move out of the way and to stop talking. That same concept applies in health care. For example, in professional associations, the period right before the board meeting is one of greater tension because the staff wants everything to flow smoothly. That is not the time to introduce a new idea unless it is a matter of critical timing to secure an answer.

Table 9.2 presents a hypothetical analysis. Let's say that Toni and Sam are having an exchange. We could analyze that exchange to determine who will influence whom. Both people bring skills to a situation and have the potential to influence each other—but from a different perspective.

TABLE 9.2 A Hypothetical Analysis of Influence

The Elements	Toni	Sam
Knowledge-based competence	Has 5 years of experience and is certified in area of expertise	Has 20 years of experience and serves as the "go-to" person on the night shift
Authority	Is licensed as an Advanced Practice Registered Nurse	Is licensed as an Registered Nurse
Status	Is the unit educator	Holds the title of RN III
Communication traits	Has basic proficiency in communicating with others in an informal situation	Is highly competent and charismatic
Time and timing	Plans a 2-minute conversation about an issue and asks the other person to come prepared to address the facts	Has "planted seeds" for the past 3 weeks and commits to free up patient care commitments to engage in any conversation about an issue

See related box below: "Our View."

REFLECTION Review Table 9.2 and consider who is likely to have the most influence in this situation. What factors sway you to choose one or the other? (Our view is presented in the box at the end of the chapter.)

The interaction of these various elements is either evident or hidden in every situation. For example, we don't often experience someone saying, "I'm the boss and what I say goes!" Rather, that thought, if held, is hidden—no one is talking about it, but everyone may be thinking about it. The attitude of being the boss can be a highly influential factor in professional exchanges. If the boss is facilitative and supportive, people look to that person for guidance and support, but if that person is controlling and generally directive, they look for the "orders." In the first case, people look for affirmation; in the second, for avoidance of rejection. Yet gaining and using influence can be a hedonistic experience. The abuse of influence is called undue influence. This means the influencer exerts so much influence or power that the person being influenced feels as if the only response is to concur with the influencer's position.

REFLECTION Using the elements identified earlier (and represented in Table 9.1 in the left column), describe how you perceive yourself in relation to each element. Ask a colleague for validation.

THE SCIENCE OF INFLUENCING

As early as 1984, Robert Cialdini identified six factors that influence people, as we discussed in the prior chapter on framing and discussed briefly earlier. In this subsequent work, *Pre-suasion: A Revolutionary Way to Influence and Persuade*, he offers ideas about what to do to basically help people be more receptive to the principles of persuasion.[5] Some examples of those strategies have to do with the following:

- Single chute: Once we are presented with a particular view, we tend to see everything in that light. Our attention is focused, and because it is, we tend to give greater importance to that view. For example, when an organization buys a new piece of equipment, we become more aware of how many other organizations also own that item—because we are focused on that equipment.
- Cold or warm beverage: Offering a warm beverage to others has the potential to make them more receptive to whatever topic we plan to discuss. The idea is that the warmth of the beverage is designed to help us feel more receptive to communication.
- Use of the word *we* instead of *me* creates a feeling of being in the discussion together rather than that you are lecturing me about something. How differently people react when their health care provider says something like "we can figure out a plan of care" as opposed to "here is what you need to do" or "I'm in charge of your plan of care."

Cialdini's point with this second book is that we have the opportunity to channel people's attention to create what are known as *privileged moments*. In those moments, people are particularly receptive to being influenced. What is really important, however, is that he emphasizes, as he did with his first book, that ethics should guide our behavior and that the intent is to help others hear our messages and not to use these strategies to exploit others. His final point is that when you use pre-suasion, you are more effective in influencing others. If the work of leaders is about influencing, we should consider how to be more effective in doing so.

Cialdini also offers the idea of the Five Magic Words: "Even a penny would help." That example, related to charitable giving, resulted in increased donations as opposed to when those words weren't used. The concept is that even something small will make a difference. Think how we could use that in meetings where people tend not to participate. We could say, "Even a basic thought would help." (Yes, we used an extra word, but you get the point of being succinct and creating the mindset that anything is better than nothing.)

OUR VIEW (RESPONSE TO THE FIRST REFLECTION [SEE TABLE 9.2]) In our view, Sam is likely to have more influence. He has sufficient knowledge, although it hasn't been validated through a certification process. Toni is likely to have more influence in the area of authority. Combining Sam's title with the status of the "go-to" person on the night shift probably gives him an advantage in the status category even though his title alone might not lead to that conclusion. What "wins" this situation for Sam is the combination of communication traits and time and timing. Having preplanned and followed through strengthens Sam's position, and having as much time as needed for the current discussion is powerful. Toni can win the timing issue only if the position of authority is used, which might resolve this current situation but will not be of service in the long term.

LL ALERT

- Don't let the ability to influence others become the end.
- Don't forget that influence is merely a means and must be done in an ethical manner.
- Don't forget to consider the targets and the agents.

SUMMARY

The most powerful tool we have is our ability to influence others—irrespective of a formal title of leadership. Using influence wisely is critical to our effectiveness. Considering Cialdini's work on persuasion (and pre-suasion) enhances our ability to be influential.

LL LINEUP

- Establish a 2- to 3-week plan to incorporate the six principles of persuasion in your work.
- Write out what you perceive to be your most likely Five Magic Words.

REFLECTION Consider who influences you. Identify them by name and then ask yourself what, if anything, they have in common. Now look again at Table 9.1 to determine which of those principles seems to influence you the most. We all are influenced by others and by those principles—so no answer is right or wrong. Now you know what the source is that influences you the most. It may be someone who does original research and you feel included in the latest information. Or you may depend on someone you like a lot to shape your opinion on something, especially if you don't have time to study the issue yourself.

10

Advocating

An advocate is a person who speaks or writes in support or defense of a person or cause. We could also advocate for nurses and for ourselves. Nurses often teach special groups, such as children and people with disabilities, to advocate for themselves and to "speak up." Groups such as the #MeToo movement and the Speak Up initiative for patients from The Joint Commission, which was revitalized in 2018,[1] are examples of group advocacy.

SELF-ADVOCACY

The basics of self-advocacy focus on proactively developing an understanding of what is needed to be successful. For example, we might focus a clear understanding on the multiple aspects of leadership described in this book. We might also include an understanding of finance, facility/state/national regulations, standards of care, and ethics. Effective self-advocacy and a deep understanding of ourselves can be demonstrated by the ability to ask for help when needed from an identified trusted colleague. Historically, women and nurses have been relegated to "second-class" status and positions. Many nurses are quiet observers in the course of important strategy or policy discussions where decisions are made. This example substantiates the importance of learning how to speak up not only for others but also for ourselves. While learning to speak up, we find the interactions will not always go as we would desire. Mistakes will be made, and learning will occur in this process. Because it is more art than science, learning to advocate for ourselves takes time and practice. The process probably varies for each leader and is dependent on the differences in character and personality. With regard to creating a plan, self-advocacy is dependent on what we want or what the desired outcome is for the plan. Then, we must execute that plan. As an example, nurses don't often advocate for themselves publicly, but we saw such action during the 2020 pandemic when expressing their concerns about the lack of protective gear.

PATIENT ADVOCACY

According to the American Nurses Association, advocacy means using one's position to support, protect, or speak out for the rights and interests of another.[2] Nurses have consistently included patient advocacy as a fundamental aspect of their practice. The *American Nurses Association's Code of Ethics for Nurses and Scope and Standards of Nursing Practice* clearly identifies nurses' ethical and professional responsibility for protecting the safety and rights of their patients.[2] We see how important it is for leaders to develop their voice and to facilitate nurses in their organizations in "speaking up," especially in support of patients and safe patient care. Additionally, the public expects it. In a 2019 poll conducted by the Commonwealth Fund, the New York Times, and Harvard T.H. Chan School of Public Health, **only** nurses were seen as trustworthy of fixing the health care insurance crisis.[3] In each question category, nurses were listed as the first (most preferred) to address the problem, and they exceeded the second most preferred by almost twice—the second group was physicians. The public expects we will advocate for them![3]

SPEAKING UP

Speaking up is a communication tool that we assume everyone learns, yet few adopt the methods of speaking up learned in basic courses. Most importantly, we often do not speak up and hold each other accountable for the rules or norms or policies of our facilities. In the early 1980s, a jetliner crashed into a bridge that connects Washington, DC, with Virginia and all but five people were killed.[4] The cause of this crash was ice buildup on the wings. The investigators discovered that the copilot, who was actually concerned about ice buildup, mentioned it to the captain, was ignored, and didn't bring it up again. Not speaking up killed 79 people in the plane crash. Now think how many patients die from hospital-caused infections because someone didn't follow policies and no one spoke up. Bonnie Pierce[5] described research documenting that commonly people do not speak up when another person cuts in line—a social norm. These people "do the math in their heads" of what the odds are that the person confronted will act out or cause a scene and decide it isn't worth it.

REFLECTION Consider your workplace social norms. Do they support silence or speaking up? If someone speaks up, are they supported by their colleagues, administrators, and those considered to have more power? What risks are you willing to take?

When nurses detect dangerous shortcuts, incompetence, or disrespect in the workplace, do we speak up? Sometimes, we do not feel comfortable or supported in speaking to such issues, and patients are put at risk. Differences in thinking among the professions—medicine, nursing, pharmacy, social work, and the allied health professions—result in difficulties in this aspect of communication and teamwork. Power differentials exist in most organizational structures, with physicians at the top and nurses holding less power in many interactions concerning patients. Nurses often must speak up regarding patient issues to people holding more power, and if the issue is about inappropriate behavior with someone holding more power in the structure, nurses can be very uncomfortable. To add to this discomfort, nurses have been taught they are responsible for the safety of patients and to advocate for them. The dilemma is the less powerful (nurses) speaking to power (physicians and administration) regarding patient safety issues. Due to this conundrum, we can see that the challenge to speaking up is in serious jeopardy.

Speaking up in health care is a major issue because communication breakdown can lead to sentinel events. The original research on the importance of communication in the patient care setting was done by David Maxfield and others through the auspices of the American Association of Critical-Care Nurses (AACN) and reported in the white paper, *Silence Kills*.[6] As the research gained notoriety, The Joint Commission placed great emphasis on communication that advocates for patients. Some aspects of communication breakdown are (1) true human errors, which are honest mistakes that occur spontaneously, and (2) the "undiscussables."[7] The three most common undiscussables are dangerous shortcuts, incompetence, and disrespect, all of which lead to shutting down discussion and nurses refusing to speak up even when patients are at risk. In one study, 17% of nurses used appropriate safety tools such as checklists, warning systems, and protocols but were unable to speak up in a way that others would attend to them and listen to their concerns.[5] We cannot depend on nurses' personal motivation to speak up. As a result, leaders must create sources of behavioral influence and social and structural processes that will influence behavior and create safety for others to speak up and to advocate for patients and safety. A part of this effort must also include the development and maintenance of a civil culture, because we will not speak up when we do not feel "emotionally safe" due to an uncivil culture.[8]

The American Organization for Nursing Leadership (AONL), formerly known as AONE, sees nurse leaders' responsibility as transforming systems in their respective organizations so patient safety and effective communication traverse across disciplines and nurses are supported in speaking up and providing critical information in advocating and protecting patients.[9] Leaders need to encourage and support professional development to focus on quality care and advocacy. Self-awareness, positivity, critical thinking, and problem solving in tough quality situations where the power is uneven or stacked against the direct-care nurse should be included in these courses. Exercises to improve or grow self-esteem and to increase knowledge of the system and the chain of command can demonstrate additional options when nurses feel unheard.

WHY PEOPLE DON'T SPEAK UP

As if the complexity of speaking up weren't hard enough, we need to consider how to know what to say or how to say it or if the timing is right.[10] Often we don't speak up because we are waiting for someone else to speak up or we are anxious about creating a breakdown and are clueless as to how to resolve it . Even worse, we are afraid of appearing hairbrained or stupid. Given those self-judgments, we decide it's better to say nothing. Kevin Daum offers five reasons to speak up, as shown in Table 10.1. Remaining silent can be interpreted as approval. In addition, not speaking up so that we maintain our comfort level puts our need to be comfortable above the needs of others and putting important issues on the table. In addition, if we are in a group or team meeting, we must have a reason for being there. Thus we need to demonstrate our commitment to the process by being actively involved, including speaking up. This is a form of honesty, and demonstrating honesty is one method of building trust within a group or team.

All of us are individuals and different from each other, so no one has the information or perspective any one person has. Consequently, individual perspectives have value, and speaking about individual thinking and perspectives is worth communicating. Our thoughts could be delivered in the form of a question to clarify what is being said. It is an excellent way to engage the group and perhaps encourage a colleague to speak up. And last, it is critical to speak up because others may be thinking similar thoughts and are also afraid to speak up. When our peers speak up, others are encouraged to share their opinions. Thus the discussion and problem solving are enhanced, and patient care may be improved.

TABLE 10.1 **Five Reasons We Should Speak Up**

Reasons	Rationale
1. Silence is deemed to be approval.	Silence is an active form of communication; people are aware of the lack of input; disapproval without speaking enables others to think you are at fault for negative outcomes. It can create resentment.
2. The greater good should be the priority.	Do no harm by offending or criticizing someone. If a person or team is on a dangerous path, do not put your own need for comfort above the needs of the others to reconsider the path.
3. Demonstrate you are invested.	If someone invited you and you have no interest, find a better use of your time. If you choose to stay, show your commitment by being involved, active, and vocal.
4. No one else may know.	Your experience and knowledge have value; no one else has your unique perspective; your piece of the puzzle may be the most important factor.
5. You may not be alone in your thinking.	It's possible that your insights and conclusions have occurred to others, but they may be unwilling to speak up. By speaking up, you encourage them to voice their opinions.

Adapted from Daum K. 5 Reasons you should speak up (even when you think you shouldn't). Available at: https://www.inc.com/kevin-daum/5-reasons-you-should-speak-up-even-when-you-think-you-shouldnt.html

One of our colleagues was in a meeting to address issues involving the cardiac catheterization services. Physicians from two different practices were present, and the discussion devolved into who would be called when a patient came to the emergency department (ED): would it be the physician group that was assigned call for the day or whoever happened to be "in-house?" The discussion became heated, and finally the nurse, who was perceived to be quiet and accommodating, said, "Is this meeting about your practices or is this meeting about patient care?" The physicians decided that whoever was available in-house would see the patient, regardless of who was next on call. All the nurse did was ask one question and it changed the discussion completely. To advocate, each of us must speak up.

REFLECTION Think about your most recent work experiences. Were difficult conversations held, or were difficult situations glossed over so that no one needed to speak up? What could you consider doing next time such a situation occurs?

Challenges When Nurses Advocate

Direct-care nurses know about and understand conditions that may result in harm to patients, both near-misses and adverse events. We learn early in our careers that we are the advocate for our patients. We understand the necessity of asking questions and raising issues especially related to safety. Although the work of The Joint Commission has challenged facilities to establish cultures of safety that promote and encourage everyone to raise issues, facilities and systems are far from perfect, and nurses may face challenges in advocating for patients.[11] Several examples of these issues are important to discuss:

- *Nurses may lack adequate communication skills to describe concerns in a manner that enrolls decision makers to respond.* A nurse who describes staffing as unsafe has not provided enough description of evidence to allow nurse leaders to respond to the concern. Nurses must be specific about concerns. A leader might emerge and say the following: "I'm worried that our current staffing didn't account for an intensive care unit (ICU) patient being transferred into the unit nor two admissions from the ED. How can we adjust staffing to accommodate these changes? Or what are some optional strategies?" This type of response to leaders identifies a problem and potential solutions.
- *Nurses may not know how to address an issue.* Nurses may not be clear about a course of action concerning a physician who fails to respond adequately to a patient issue at 2:00 a.m., or who might make corrections for a chronically late medication delivery from the pharmacy, or what to do about a medical device that repeatedly fails during the night shift. Policies and procedures for such situations may not be clear, or unwritten rules for coping with issues on the night shifts may squash the desire to speak up. And direct-care nurses

may not be adept at negotiating within the formal or informal hierarchy existing in health care organizations. Leaders emerge to learn how to be effective.

- *Nurses may lack knowledge about established processes and protections and may fear retaliation when advocating for a patient.* Raising a concern disrupts the status quo and challenges the organization to confront problems. If identifying concerns or opportunities for improvement is viewed as complaining, those raising concerns may be labeled "troublemakers." Yet leaders can convey messages that don't sound like complaints.
  - An extreme example of retaliation for patient advocacy activities occurred in Winkler County, Texas, when two nurses were criminally indicted by the county attorney for reporting a physician to the Texas Medical Board due to patient safety concerns. Charges were dropped against one of the nurses, and the jury found the second nurse not guilty. Subsequently, the Texas Medical Board took action against the physician for witness intimidation and medical practice violations. Further, the Texas Attorney General's office indicted the hospital administrator, Winkler County sheriff, county prosecutor, and physician for retaliation and other charges.[12] (See the Texas Nurses Association for more information.)
- *Nurses may be hampered in advocating for patients in organizations with no shared decision-making processes in place.* If these shared decision-making committees, such as performance improvement, staffing committees, and product evaluation teams, are absent and the opportunity for improving patient safety is absent, what is the structural support for advocates? The lack of structure certainly dampens the potential for a leader to emerge.

The nurse's duty to patient safety and the role in patient advocacy are well established. The value of nurses advocating for patients actually supports an organizational culture of safety. Nurses speaking up isn't always appreciated, yet the acknowledgment and response to nursing concerns about patient safety can make a powerful contribution to patient outcomes. As leaders, we have a responsibility to advocate for those who are yet unable to speak up for themselves.

COLLEAGUE ADVOCACY

Nurses not only advocate for patients but also for nurse peers, colleagues, and the profession. This broader type of professional advocacy is often tied to patient care issues. As nurses we work on such issues because it is the right thing to do for the profession and for patients.[13] For example, in 2013, the Colorado Center for Nursing Excellence (the Center), the nursing workforce center for the state, was collecting information for a white paper on the status of advanced practice registered nurses (APRNs) in the state when phone calls came from APRN students who were just completing the final year of their programs. They said they could not find jobs because physicians were unwilling to provide the 3600 hours of supervision required for the new graduates to obtain prescriptive authority. The Center documented 60% of the new graduates were leaving the state. Clearly, a problem existed for new graduate APRNs and for health care in the state. The law, which had been part of a compromise to obtain independent practice for APRNs, needed to be changed. Through extensive data collection, a health care collaborative was created to advance the legislation addressing the issue. Rather than focusing on the restrictive APRN regulation, the Center reframed the issue as one focused on "access to care" for the rural areas of the state. These APRNs could be the providers of care for rural areas of the state.[14] Efforts were successful, and the law was changed to 1000 hours of supervision by either a physician or an APRN with prescriptive authority. This would work! The nurses had advocated for the APRNs and for the nursing profession and advocated for a solution that supported access to care for the rural population of the state.

What other APRN issues existed? More than 50% of rural providers were over the age of 60. What could be done to ensure access to care for the rural population? The Center advocated for using APRNs. A recruitment program for rural nurses who were embedded in their communities and were committed to returning to those same communities after completing APRN programs could be more effective than the current approach. Since 2015, the Center created scholarship funding for over 100 nurses from these rural areas. Unlike many new physician graduates who go to these rural areas and serve for only 2 years to achieve student loan forgiveness, these APRNs return to the rural areas, to their home communities, and provide primary care for these communities.[15] The Center advocated for nurses who then advocated for their patients and rural communities.

Advocacy needs to benefit patients, colleagues, the profession, and even ourselves. It is a key aspect of leadership.

LL ALERT

- Don't remain silent when the actions of colleagues or patients have the potential for harm.
- Don't avoid the larger impact of speaking up for the profession. Changing something for yourself only is insufficient.

SUMMARY

To be an advocate for ourselves, for colleagues, for patients, or for the profession, leaders must first be able to problem solve. This includes taking time to develop a compelling request to address the issue, devoting time and energy to learning effective communication skills, and being willing to speak to the issue clearly and concisely. As leaders, we influence others through demonstrating competence, credibility, and trustworthiness. In addition, leaders can collaborate with like-minded people by focusing on goals, modeling positive professional behaviors and helping novice nurses to acquire these behaviors. Effective leaders advocate for others by protecting nursing resources in difficult times and by increasing staff skills through role modeling, speaking up, and resolving conflicts.

LL LINEUP

- Speaking up is a critical aspect of advocating for yourself, for others, for the organization, and for the profession. Identify how you believe an "ideal leader" would speak to specific issues.
- If need be, practice speaking up about an issue before you must do so.
- Identify colleagues with comparable values to support you.

REFLECTION Think about the last group meeting you had and reflect on how you participated or not. Did you speak up about issues? How did you convey your message? Was it heard? Did some members say nothing? How would you encourage them to speak up at future meetings?

11

Coaching

When many of us first hear the word *coach*, our thoughts turn to sports. We think about the famous coaches we've known or heard about. It might be Coach K (basketball coach at Duke University and coach of the 2008, 2012, and 2016 Olympic basketball teams—all gold medal teams) or Lou Holtz (football coach for the Fighting Irish of Notre Dame and for the University of South Carolina). In such roles, a coach provides special teaching in the respective subject, especially to prepare the athlete for a specific competition or goal such as a gold medal.

The term *coach*, which originated in the early 1800s at Oxford University, described an instructor who "carried" a student through an examination or the processes used to guide learners from their current situation or where they are now to where they want to be. Historically, coaching has been influenced by various fields of activity, including psychology, leadership research, personal development, the human potential movement, and others.

As leaders we are responsible for other people, whether it's a team, a unit, or an organization. The key responsibility to these people is to facilitate their growth and to encourage them to be more than they ever thought they could be. The nurses we grow or nurture become a part of the legacy we create. They value what they learned about themselves and about leadership and use us as role models. One of the key tools we can use when working with and growing people is coaching.

Coaching is done by leaders to encourage and support people to attain professional and personal goals. Some people would say that effective leaders need to spend as much as 40% of their time coaching people.[1] Organizations such as Gallup, which developed the StrengthsFinder tool, believe everyone could benefit from a coach—both adults and children.[2] Coaching is an approach that supports human beings to adapt purposefully to change. And most leaders would like their followers to embrace change, learn, grow, and advance in the workplace. Very little is more fulfilling than watching people learn and grow—it is reminiscent of flowers blooming.

At the same time, to be a good coach, it helps to have been coached—to understand the power of discovering motivations, behaviors, "blind spots," patterns, beliefs, and values. One of us first met Pam, the coach, in the late 1980s in a workshop focused on personal growth

"I noticed Pam asked really great questions, but she was functioning as a support person to the chief facilitator. She continued that work until she was convinced (perhaps via some unconscious coaching) that she should be in the front of the room presenting. She worked very hard and became an excellent presenter. She also worked with me to help me focus on accomplishing goals. She coached me for a dozen years. We talked on average every 4 to 6 weeks. Sometimes we were physically together; most of the time we talked on the phone. She was a master at asking questions—a signature skill of a good coach. When coaching, she worked using the philosophy that I had the answers inside me. She said I just needed to sort and pull them out. She never let me off the hook but consistently asked me to learn from my experiences and to delve deeper to understand what motivated my behavior or reactions to difficult situations. She also kept very good notes and would check on commitments I made and the process I used. She used many of the areas of development identified in this book. I am clear I would never have grown as I did without her excellent coaching."

TYPES OF COACHING

Within organizations, multiple types of coaching have been identified. Table 11.1 summarizes each. *Executive coaching* is available usually by external coaches from established coaching firms. Many organizations find it quite expensive to take this in-depth, one-on-one coaching to individuals beyond the top-level executives. However, organizations can internally train coaches, who are usually managed by the human resources department. This approach is identified as *developmental coaching* and is dedicated to the improvement in leadership skills of the midlevel leaders. Coaching is a methodology that is quite complex when done well. Therefore it is important that the internal coaches receive adequate training. Internal

TABLE 11.1 Types of Coaching	
Executive	Focuses on top-level leaders in an organization and provided by an external resource.
Developmental	Focuses on other leaders in an organization to grow their leadership talents.
Administrative	Serves to address performance issues for corrective action. Note: This is a misnomer for a coaching strategy.
Group	Provides support to a group (team) working on a task. Used to enhance performance.
Just-in-time	Provides feedback as close to an event as possible and designed to strengthen or correct a performance.

coaches need a strong skill set; they also need to address issues of confidentiality. One of the negative aspects of internal coaches is concern about who else will know about the content of the coaching session. Very clear guidelines must be established for internal coaches.

Administrative coaching may be a misnomer. When leaders are attempting to address performance deficits, they need to be clear about when an interaction is corrective action and when it is coaching. These are two different uses. Tools exist for managers and leaders to use in coaching for performance, which is focused on improving work results. *Group coaching* for identified teams is also widely used. One coach can work with a team or a workgroup to follow up on any commitments made or to support them in working through the group process. *"Just-in-time" coaching* is done in the moment with particular events or issues; it is brief and to the point and usually begins with a question such as, "May I give you some coaching/feedback?" This is an approach that can be very helpful because it is timely and connected directly to observed behavior.

REFLECTION Consider what type of coaching you might have received. Were you clear about the intent? If you experienced a situation where you wanted someone to help you think through an issue, did you know how to secure a coach? Can you see the value of being coached and coaching others?

We have discovered that coaching is a powerful tool that can accompany adult education. For example, at the Colorado Center for Nursing Excellence, most of the educational workshops are followed by one-on-one or group coaching sessions. This supports follow-up on the participants' learning and discussion/feedback about the implementation of new skills and tools. If the person has difficulty in the implementation process, this can be discussed and optional strategies explored in support of improved performance. Feedback from workshop participants indicates that the follow-up experience successfully changed their behavior and allowed them to be more successful. One coachee indicated the experience completely changed her personal and professional life. She was able to use the tools she learned in the workshop because she had support and analysis about what worked for her and what didn't. Consequently, if the goal is to support others to attempt new or different behaviors, coaching is an essential part of the process. This could be a valuable aspect of professional development departments.

WHAT IS COACHING?

Coaching empowers others to establish their own goals and to find their own answers. Effective coaching is an approach that emphasizes respect, openness, empathy, and a true commitment to speaking the truth with compassion. Coaching conversations are about collaboration and possibilities rather than about authoritarian or superior–inferior discussions. At the same time, coaches must hold coachees accountable in a nonjudgmental manner for what they want or for what they say they will do.

Because coaching is not a common resource available to many of us, we need to be aware of legitimate resources. The International Coach Federation (ICF) is the leading global organization dedicated to advancing the coaching profession by setting high standards, providing independent certification, and building a worldwide network of trained coaching professionals.[3] The ICF defines coaching as partnering with clients in a thought-provoking and creative process that inspires them to maximize their personal and professional potential, which is particularly important in today's uncertain and complex environment.

PHILOSOPHICAL APPROACH FOR COACHING

Coaching is not therapy. Consequently, we must consider the framework for coaching. We believe that coaching honors the individual as a human being who is naturally creative, resourceful, and whole and who can discover solutions to problems and issues.[4] Solutions are inside of them. Human beings want support in discovering additional pathways to reaching professional and life goals.

This is why coaching can be so helpful to many people. It reaffirms who they are and that they are "OK" as they are. How does this apply to leaders? The following example is one demonstration.

Let's say Joe is serving as a coach from a perspective of human beings are "naturally creative, resourceful, and whole."[4] Joe believes people can choose, discover answers, take actions, learn, and experience resiliency. In the face of incredible stress, difficulty, and even tragedy, people are still capable human beings who will survive. Coaching is *not* about fixing the situation for the coachee. The conversation Joe might have with Sam (a coachee) is about a powerful interchange that creates a mood, a tone, and nuances that focus not just on words but also on the unspoken message with the corresponding meaning or interpretation. This interaction requires that Joe be 100% present in the moment and through intense listening, often intuitively, asks the "right" questions, which lead to a realization or an "a-ha" moment for Sam. If Sam is really committed to learning through the coaching process, he, too, is equally committed to being present and listening intensely.

THE IMPORTANCE OF LISTENING

Listening is one of the most important skills a leader can develop. Typically, we have been taught to speak. We might even have engaged in courses beyond basic grammar to learn how to deliver effective messages or provide the proverbial "elevator speech" (a speech that can be given on a topic in about 1 minute). We seldom learn how to listen. Hearing is taken for granted, and it is as much an active part of communication as talking. Leaders need to be even more astute in listening because many people assume that because they told someone else something that it was heard and understood. Leaders need to be able to reflect what they hear, seek clarification, paraphrase, and summarize just as we might do with our patients. We need to be able to then translate whatever the message was into the message that can be heard in different circles. The same message given to us by a nurse colleague may need to be translated into legalese for an attorney or into a specific style for different socioeconomic groups or into "C-Suiteese" or business terminology for the designated leaders of a health care organization. Obviously, if we didn't hear the message accurately, we won't be able to represent it appropriately.

When coaching, listening makes all the difference. The Coaching Training Institute[4] describes three levels of listening. Level 1 listening is a form of partial listening, which is interspersed with self-talk such as "I had an experience like that once," "I know how it feels," "How should I respond to that comment?," or "I'm anxious about saying the wrong thing to this person and looking stupid." In this way, coaches are primarily interested in their own opinions, thoughts, and feelings. This is a normal response and makes perfect sense for when you are selecting a movie to see. And it is the level at which coachees should be thinking and listening. The coaching is about them.

TABLE 11.2 Levels of Listening

Levels	Description
Level 1 listening	Listening and thinking about how the coachee's comments relate to the life stories of the coach: "Oh, I experienced the same thing."
Level 2 listening	Completely focused and intent on the coachee. No extraneous thinking. Intent on the content and the story being shared.
Level 3 listening	Moving back to a softer focus so that the coach is listening not just for content but also for tonality, facial expression, and emotional aspects (anxiety, fear, sadness, pain, etc.).

Level 2 listening occurs when a coach is focused on the coachee like a laser. This intense focus is similar to the focus an athlete has in an intense performance such as track and field or in ice skating when the athlete is said to be "in the zone." Level 3 listening is when the coach softens the focus and can detect changing energy such as sadness, lightness, or any other change in attitude. A keen awareness of the surroundings and environment supports the coache to be conscious of mood, tone, hesitancy, and silence.

Effective listening requires considerable energy, and yet it is often the case that such sessions are some of the few times when a coachee can feel truly "heard" and understood. This discussion underscores the importance of a coachee being 100% present and listening at Levels 2 and 3. Table 11.2 summarizes these levels.

THE IMPORTANCE OF QUESTIONS

Questions stimulate the brain and mind. When a question is asked, the brain goes in search of an answer, causing the person to think and seek possible, believable answers. Questions can also motivate a person to experiment with these possibilities.[5] Questions stimulate an interchange between the coach and coachee and create a dialogue and a relationship. Questions create more of a peer relationship and less of an educator/learner dyad where one has the power and the other is at the mercy of the leader/coach. Questions honor the coachee as a person and communicate the value and equality of the coachee with the coach.

Questions can reveal the data and experiences of the coachee's life. They stimulate the coachee to remember what has worked successfully in relationships and interactions in the past and what skills might be used in current situations. Such questions can serve as great motivation for the coachee, creating "buy-in" and leading to appropriate action. Action leads to results.

Asking questions can empower the coachee. Nearly all coachees have the solutions to their issues inside of them. They often do not have the confidence to risk acting on these solutions. The coach empowers and supports them through affirming their good ideas discovered by asking questions and encouraging them.

Returning to the Joe and Sam example, we might find Joe asking enough questions so that Sam can see his own answer of what to do. Joe might then ask: What might prevent you from taking that action? This question can direct Sam's focus to practical obstacles such as timing, money, and confidence. At that point Sam might give an affirming message that gets to the core issue of the communication.

Some people believe that leadership is about taking responsibility. The sign on President Harry Truman's desk said "The buck stops here" to indicate he was ultimately responsible for whatever happened throughout government, including the delivery of the atomic bombs that ended the war with Japan—an awesome responsibility. Asking a question such as "What can *you* do to solve this problem?" shifts the responsibility to the coachee and supports him or her to take responsibility for making something happen.

In coaching, a major goal is to create trust and transparency between the coach and coachee. Asking significant questions and listening to the responses creates a bond or relationship because it becomes clear that the coach is truly interested in this person. The interest is authentic. Discussing the issues dearest to coachees—their thoughts, feelings, and concerns—can lead to transformational behavioral changes in their lives.

A general rule for coaches is to create an environment in which the coachee speaks 80% of the time and the coach a maximum of 20% of the time. Just the focus on the coachee and the intense listening convey the value of the coachee as a human being and creates a meaningful relationship.

REFLECTION Consider the last time a colleague confided in you. How much of the time were you talking (maybe even offering advice)? If it was a majority of the time, consider what general questions you could ask to focus the conversation on the other person. List the words and use them the next time.

This kind of interaction requires that a relationship be developed that includes great trust. A trusting relationship can be developed through establishing an approach of respect, valuing the individual, and being nonjudgmental and supportive. Interactions such as the one with Sam are more likely to encourage Sam to take risks and attempt to address issues using various strategies. A nonpunitive milieu of safety supports trust and encourages professionals to step outside their comfort zone.

Many of us have an "a-ha" moment, when we suddenly gain insight into something. As an example, one of us was involved in the personal growth/human potential movement when it was popular a few decades ago:

"During a personal growth seminar entitled 'Money and You,' I observed the following. The businesspeople learned, to their surprise, that the primary purpose of the 3-day seminar was focused on understanding 'you' and not on creating money. In an advanced course, a participant was clearly upset because she sent her entire office to the basic workshop expecting a monumental change in their behavior and attitudes. Yet they didn't seem any different. Her angry question to the presenter in front of the entire group was something like, 'Where do you get off charging these outrageous fees for the basic workshop and there is no positive outcome or change?' It would be easy to become defensive and reactive to this kind of attack. (Haven't we all been in situations where difficult people were angry and attacking?) The presenter replied, 'It sounds like you are distressed over the lack of results from sending your people to the basic workshop, with no perceptible changes in them?' The response was, 'Yes, and I've wasted a lot of money.' He paused and then said, 'We are here in Vermont for 4 days. Do you think it snows a lot here in the winter?' She responds affirmatively. He nods and after another pause, 'We have separate meeting facilities from the condos and have to travel to get back here for the meeting, right?' She says yes. He nods and asks, 'So if we got a foot of snow, what would you do to be able to drive to the meeting place?' 'Well, the driveway would have to be cleared.' Presenter, 'Yes, and there is a shovel in the garage that you could use. So, what is the shovel?' The participant

breathes deeply and says, 'OK, I get it,' and sits down. What she got was an 'a-ha' moment regarding the shovel being a tool."

In these kinds of workshops, participants were given a set of tools. What they did with the tools was up to them. In addition to thinking about choosing to use tools or not, the woman who asked the question could consider what the impact of her leadership was with the people in her office. If she employs anger and reaction, the employees may not feel safe to try out new tools. The presenter simply led the woman through a process of discovery. The use of questions in situations where anger and upset dominate is to support the learner to discover answers to issues and concerns for themselves. For us to become defensive or allow the confrontation to escalate is counterproductive. Instead, just ask questions.

THE IMPORTANCE OF FEEDBACK

According to Douglas Stone and Sheila Heen, for many years, leaders cringed whenever others said they wanted to share some feedback. In some cultures, feedback is usually interpreted as negative when, in fact, three types of feedback exist: positive or acknowledging feedback (thanks), coaching or constructive feedback (a better way to do it exists), and evaluative feedback (here is where you stand in relationship to your peer group or the expectations). What frequently happens with feedback is we get "triggered." The triggers include (1) the feedback is wrong, unfair, or unhelpful; (2) the feedback is delivered by a person we do not like, respect, or trust and therefore the feedback is invalidated; and (3) the feedback is threatening, puts us off balance, and is tied to how we see ourselves or our identity.[6]

From another perspective, feedback can suggest that how we are is not OK. Yet we struggle with a drive to learn and grow while we also yearn to be loved, accepted, and respected just as we are. The drive to learn juxtaposed with the longing to be accepted creates an anxiety-producing tension, which we then attempt to reduce. If feedback is not handled well or it comes from someone we do not like or respect, it becomes a juggling act of learning in the face of fear. The purpose is to learn not to become defensive and "shut down."

We learned a lot from Douglas Stone and Sheila Heen's work,[6] which focuses on the science and art of receiving feedback well. Their work does not mean we must internalize all aspects of the feedback. Instead, we can choose whether and how to use the information even if it comes from a person we do not like. We can choose to listen rather than to react or be upset. That said, one of us has to admit she often considers the source when accepting a compliment. She probably does that with feedback too. We really want to know the other person is perceptive, smart, better informed on a topic, or more connected to the issue or the people we need to be concerned with.

Each of us can choose how to use feedback. A good response would be, "I'd like to think about what you've said. Can we talk more later this week?" If the person conveys the discussion must occur immediately, ask for examples and more clarification to have several seconds of processing time. The benefits to listening and making our own assessment may reveal some "blind spots," or aspects of what happens and our response that we haven't seen before this event. For example, one of us was unaware her emotions, such as fear, anger, upset, disgust, or joy, could readily be seen on her face. This was important information to have.

The benefits in asking for feedback and controlling the triggers include richer, more rewarding relationships; a growth in self-esteem; and the ability to focus on learning from the feedback. The positive mindset of requesting feedback can make it feel less threatening. People who are willing to look at themselves and their behavior are easier to work with and less defensive, and this positive behavior can be linked to increased job satisfaction, greater creativity, and lower staff turnover. Positive behavior contributes to a strong, productive coaching relationship. The leader is the person who establishes a culture in which feedback is valued rather than feared.

COACHING FOR PERFORMANCE

Most every leader has had a meeting go awry due to a specific person's less-than-optimal behavior. The coaching approach to such situations is to choose to have a private conversation or follow up with the person to provide constructive feedback. This interaction can begin with a question such as "How did you think the situation went?" In our experience, most people know when they have blown it or made a major misstep. The question starts the discussion, and we might even add humor and are careful that no judgment about the person can be perceived in the conversation. For example, in one of our early positions in nursing, a patient left the hospital in the middle of the night.

"The chief nursing officer called a hospital-wide meeting to discuss what we thought about the situation. After asking that, she introduced some humor by saying, 'At least we didn't document something like the patient slept well!' That statement created a more relaxed atmosphere so that we all could look at ways this situation wasn't repeated."

When attempting to implement performance coaching, coaches need to remember the general guideline about the ratio of positive to corrective coaching. Remember to find two to three positives to every corrective item of coaching feedback.[7] For positive coaching, being specific about the observed action helps the coachee return to the situation mentally. Additionally, delivering acknowledgments directly or eye-to-eye can help convey the idea of nonjudgment. An example of acknowledgment is:

- I want to acknowledge the interaction you had with Bob's (patient) family. Your concern and authenticity when responding to their concerns were exemplary.
- I noticed that you were almost 15 minutes late this morning and I feel concerned. Can you see that being late for report affects the rest of the team? How would you like to address this problem in the future?
- I appreciate your commitment to addressing lateness, and I want you to let me know next week how your plan to avoid being late is working.

When coaching for improved performance, clearly identify the situation, issue, or problem. Preferably, leaders should actually observe what happened and that the observations are direct rather than thirdhand from another person. For example, Joe in his interaction with Sam might begin a conversation with the following examples of questions found in Table 11.3. These examples can help show how to probe more deeply about a conversation—something we don't always do.

TABLE 11.3 Examples of Questions the Coach Might Ask of a Coachee

"Describe for me in as much detail as possible the interaction you had with Sally on the night shift."
"What didn't work as well as you would have hoped?"
"What was your desired outcome of the interaction?"
"How would you handle the situation differently in the future?"
"What did you learn from this?"
"What is the conversation you would like to have now with Sally about this interaction?"
"When will you talk to Sally about this? Is there anything else you need before the conversation with Sally?"
"When would you be willing to meet with me after you see Sally?"
"Shall we plan to talk about how the interaction went with Sally the next time we meet?"

REFLECTION Assume you cannot currently afford a coach for yourself. Look at the example questions in Table 11.3. Which ones would work well if you asked them of yourself? Would you use them if you were Sam?

This type of interaction is much more apt to lead Sam through a process of discovery than to have him feel denigrated or punished about the problem interaction. This coaching conveys that Sam has the responsibility to manage the situation with Sally, a coworker with whom Sam had a disagreement. Joe is not going to make judgments about what happened. He will have the same or similar conversation with Sally. The expectation is that everyone behaves as adults and handles and cleans up their own communication breakdowns.

LL ALERT

- Avoid selecting someone as a coach because that person is most convenient.
- Don't merely pick a name out of a list of coaches. A coach needs to fit with you and your style.

SUMMARY

A positive philosophical approach to coaching uses questions, intense listening, and positive feedback. Creating a culture where coaching for performance and coaching in the moment are viewed as supportive focuses the nurses on learning and growth. Emphasizing the growth of your people serves to enhance their development and excitement about being part of creating a legacy.

LL LINEUP

- Learn a skill set around coaching.
- Practice using questions when interacting with others.
- Listen attentively and be totally focused on the other human being.
- These are the first steps to developing a coaching approach.

REFLECTION Think of a time when you have been working with someone and practiced only Level 1 listening. How do you think the person felt? Were you busy in your head and not really understanding what that person was attempting to communicate? What can you do to move to a higher level of understanding?

12 Mentoring

Mentoring is a process for the informal transmission of knowledge, experience, and psychosocial support from a more experienced person to a less experienced person. Often, mentoring occurs when a more experienced leader shepherds the younger professional through the "mine fields" consisting of people and structures within organizations and the profession. The mentors have an area of expertise, knowledge, or success in health care and know how to help mentees advance within a system or the profession. Typically, mentoring encompasses informal, face-to-face communication over a sustained period. The mentoring experience and the various aspects of the relationship affect the amount of support, career guidance, and role modeling that transpires in mentor–mentee relationships. Also, a graduate nurse may mentor a nursing student and help the learner decipher issues such as study habits, school finances, or emotional support around the stress of school. Often in culturally diverse student groups, any kind of family upheaval or stress can precipitate students leaving school. We have found that a mentor can support students working through issues and manage to stay in school.

"I have fond memories of one of my most important mentors Dr. Ingeborg Mauksch. I was in the master's program when I first met Inge, a visiting professor who taught the first course in the program, a 5-week Issues in Nursing course. Eighty students were in the class, and Inge had a creative way of getting to know us. She invited us in groups of eight to her little apartment for wine and cheese (it was the first time I realized faculty consumed alcoholic beverages!) and asked us the question of the evening: Why are you in graduate school? Everyone else gave heart-warming, altruistic reasons for being in school, and when my turn came, I truthfully said I was in school for more money and better hours! The room got very quiet and after what seemed like an interminable pause, Inge said, in her thick German accent, 'Nursing is in desperate need of leaders. If you are only here for more money and better hours, you had best reconsider.' It was a bonding moment for us. Inge liked my spirit, and I liked her frankness. I spent the remainder of my master's program reconsidering. For many years, Inge came back to Colorado each summer for Chautauqua, the nurses' association summer conference/vacation in Vail. I always volunteered to pick her up at the airport and drive her to Vail. Consequently, we had nearly 3 hours in the car together each way. It was an amazing time in which we often talked about my career and education (Inge insisted I return to graduate school for a doctoral degree as soon as possible). Even though Inge lived in Tennessee and then in Florida, whenever I had a crucial career decision to make, I called Ingeborg, who offered counsel, asked important and revealing questions, and cared about me and my contributions to nursing. That's what mentors do."

REFLECTION Consider the various people who have helped you become who you are. Did any of them serve as a mentor? What specific behaviors/activities represented a mentorship to you? What will you do to pay this gift forward?

ASPECTS OF MENTORING

Mentor can be defined as a "trusted counselor or guide." As described in the story earlier, mentors are people who help with the mentee's career or advise in the workplace because they enjoy the relationship and are dedicated to growing people. Some of us have had no mentoring relationships; others of us have had several mentors. For those of us among the latter group, we may have experienced various behaviors. Mentoring can consist of informal communication over an extended period and can be face to face or via telephone, teleconference, or other technology either in the workplace or in professional organizations. Often this relationship develops into a friendship.

Mentoring can also be a clinical or academic assignment. A clinical leader may be assigned a nurse manager who is new to the system. An experienced faculty member could be asked to mentor a new faculty member. Or a direct-care nurse could be developed as a mentor and asked to mentor a student. Most students love these relationships because they are in a mentoring relationship with a person they would describe as a "real nurse." The critical issue is to develop a positive and meaningful relationship with the mentee.

One of the most important aspects of mentoring is for the mentor to clearly understand himself or herself. To be a successful mentor, John Maxwell believes that you must first seek to understand yourself and then others.[1] This idea correlates with being a successful leader, which also focuses on knowing and understanding yourself. Tools are available to facilitate this effort, such as those described in Chapter 6. The DiSC workstyle profile, Myers-Briggs, the EQi (or emotional intelligence), and Gallup's Strengths-Finder 2.0 are all tools that can be used to gain insight and perspective about yourself. Such tools can identify what you do well and how you interact with coworkers, with a primary focus on behaviors. In other words, what do you do or how do you act in certain situations? Are these unconscious behaviors helpful or distracting?

Mentoring is not about "what's in it for you." Mentoring comes from a more selfless perspective. It is important to consider your purpose in mentoring. Do you do it as a task to be completed for promotion or to benefit you in some other way compared with mentoring because you want to support others in learning and growing, to raise them up to a higher level, and to support them to be all they can be?

DIFFERENTIATING MENTORING AND COACHING

Some people use the terms *mentoring* and *coaching* interchangeably, leading to confusion for prospective mentors and mentees. These two roles are similar in their support of someone's development; however, they involve different perspectives and skill sets. Mentoring tends to focus more on relationships, whereas coaching is focused on changing behaviors or approaches to situations and issues. Coaching is goal focused in terms of reaching a specific professional or personal objective over a period of time, with observations and feedback around what worked for the coachee and what didn't.

Mentoring usually looks like the story about Ingeborg and her career advancement over support many years. They communicated in person, via telephone, and in written notes. Ingeborg supported Karren's growth and development, particularly as it related to leadership. She was a source of wisdom, teaching, and facilitation, but she did not observe or advise the author in performing skills either clinically or in leadership. Nor did Ingeborg provide instruction in specific behavioral changes in daily work.

> **REFLECTION** Return to the earlier reflection. If you said you did not have a mentor, how would you find someone now at this point in your career? If you did have a mentor, now consider the behaviors you cited in the first reflection. Have any of those behaviors been incorporated into your professional behaviors?

In comparison, coaching typically involves an association of a specified duration that focuses on the accomplishment of specific goals or objectives identified by the coachee. The coachee sets the agenda for coaching sessions. The coach asks questions to stimulate thinking and problem solving by the coachee.[2] Sometimes issues are behavioral or situational, where the coachee didn't obtain the desired outcome. With the support of the coach, the coachee can review, reflect on, and analyze what worked and what didn't and consider how to create the situation differently in the future. Coaches do not provide advice or suggestions but lead the coachee through a process of discovery to help coachees identify a different approach to difficult situations and strive for different outcomes. A special way to employ mentors is to mentor students, especially ethnically diverse students. We have found that mentoring these students increases the graduation rate.[3] These mentor–mentee relationships usually last for a year or until the students graduate—or a lifetime if a lasting relationship is developed.

MENTORING AND PRECEPTING

How do mentoring and precepting differ? Many organizations have programs for new graduate nurses and for new employees that support the newly hired to be successful. A nurse employee new to the institution is paired with an experienced nurse from the unit where he or she has been hired to work. The experienced nurse has a checklist of activities and competencies, which must be successfully completed by the end of the designated period.

These behaviors are a precepting process in which one might precept a new nurse and help guide that person in learning the specifics of working in a certain area. This is a time-limited process and usually ends when nurses complete "orientation." New nurses could continue to use

TABLE 12.1 Distinctions Between Coaching, Mentoring, and Therapy/Counseling

Coaching	Mentoring	Therapy/Counseling
Goal: Increasing performance	Goal: Career development	Goal: Healing from psychological injury
Sustained for a mutually agreed period	Time frame set by the mentor and the mentee in recognition of the mentee's career goals	Agenda set by the client in recognition of the client's psychological needs
Coach need not know anything about the coachee's industry	Mentor is an expert in the mentee's field (some aspect of nursing)	Therapist need not know anything about the client's life before therapy
Allows coachee to find their own answers through a pattern of questions	Sometimes highly directive	Allows client to find their own answers through a pattern of questions
Asks "what," "how," and "why" or "why not"	Tells "how"	Asks "why"
Focus is on addressing the present and creating the future	Focus is primarily on creating the future	Focus is on healing from the past
Accountability is an explicit feature	Accountability is an implicit feature	Accountability is not necessarily a feature
Seeks to build on coachee's strengths and facilitator's personal skill development	Seeks to provide a model for career development	Seeks to build insight and possibly develop capacity
Parties in the relationship are equal—little power differential	Mentee is considered competent and capable of creating a powerful professional portfolio and career path	Client needs healing
Coachee is considered healthy, creative, resourceful, and whole; focus is on problem solving or generating a powerful future for the individual	Mentee is considered competent and capable of creating a powerful portfolio and career path	Client needs healing
Confidentiality is essential to the relationship	Confidentiality may not for an element of the relationship	Confidentiality is essential to the relationship

Adapted from the Diversity Mentoring Toolkit, Colorado Center for Nursing Excellence.

these preceptors as "resource" nurses, someone who has considerably more experience and knowledge regarding a specific patient population. Hopefully the preceptor and the preceptee become friends, and the preceptor facilitates the preceptee into the more social side of the unit, such as introducing the nurse to any specifics that are distinctive to the area, as well as all the providers and support personnel. A good preceptor also orients new employees to the unwritten rules and expectations of anyone joining the area. For example, working toward certification may be an expectation.

Both mentoring and coaching offer incredibly valuable developmental support. However, one offers high-level guidance for long-term development (mentoring), whereas the other (coaching) helps provide more immediate improvement in targeted areas. Significant differences exist among coaching, mentoring, and therapy (see Table 12.1). For example, the goal of mentoring is to facilitate professional development and targeted career goals, whereas the goal of coaching is behavior specific and immediate job-related development. The goal of therapy is healing from a psychological injury. Similarly, for coaches, the coachee is considered healthy, creative, resourceful, and whole. And the focus is on problem solving for the individual or organization. The mentee is considered competent and capable of creating a powerful career path and "professional portfolio." In therapy, the client needs healing. Clearly significant differences exist in these roles.

THE MENTORING ROLE

Some people are intuitive mentors, whereas others are assigned as mentors; for example, in academia, when a new faculty member can be assigned to a senior faculty member. A nursing leader in a health care facility could be a mentor for a select group of nurses in guiding improvement in the quality of care provided to patients.[4] Academic mentors for students could be effective direct-care nurses or faculty members who work closely to support the advancement and success of students at all levels. In a different situation, a strong leader can be a professional mentor, one who supports and encourages other nurses in their professional advancement through their careers.[5] Some facilities have courses or preparation for mentoring. Toolkits are available for mentoring both in service and education.[6,7]

Both challenges and rewards come with the role of mentor. Framing the role of mentor as a process whereby the mentor can mold their mentees into leaders, rather than just good followers, is a laudable ideal. Furthermore, they can be molded into leaders who can mentor others in leadership. Talented mentors can have a long-term impact on the lives and careers of their mentees, such as Ingeborg in the opening story.

Mentors provide guidance based on their knowledge and experience. They create a positive relationship and a climate of open communication with the mentee. The mentor helps the mentee identify career goals, both personal and academic, and leads them through a problem-solving process—a process of discovery. For example, Ingeborg strongly encouraged returning to school.

The mentor offers constructive feedback in a supportive manner, in a way that it can be received and integrated and does not create defensiveness. For example, Marcus Buckingham and Ashley Goodall suggest saying something like, "Here's my reaction to the situation" instead of asking "Can I give you some feedback?" Rather than saying "Good job," say "Here are three things that really worked for me about that situation. What was going through your mind when you did them?"[8]

The mentor shares examples of both successful and challenging clinical and personal experiences, as well as serving as a professional role model. The mentor can discuss learning that occurred in such situations. This approach serves as an example of the mentor not being perfect or all-knowing, but rather a role model for a learner throughout life. This openness and vulnerability can also increase the trust level between the mentor and mentee. It is easy to see that mentors cannot have dishonest communication or feedback with the mentee. Such behavior destroys trust and inhibits any effectiveness in the relationship. It would negate the ability of the mentor to be a cheerleader for the mentee, enthusiastically acknowledging positive behaviors and outcomes. If the mentor is dishonest about communication and feedback, he or she is probably dishonest about acknowledgment. A heartfelt acknowledgment can be very positive for a learner and reinforces essential learning and behavior.

At the same time, mentors ask mentees for feedback as to how the mentoring session went and what could be done differently or what would work better for the mentee. The goal is to meet the mentee's needs. In addition, mentoring is about being trustworthy and serves to help the mentee realize his or her potential. On the other hand, if the mentee does not honor commitments or misses agreed-on meetings, it is an opportunity to relate such events to professional responsibility and to support the mentee in developing a more effective set of skills and commitments.

The mentor–mentee relationship is about support and development and increasing knowledge and skills. Mentors understand different and conflicting ideas due to their excellent listening skills and their ability to be a sounding board for the mentee. A mentor's skill set includes creating clear expectations for the mentee. A mentor does not impose personal views on the mentee but often makes suggestions. Mentoring is not precepting, counseling, consulting, or coaching.

Mentoring in academic settings can produce decreased turnover in faculty due to the structured integration of new faculty into the educator role,[5] support for the implementation of evidence-based teaching, and encouragement for teaching scholarship. A mentor program that focuses on these areas of development leads to increased success in adaptation to the role.[4] Some institutions have a mentoring network, which increases resources to the mentee and allows for the occasional incompatibility of mentor and mentee. This is positive because the initial mentor typically has no backup, and having options is important.[9]

Leadership authors James Kouzes and Barry Posner[10] advise mentors to look for "teachable moments," which can identify, expand, or realize the potential of the mentees with whom they are working. Such moments can emphasize the importance of personal credibility as essential to quality mentoring skills. As described previously, Ingeborg found every moment possible to provide encouragement to encourage doctoral education because she viewed advanced education as a significant step in personal credibility and emphasized Karren's potential to make a difference in nursing leadership and to influence other nurses to become leaders.

> **REFLECTION** We all have teachable moments. Have you thanked the person who made that moment memorable? What teachable moments have you witnessed where a major learning experience occurred?

PHASES OF MENTORING RELATIONSHIPS

In a formal mentoring program, the first phase is the orientation phase, which involves getting to know each other, including sharing aspects about ourselves as mentors. This could include family, pets, and hobbies such as a love for cooking, reading, or sports. The focus is about building rapport and finding commonalities. It is also helpful to establish roles and expectations, as well as the purpose and benefits of the relationship. The mentor may see considerable potential in the mentee.

The second phase is the working phase, which involves identifying specific needs and goals and beginning to work on these:

"I became the nurse manager of labor and delivery and began implementing significant changes. Calling my mentor precipitated Inge asking questions about goals for each idea or innovation considered in the new position. What do you want to accomplish? She almost always asked me questions that proved critical to the decision-making process and to reviewing and revising outcomes and goals."

The third phase is the separation phase in which the goals have been achieved and sometimes the mentoring relationship transitions to ongoing friendship. If an ongoing friendship does not occur, it is valuable to discuss what has been learned or achieved through the relationship and to express gratitude on the part of the mentor and the mentee. This change would be important to a structured mentoring program such as mentoring students until graduation or new faculty members through their first semester or year. Remember, however, that mentoring doesn't necessarily stop when a student graduates or a faculty member is promoted or moves on. One of us often has former colleagues tell her something they are doing, and they attribute that action to her discussing something with them. The influence of a mentor can exist for years, even if the interaction has dwindled or ceased.

ESTABLISHING SUCCESSFUL MENTORING RELATIONSHIPS

Getting to know each other requires time and engagement and is worth the investment because it builds trust. Becoming acquainted with another's interests, values, beliefs, and personal goals can be a process that is often omitted due, in part, to beliefs about time constraints. Creating time specifically for focusing on this aspect of the mentoring relationship can create a safe environment for the mentee. Getting to know each other and feeling comfortable with each other provide a venue for open and honest dialogue.

Focusing on good communication skills and a positive feedback plan enhances the relationship. Poor communication or communication breakdown creates a barrier to healthy relationships. Both the mentor and mentee must focus on effective communication, which involves active listening (discussed in the coaching chapter) and can involve verbal feedback. One effective approach is paraphrasing what the mentor heard the mentee say: "What I hear you saying is…" and then the mentor rephrases the mentee's ideas in the mentor's own words. Through this active listening approach, the mentor demonstrates that she or he both heard and understood the communication efforts of the mentee. The mentee can then confirm or clarify the communication.

"I" and "we" statements—as opposed to "you" statements—are critical in these conversations. In listening to the mentee, reduce emotional reactions and refrain from drawing conclusions prematurely. Listen for the main points and construct a mental outline of the other points. Reduce distractions and attend to the mentee's facial expressions and a sense of the emotional content of the communication. Gather a sense of feelings, as well as facts, or the story.

Listening to the mentee is critical to establishing effective mentor–mentee relationships. The quality of the relationship can be pivotal to problem solving when the mentee has a serious problem, which might involve learning to lead, success in school, or successful orientation to a new clinical role.

LL ALERT

- Avoid behaviors that are not role models for desired mentee behaviors.
- Don't confuse the roles of mentor and therapist.

SUMMARY

A mentor must be well prepared to maximize the mentoring experience for the mentee. Each mentor has a personal style, and yet the basic mentoring foundational information is the same. A course also instills a specific philosophy or approach to mentoring. To be effective, mentors must be willing to invest themselves in others—not merely hold discussions. Similarly, the mentee must have that same investment if growth is to occur.

LL LINEUP

- Seek out a mentor if you have never had one.
- If you have a mentor, discuss what you are learning. If you have never mentored or helped someone, think about how you could do so.
- Consider attending a mentoring workshop.

REFLECTION Think about a mentoring relationship you have had. It could be clinical, academic, or professional. Can you identify significant conversations or approaches to situations that influenced the mentee? How do you know your approach worked? What did you find worked in specific circumstances? What didn't work as well? Did you take a few minutes after each mentoring experience to assess the process and identify what could have worked better? If you haven't had a mentoring experience, consider who might be a good candidate for such a relationship. And, as a leader, whom can you mentor?

13

Visioning

President Kennedy created a vision. That vision captured a nation. Few people alive at the time will ever forget where they were when Neil Armstrong walked on the moon, July 20, 1969. People had been dreaming of going to the moon for centuries. President Kennedy galvanized a nation to take action. When JFK gave this speech, we knew less than 10% of what we needed to know to travel to the moon.

> *We choose to go to the moon in this decade and do the other things, not because they are easy, but because they are hard, because that goal will serve to organize and measure the best of our energies and skills, because that challenge is one that we are willing to accept, one we are unwilling to postpone, and one which we intend to win, and the others, too.... Many years ago the great British explorer George Mallory, who was to die on Mount Everest, was asked why did he want to climb it. He said, 'Because it is there.' Well, space is there, and we're going to climb it, and the moon and the planets are there, and new hopes for knowledge and peace are there. And, therefore, as we set sail we ask God's blessing on the most hazardous and dangerous and greatest adventure on which man has ever embarked.*[1]
>
> ***JFK Moon Speech at Rice University in Houston, Texas, September 12, 1962***

CREATING A VISION

Clearly, most leaders do not create a vision of a global scope, yet the principles for creating a vision are the same, whether it is a small business or a nation. Regardless of the scope of the vision, nothing happens until it happens in someone's mind. Visions are a big picture of the goals or where the leader wants the group or organization to go. Visions are not mystical. They usually contain some big ideas that excite and enroll people, and they often relate to what we earlier called *purpose*. Visions and purposes answer the question: Why am I here?

Dreaming is the first step and suggests that the leader must allot time to dream. Dreams evolve from astute observation. To be effective, we immerse ourselves in watching, listening, and wondering. This process requires that we attend to the world around us, including talking to people, asking questions, reading, probing, and gathering information. As Walt Disney said, "If you can dream it, you can do it." That means that if we want to do something great, such as being part of a legacy, we need to be able to dream what that legacy might be. To do that, we have to dedicate time to our dreams. Bernadette Melnyk, Dean of the College of Nursing, Vice President for Health Promotion, and University Wellness Officer at The Ohio State University, says we must dream big. In other words, we strive toward what we dream, and if we dream in a limited way, we won't achieve all we could. Think what might have happened if President Kennedy hadn't created the view that we could go to the moon at a time when we knew very little about how to get there! To turn a dream into reality requires that we are clear about what the dream is and that we direct our energy toward making it a reality.

Next the leader reflects on information gathered that suggests the dream could become a reality and what has been learned about the challenges that facilitate or limit the potential for reality. Important events or goals within the facility need to be reviewed, and learnings need to be examined. During reflection, the leader can identify examples and some stories about a vision. The important point is to be able to speak authentically to these ideas as they relate to the vision.

As Warren Bennis said, "Leadership is the capacity to translate vision into reality."[2] The translation involves sharing the vision and enrolling employees in the vision. Some people have difficulty with an abstract concept, such as a vision statement. Thus, leaders throughout an organization can help translate the vision because they can say what the organizational vision means to a particular unit or service, such as "To those of us working on 3East, we can see we need to institute several strategies designed to help our dialysis patients see this unit as their home away from home."

Personal stories are a rich source of material. When selecting stories, we need to use broad categories, both positive and negative. Such stories, including personal challenges, major changes, new experiences, lost opportunities, awkward situations, failed attempts, and turnarounds, help to communicate both the vision and the values. Our goal in telling these stories is to touch something in people, to inspire people, and to encourage them to reach for remarkable achievements. Enthusiasm about a vision is paramount. Passion and enthusiasm are contagious.[3] One of us, as an example, has served in several volunteer leadership roles:

"I would say the president's role is to advance the mission of the organization, not to achieve some personal goal. To engage others in seeing the impossible as possible, I often ask two questions: What if? and So what? The first question is designed to think differently; the second is designed to determine whether whatever is being done will make a difference. Both questions can stimulate new ways of fulfilling the mission and serving society."

REFLECTION Look at your organization's vision statement. Does it pose a challenge? (What if?) If the vision were not achieved, what difference would that make? (So what?) If you are unable to see that the vision statement poses a challenge and that failing to achieve it would leave the organization in a less than desired place, how would you change it?

ENROLL IN THE VISION

When the leader has clarity about the vision to be conveyed, three simple rules apply to enrolling the employees in the vision (see Table 13.1): (1) The leader must create a Brightness of the Future, which translates into what the employees will have in the future that is important to them, something they do not have now.[4] (2) The leader must have frequent interactions with the employees to remind them of the vision and where they are on the road to obtaining it. (3) A believable alternative must be identified: What happens if they do not achieve the vision? What do they lose by not realizing the vision? This is the "why" that Simon Sinek advocates as the motivator to change.

TABLE 13.1 Enrolling in the Vision

Stages in enrolling followers in the vision
1. Create a Brightness of the Future—what will the follower have that they don't have now
2. Ensure Frequency of Interaction—the leader must frequently see and interact with the followers and stress the importance of the vision and remind them what will be gained
3. Create a Believable Alternative—followers must know what they will lose if they fail to engage with the vision

Data from hubspot.com. Getting buy-in for your vision. Available at: https://www.hubspot.com/leadership-tips-crafting-a-team-vision. Accessed May 28, 2020.

Another one of us, as a new PhD, was hired into her first director-level leadership position:

"The physicians insisted I be hired (the chief executive officer [CEO] was resistant) because the obstetrics (OB) area was one of the first four LDRPs (labor, deliver, recovery, and postpartum stay all in the same room) in the nation, and it was floundering. I was so busy working on methods to make the new concept work that it took 90 days before I ever looked at a budget. By the time the financials were reviewed, only 6 weeks remained until the end of the budget year. To 'make budget' and not forfeit staff positions, the unit had to have 150 births for the last month of the fiscal year. The last time that had been achieved was 5 years before! My crazy idea was that everyone would 'visualize' 150 births for the month, and to that end, I had stickers made that said '150 Births.' They were everywhere—next to phones, on charts, in the nurses' station. In addition, I put a large paper barometer next to the delivery board and had it divided into 31 days with the number of births each day to reach 150. I was very enthusiastic! After being home for the weekend, I arrived early Monday morning to find graffiti on the barometer and realized the staff were not enrolled. I sat down in the nurses' station with the night shift and had a discussion with them. We talked about the finances and what it would take to have 150 births. One crusty old night nurse said, 'What's in it for us?' In reality, 150 deliveries was more work for them, but thinking very quickly, I said, 'If we have 150 births next month, I'll bring in fresh gulf shrimp for all three shifts with all the accoutrements.' The response was a 'Harrumph.' Needless to say, I was very nervous and totally clueless as to the possibility of success. We did 165 births for the last month of the fiscal year. Where did they come from? Physicians also used the hospital down the street for some of their deliveries in addition to this LDRP unit. The staff enrolled the physicians in shrimp. The physicians simply brought more of their patients to the unit!"

The Brightness of the Future was shrimp: the staff also knew positions would be cut if they missed the numbers, but it was more fun to think in terms of shrimp. Frequency of Interaction was created by rounding morning and afternoon every day and talking with staff, asking for additional ideas, and having fun. The Believable Alternative was no shrimp and some people being laid off. Due to the possibility of positions being cut, the motivation was high, and it was still more fun to think in terms of shrimp.

"The staff celebrated as the shrimp arrived. As we ate, the crusty old night nurse asked, 'So what does it take to get lobster?' Again, I was thinking fast and said '200.' When they did 180 a couple of months later, I became very anxious—lobster was expensive! It was time to talk to the CEO! I told the CEO the story, and he looked at me very intensely and then said, 'If they do 200 births, I'll buy the lobster.' He was enrolled in the vision!"

We likely couldn't provide shrimp or lobster every month as a tangible reminder of the vision, but sometimes the expense of such a luxury makes a vision possible in the short run while the team is buying into the long-term vision, in this case more deliveries.

In the crisis of avoiding losing positions, shrimp worked. However, the real long-term vision was much bigger than shrimp. The dream grew and expanded and was adopted and adapted even more by the staff. The obstetrical service for the facility became a national model that evolved into research projects and publications and the sponsorship of successful national symposia on the implementation and utilization of LDRPs. One of the first Women's Resource Centers was created, including education and a speakers' bureau, a breast center, a lactation program, a mother's milk bank, a 90% breastfeeding rate in discharged mothers, and healing touch practitioners who were available for patients throughout the facility. This all occurred in the 1980s, when intensive care unit (ICU) visitation was 10 minutes per hour and families were viewed as a burden. It takes a leader to be open, imaginative, and supportive of staff to dream and to have visions of how care might be if the focus is on the patient.[5]

To create a longer-term commitment to the real vision (increased service in this example) requires additional strategies other than what to feed a group. What seems to be important is to translate individuals' views of themselves and their purpose in life (or at least in working where they are) into how their views and purpose fit with the vision. If the vision statement doesn't mean anything to individuals other than to be able to recite it if asked, they will likely not be engaged employees who are contributing toward making or sustaining a legacy. This means that leaders can simply hold a meeting and talk about the new vision statement. Leaders must be able to relate to employees on a one-to-one basis by knowing what each person sees as his or her purpose. Knowing that allows leaders to translate what someone does on a unit into a contribution to the vision.

REFLECTION What is your dream? How will you enroll others? Seriously, stop and write it down.

VISIONS THAT WORK

Some visions excite people and move them toward great achievement. Other visions can create that glazed-over numb feeling. Effective visions create a sense of where we are going, a desirable future. In the example earlier, the vision was to make budget and maintain staffing. But it was disguised in "shrimp" and having fun. That might not work today, but it is an example of joy at work!

Great visions answer the question: What is our purpose or why do we exist? Do we serve a greater good? If we haven't thought seriously about these questions, we haven't gotten to a solid vision.

What values or principles guide us on the journey or in the process of achieving the vision? If these aren't aligned with the organizational vision, we may have a great idea—for a different place where a better fit exists between our values and the organizational values. Our goal in creating a leadership vision in an organization is to capitalize on the talents and distinctions of the organization to be even better at what we do or to reconsider the business we are in. Think of some of the businesses that have changed their mottos to reflect the bigger picture of how they are seen in the global market. One example might be Starbucks that started as a "coffee house" and is now a neighborhood gathering place that serves coffee, other beverages, and food. One of us has provided consultation services in the Middle East and heard repeatedly that many natives prefer Arabic coffee but go to Starbucks because that is where informal business is done. In other words, Starbucks is a gathering place first—the coffee is secondary.

According to Jesse Lyn Stoner,[6] visions that address three of these components—destination, purpose, and values—create a tremendous amount of energy. A higher level of employee commitment is generated due to the ability for them to see the relationship between the unit purpose and goals, the path to the destination, and the connection to their own beliefs and values. Each staff member is clear about what they are doing, why they are doing it, and how their work contributes to the purpose.

LL ALERT

- Don't be afraid to dream. Avoid what destroys dreams.
- Avoid being negative.
- Don't associate with people who "rain on your dreams."

SUMMARY

Dreaming about how the world or the organization can be a better place is critically important. Dreaming requires dedicated time, talking to others, working with them, and gathering thoughts and ideas. Then everyone must be enrolled in the vision, including the ability to see the Brightness of the Future, being the cheerleader for the vision, and clearly communicating the Believable Alternative. Leaders in any role have the obligation to make the future possible for others and to translate individuals' purposes/dreams into contributions to the organization.

LL LINEUP

- Set aside 15 minutes, three times per week, and think about a serious problem or a major issue that affects you as a leader.
- Collect information between sessions by talking with others about the issue.
- Focus your thinking on creating an opportunity and who would enroll in the effort to make the dream a reality.

REFLECTION Consider a time when you dreamed about a change or a goal that made a difference for others. What was your process? How did it work? Did you omit any steps?What did you do to make the dream a realization? How would you do it differently today?

14

Wisdom

In 2006, the Robert Wood Johnson Foundation (RWJF) released its report, *Wisdom at Work*, to acknowledge older, experienced nurses' contributions to the workplace.[1] Although that view is likely true, not all nurses with wisdom are older, and not all older nurses have wisdom. In fact, Chip Conley, author of *Wisdom at Work: The Making of a Modern Elder*, says studies have shown wisdom does not correlate with age.[2] He goes on to say that wisdom is really about seeing patterns. That is what makes nurses valuable! We see patterns in patients and know they either are getting better or are about to be in trouble. We see patterns in our profession and have made improvements in the way nursing care is organized and delivered. We see patterns in our organizations and have made improvements in the way the organization operates. Unfortunately, those problems have persisted to the point that physicians saw the desirability of creating the fourth component of the original Triple Aim. The Quadruple Aim is composed of enhancing patient experience, improving population health, and reducing costs (the original Triple Aim) and improving the work life of health care providers.[3] The Quadruple Aim makes sense because it actually is built on decades of research related to the Magnet Recognition Program®, which started with looking at why nurses stayed or left certain organizations.[4] Over the years, the research has continued to evolve, but the core message has remained the concern for the quality of organizational life for nurses and others because it is related to the quality of care for patients.

All of us in health care have been less effective at the organizational level in correcting the multitude of patterns we observe on an ongoing basis that prevent us from being great. We have the opportunity to change that.

WHAT IS WISDOM?

Wisdom can be defined as having experience, knowledge, *and* good judgment.[5] Although one normally develops better judgment as one ages, the fact remains that we know we have many younger colleagues we would describe as having great judgment. They also have great knowledge. What they lack is the years of experience to be seen as wise. This most likely comes from the idea that time generally allows experienced nurses to reflect on their practice. This reflection on practice results in new insight from those experiences, which leads to gaining personal knowledge.[6] Susan Matney, Kay Avant, and Nancy Staggers compared various models of wisdom, the simplest of which is known as the Model of Wisdom Development.[7] This model suggests that our experiences and the intent to learn from them and our interactions with others allow us to learn from life and that leads to wisdom. Logically, the way to capitalize on our experiences and interactions with others is to reflect actively on what is happening to us and how we can improve on what we do. Again, wisdom is not solely age related. Consider some people who repeat the same mistakes over and over again. Perhaps they didn't stop to learn from their experiences to visualize a different approach to a comparable problem.

As nurses gain experience, including in leadership, they tend to be seen as wiser than when they first took a position or joined the organization. This view of wisdom is critical for leadership. People want to follow others who know what they are doing and who are more often right than wrong.

REFLECTION Who are the people most influential in your learning about leadership? Can you attribute some specific knowledge or ability you have as a result of being influenced by these people? Would you describe these people as influential or as wisdom workers? (Remember that wisdom doesn't mean older, it simply means wiser.)

STRATEGIES FOR RETAINING THE OLDER WISDOM WORKER

The RWJF report offered several strategies for retaining older, experienced nurses.[1] The reasoning was that it would be foolish to lose decades of knowledge because an experienced, smart worker couldn't meet certain physical demands. One of the recommendations was *changing personnel policies to provide greater flexibility in scheduling and creating positions where physical stamina wasn't critical to the position*. That recommendation benefited not only older nurses but also those with time demands from other sources, such as family, or those whose physical limitations required accommodations. Those policy changes likely also benefited patients who received care based on the wisdom these nurses held.

Somewhat related was the idea of *better ergonomically designed equipment and furnishings*. That emphasis has benefited all of us. Although we often can't readily change the layout of a clinical area, the chairs, counter heights, access to equipment, and so forth have been changed to benefit all of us.

Improved introduction to and use of technology was another recommendation. If you weren't in health care when computers were introduced, you have no idea what havoc erupted. Even with practice runs for weeks in advance of a "go-live" date, chaos still ensued. We (the authors) have never heard any nurse say going from paper to electronics was a smooth transition. That change, however, has brought many benefits to us and to our patients. Living through the transitions, however, was (and still is) a challenge. The idea of how to introduce technology—of any kind—can only improve the transitions we make on a regular basis. When the American Nurses Credentialing Center elected to have a full-fledged exhibit hall for its Magnet® conference, it wasn't just to provide revenue to support this magnificent event. It was also to provide the opportunity for nurses to interact directly with the exhibitors to help them understand how their modifications could benefit nurses and patients.

Changes in organizational culture is a recommendation that we can't say has been wholly successful. Actually, the idea of an unhealthy workplace may have worsened because now physicians report they, too, are suffering from the effects of the culture in which they work, as stated at the opening of this chapter. To exert wisdom on this issue is a huge challenge. Attempts to address organizational culture can be found in a document published by AACN (American Association of Critical Care nurses), which evolved from the original work, "Silence Kills."[8]

The next recommendation related to a *commitment to training and education*, especially considering we were simultaneously creating new positions to accommodate the needs of older nurses. Continuing to learn is what helps all of us remain relevant to our workplaces. When new roles are created or nurses who were assigned in intense clinical areas were moved to positions that were less physically demanding, new learning opportunities had to be created.

Together these five recommendations converted the workplace we knew from the past. Now we all had to be equally concerned about retaining the talent we had; changing the physical and psychological climates was just a piece of that overall reform.

REFLECTION Look at the words formatted in italics earlier. These were key recommendations focused on older, experienced workers as strategies to retain them. Consider which of those recommendations would not be appropriate for any nurse. (Hint: If you can't see how these apply to all positions in nursing in any setting, please look at those words again.) Now think about where you work. Can you describe what your organization does that is reflective of those recommendations? Which one(s) are well established in your organization? Which one(s) need the most work? What can you do to move the work ahead on the recommendation needing the most help in your organization?

COLLABORATION

In 2019, the American Nurses Association (ANA) joined the TIME'S UP Healthcare movement. What does that have to do with wisdom? Here is our thinking on this strategy. First, it is dealing only with the issue of sexual assault, harassment, and inequity—*and* we could imagine if these issues were solved what a difference could occur in workplaces! For at least two decades we have talked about and acted on the issue of unhealthy workplaces, and one of those issues had to do with harassment and its associated behaviors. The TIME'S UP Healthcare movement is one more strategy to evolve the workplace into somewhere people feel safe and welcomed. The Magnet Recognition Program® has expectations about making places better. However, only a handful of hospitals in the world have achieved this designation. What about the others?

We also have had strategies around healthy work environments. Many organizations, including ANA and the American Association of Critical-Care Nurses, created programs specifically designed to improve the workplace. Although these efforts have made improvements, we haven't really made a global, dramatic change. Now the TIME'S UP Healthcare movement, as a collaborative effort about all health care workers, has the potential to increase our voices.[9,10] That is an example of a wise approach. Everything that affects nurses affects other disciplines in an organization and vice versa. When we can make a bigger case for something, we have more potential to bring about change. From our perspective, the big payoff is that if workplaces were healthier, we could be using our talents directed toward solving delivery and care issues rather than basic workplace issues. Think what a dramatic impact a change such as that advocated by TIME'S UP Healthcare could have! Our wisdom workers could now focus solely on issues that improve care, and our less experienced colleagues likely will have better employment experiences and thus have the potential of staying in the profession and in the organization for a longer period, which, of course, creates the wisdom workers of the future.

Our greatest concern right now is the short period many nurses at the point of care have had in the profession. Turnover has a cost to organizations, as well as to the profession's wisdom. According to the *2018 National Health Care Retention & RN Staffing Report*, "the average cost of turnover for a bedside RN is $49,500 and ranges from $38,000 to $61,100, resulting in the average hospital losing $4.4M-$7.0 M. Each percent change in RN turnover will cost/save the average hospital an additional $337,500."[11] Nurses can't exert wisdom if they haven't gained the experience to reinforce the patterns that lead to being wise. Organizations must increase their investment in the development of staff. This situation must change for the health of staff and of the bottom line of the organization.

BECOMING WISE

Harking back to what James Kouzes and Barry Posner say about reflection, it is clearly a strategy to use to increase our wisdom.[12] Whereas nurses who have been in the profession might not say they used reflection, we would argue that they did—and still do. Older nurses typically called this reflection something like rehash. They rehashed what happened at work and figured out what went wrong and maybe even what went right *and* they then capitalized on this information in the next situation and repeated the process. Today we have a more formalized approach and a different name for what we have done. Even nurses who didn't participate regularly in formal learning activities (earning additional degrees or attending continuing education events) used the rehash technique. Clinical reasoning is critical to the care of patients and the success of a nurse's career.

In addition to reflection, we have so many more tools available to us to increase our wisdom at work. We have journals and books, websites and journal clubs, grand rounds and professional development, and continuing education, including local, state, national, and international conferences. Some of those activities are solo events. Although that approach is good, it is even better if we can then discuss with someone else what we think we learned. In other words, we are validating our perception of knowledge through reflection with others before we engrain it in our practice.

Finally, for those who wish to advance in leadership, we can use a mentor or a coach (they do different things). These trusted advisors can help us learn from their wisdom, especially on topics that we likely would not put in print. One of us teaches in a national leadership academy, and we start by talking about the "cone of silence." The common translation of that is "what happens in Vegas stays in Vegas!" In other words, we can share experiences with the expectation that no one leaves the room and shares that story elsewhere. That is the kind of advice you can get, for example, from a mentor. Another aspect of thinking about mentoring is to create a Circle of Advisors, which basically means to create key contacts across a spectrum of issues so that you can get more than one opinion or story on a given topic.[13] Each of these external resources allows us to gain a broader perspective than what we can gain within the organization and within our current roles.

LEADERSHIP MATURITY

One other thought about developing wisdom derives from action-logic theory.[14,15] Leaders can be seen in one of seven developmental stages, which are presented in Table 14.1. One of the more important things to know about this way of thinking is the importance of the postconventional styles, which are more often associated with maturity in a profession. They are what correlated with the most successful businesses.[15] In today's health care environment, we all have to be able to transform ourselves and our work to remain relevant. (Please note that we did not list the MAP tool [Maturity Assessment Profile] in the tools in the chapter on self-assessing. That omission has nothing to do with the value of the information you can obtain from this tool, but rather the cost, which is substantial.)

TABLE 14.1 **The Action-Logic Stages**
Conventional (reliance on social structures and norms and power structures) (value on stability)
Opportunistic
Diplomat
Expert
Achiever
Postconventional (value on diversity and creative personal transformation)
Individualist
Strategist
Alchemist

Based on Torbert WR, Cook-Greuter S. Action inquiry: the secret of timely and transforming leadership. San Francisco: Berrett-Koehler; 2004; Rooke D, Torbert WR. 7 Transformations of leadership. *Harv Bus Rev.* 2005;83:66-76.

LL ALERT

- Don't assume wisdom relates only to age.
- Don't accept positions where you cannot capitalize on your talents so that you can become wise.

SUMMARY

Wisdom doesn't just happen. It is a deliberate process of learning and translating. It has the intended goal of providing the best that nursing can offer. Many resources are available to help us gain wisdom, and our ability to reflect on each day helps ingrain solid thinking and behaviors into our work.

LL LINEUP

- Create a plan for reflection that is done in a timely and regular manner.
- Create a Circle of Advisors.

REFLECTION Consider what you are doing with what you learn. Do you simply check something off a list or say you are done with a journal and toss it? Or do you create a major learning experience to improve how you function professionally? If you are not doing the latter, how will you change what you do to become wise?

Personal Overview

Although each element of the model is important, the literature about leadership would support the idea that the most important element is understanding yourself. Without that, we can layer on strategies and tasks and not change or be able to integrate that new information with who we are. Once we understand who we are and what our purpose in life (or in nursing) is, we are able to adapt to new environments, quickly assess others individually or in groups, or understand what inhibits that adaptation or assessment. Without that understanding of ourselves, we miss the most valuable resource we have—ourselves.

Please recall that we said we distilled the numerous ideas we garnered from the literature and the Circle of Advisors into a limited number of words to keep the idea of self-development reasonable. If you don't see your favorite word or concept here, it doesn't mean that it isn't important. It is important—at least to you—and likely to others. Add that word or concept (at least conceptually) to the model so you remember how important that is to you.

You will find several chapters, each focusing on some individual ability or concept important to leadership. Each chapter explains the essence of what the word(s) and concept mean. No attempt was made to provide a comprehensive review in any chapter. What we don't present is the integration of various elements. For example, accountability typically requires courage to speak up for accountability. To be able to speak up often feels as if it is a risk. And as a result we feel vulnerable. The integration of those four concepts creates a strong personal ability to be an effective leader. Now, as an example, think how much trust you need to have in another person to be truthful. And even with the most trusted colleague, feeling vulnerable is common. Helping someone learn a procedure or a concept is far easier than discussing personal habits that can be viewed as offensive or less than needed. As a result of the challenges we face daily, we need to have resilience or we wouldn't return.

Because no one personal concept is more important than another, each is presented in alphabetical order. As a result, accountability is the first concept discussed, and we could argue that it might be an aspect worth prioritizing. Yet without those other elements, being accountable might be more challenging.

Note that the words are "jumbled" in the personal triangle. That is a deliberate presentation choice to help you recall that we have all of these concepts available to us, and some rise to prominence in certain situations, whereas others may be more prominent in other situations. Where the words are placed doesn't matter because you pull on what you need when you need it. These 18 concepts provide the platform from which we can add others to achieve specific goals in specific situations.

Our advice: As you read each chapter, consider what the concept means to you. Consider how you could use it. Consider if you have limited or great experience in using the concept. Think how each concept relates to your purpose. And perhaps, most important, consider what the concept will do to strengthen your potential to succeed as a leader.

15

Accountability

When was the last time you had a campaign for handwashing? This campaign was initiated because we connect hospital-acquired infection (HAI) rates to handwashing. We have known handwashing and HAI are connected for decades (or centuries if we wish to recall Florence Nightingale's work!), and yet nurses frequently see others fail to wash their hands or use sanitizer (although this may be a questionable practice also). Do nurses speak up, especially if the other people are physicians? This is but one example of the failure to hold another accountable for safe practice. The observers might think the other people probably washed their hands in another room after they saw that patient, or they say to themselves: "I don't really want to say anything in front of the patient." Consequently, we fail to hold others accountable for meeting the agreed-upon norm or policy regarding handwashing. What prevents a conversation with others? It may be a failure to speak up due to unequal power. Those violating the policy may have more power in the organization than the observer. Or it could be we haven't been taught to speak up. Or maybe we don't have time for what might become a "scene" should those who violated the policy choose to be upset if reminded about handwashing. Regardless of the reason, the lack of accountability influences the safety of patients and health care workers. Our greatest challenge might be in holding ourselves accountable. We often see a problem in others without acknowledging we too have that problem!

NURSING AND ACCOUNTABILITY

In the nursing literature, accountability is described as the heart of nursing, and it can be found throughout nursing practice.[1] It can be an energizing force in which people do what they say they will do. Some common concepts can be found, such as a feeling of obligation to patients and to each other, which comes with consequences if this duty is violated. Nurses exhibit a willingness to perform their duties without reluctance. They have a clear intent or purpose that guides them in fulfilling their work. Nurses "own" this work and have power and control over actualizing it. Nurses have a commitment to the work, which includes a feeling of being emotionally compelled or obliged to do the work.

Marcia Rache[2] believes that three elements are crucial to accountability: clarity, commitment, and consequences. By clarity she means goals are clear and specific, such as "lower the catheter-associated urinary tract infection [CAUTI] rate to below the national benchmark." That goal is very clear and specific and easy to monitor, and the "why" is also clear: improved patient care.

The second aspect, commitment, refers to asking for a commitment to some part of the work. The person must listen, understand, and agree and then commit to the goal. This means if asked, we must respond affirmatively. If the response is "I'll try," that is not commitment. Think of Yoda in *Star Wars*, when he is teaching Luke to be a Jedi Knight and he says, "Do or do not, there is no try." *Try* is a word that promotes an excuse or justification if the individual decides not to complete the promise or agreement. This justification serves to avoid negative consequences when in reality nothing was done.

The third element is consequences. Without consequences, accountability is merely an idea. As an example, when a meeting is scheduled to begin on the hour and people drift in for 10 minutes after the hour without any consequences, we begin to think 10 minutes late is acceptable, so why show up on time? What are the consequences of not doing what you say you will do? Lack of follow-through erodes trust because others are unsure about what will be done and if the person who fails to follow through is trustworthy or has values compatible with a quality focus. The new head coach of the Denver Broncos, Vic Fangio, told the press (and probably also told his players), there would be no "death by inches."[3] Many games in the previous season were lost by inches, or small details. Translated, that means being 30 seconds late for a team meeting, if not addressed, turns into 2 minutes the next day and soon it's 10 minutes. He transfers this to not attending to details, and lack of attention to details loses football games. Lack of attention to details in health care can cost lives. Being accountable for what you say you will do in a timely fashion is important. "Death by inches" can lead to patient morbidity and mortality.

What are the consequences of failure? Does failure lead to what one of us calls "correction by crucifixion"? Are people castigated and even terminated when a significant project fails? For example, what happens when an organization has dedicated effort, time, and money to constructing an organizational culture for which Magnet® designation is sought and the written document is returned because it does not meet the standards? Do people lose their jobs because of this failure, or do leaders bring the team together and demonstrate accountability by identifying what could have been done differently or better? Leaders acknowledge weaknesses and personal mistakes and ask others to identify what could be improved so that a subsequent submission will be approved. When one of us was director of maternal-child services at a major community hospital, we created a national conference focused on the labor, delivery, recovery, and postpartum (LDRP) concept of obstetrical care.

"Although the conference was a success, major problems and issues occurred. Staff were distraught. At the debrief of the conference, several staff members wanted to dump their frustrations on the conference coordinator. We structured the debriefs in a way that encouraged everyone to speak, one person at a time, with no interruptions, until the speaker was complete and voluntarily turned to the next member in the circle. As the leader, I chose to begin by discussing my own accountability and responsibility for the problems. I apologized to the team for several things that fell through the cracks. This approach served to defuse other members of the team, and each person took responsibility for their failures in relationship to the conference. Although I was not conscious of the implications in the moment, I was role modeling constructive problem solving and an accountability mindset rather than beating up on team members who had failed at some aspect. This discussion became a learning experience about how we could improve, and everyone left the debrief feeling positive and ready to take on the next challenge. Here the focus was on continuous improvement, or how to execute the next conference or project incorporating what we learned from this conference."

REFLECTION Consider the last time something went awry. Did you identify your role in what happened? If you did speak up, did you use "I" statements as opposed to "things" statements, which convey observations but no accountability?

THE PROFESSIONAL ACCOUNTABILITY MINDSET

Rose Sherman describes professional accountability mindset as internally driven, a commitment made to yourself and to your career to advance, grow, and improve the patient care you provide.[4] The American Nurses Association (ANA) Code of Ethics for Nurses states that nurses are "accountable and responsible for the quality of their practice."[5] This statement indicates that nurses must take accountability for their actions and for those of the health care team as they relate to patient care and to other projects within the facility. Nurses must develop a mindset, a perspective, in which they evaluate patient care through evidence-based practice (EBP), including peer review, research, and continuous quality improvement. This kind of perspective mandates that each nurse be accountable for patient safeguards and the consequences of all patient care decisions. This emphasizes the importance of current EBP policies and procedures and the personal responsibility of the nurse to be knowledgeable about the current literature, as well as the policies and procedures. This accountability mindset requires a focus on continuing learning through reading, attendance at professional conferences, and active involvement in professional groups that support learning and growth. We would argue that all we do in nursing—even if patients aren't involved—could be couched in the concept put forth in the Code. Sitting in a meeting has the potential to affect patients, even if they are several layers away from the topic at hand. Any policy—even those related to benefits—influences the environment in which we work and thus the care of the people we ultimately serve.

Leaders commit to an accountability mindset and role-model that for others. If an informal leader behaves in this manner in situations where a formal leader (headship) does not, this behavior may be threatening, or the formal leader now has what one of us calls the "designated blamee." Even though we have theoretically moved to a just culture that is supported by such groups as The Joint Commission and the DNV-Healthcare, many of us work in situations where affixing blame seems to be the goal.

ACCOUNTABILITY VS. RESPONSIBILITY

Many people use the term *accountability* interchangeably with the term *responsibility*. Accountability is described as obligated to report, explain, or justify something, and responsibility is defined as answerable or accountable for something within one's power, control, or management.[6] One difference between the two is responsibility can be shared, whereas accountability cannot.[7] For instance, in an

TABLE 15.1 **Comparison of Accountability with Responsibility**

Basis for Comparison	Accountability	Responsibility
Meaning	Obligation to report, explain, or justify an outcome or lack thereof	Answerable for something within one's power or control; duty
What is it?	Answerable for the consequence of the delegated task	Obligated to perform a delegated task
Nature	Accepted	Assigned
Arises from	Feeling responsible for an overall project or goal	Authority
Delegation	Is internally generated, not delegated	From supervisor and job description
Performance	Measured	Not measured

Adapted from Surbhi S. Difference between responsibility and accountability. 2016. Available at: https://keydifferences.com/difference-between-responsibility-and-accountability.html. Accessed March 7, 2109.

organization or team, success related to responsibility may be focused on reducing the central line–associated bloodstream infection (CLABSI) rate in the intensive care unit (ICU). The team is responsible for knowing the policy for management of central lines, and each nurse is accountable for following the policy in managing their patient with a central line. The team works together in devising the best approach to safe patient care for their individual patients related to reducing infections in central lines. As a team, they strive to improve on the national benchmark for CLABSI. The ICU contributes to the overall CLABSI rate, but they cannot be accountable for the entire facility because they have no control over the remainder of the units. An excuse/blame mentality denies everyone working toward positive outcomes overall. An attitude of self-protection could exist, such as "I did my part, my patients don't have infections." Such an approach justifies behavior focusing on self-protection.

Furthermore, leaders have the duty to complete certain tasks as part of the job, such as rounding in the ICU and talking to clinical nurses about the CLABSI rate and what it means not only for patients but also for the facility and the ability to be financially solvent. When leaders take ownership of their actions or decisions (such as supporting a new evidence-based approach to CLABSI), leaders are being accountable for stimulating action around an unsatisfactory patient situation. Responsibility is the obligation to perform specific tasks such as making rounds and talking to the nurses. Being answerable for the consequences of these tasks is being accountable (making sure that another strategy is used to decrease the CLABSI rate). Responsibility is assigned, whereas accountability is accepted—the chief nursing officer (CNO)/leader feels accountable for the CLABSI rate. Although responsibility can be delegated, accountability cannot be delegated. Performance is measured by outcomes when people are accountable. Responsibility is not necessarily measured or assessed for quality.

We attempt to solve problems and issues in an organization by redefining responsibilities for various roles and restructuring the work that needs to be done. Unfortunately, changing organizational positions does not change the way people think and perform. When increased accountability is supported, the blaming and justification decrease dramatically. Encouraging people to step past responsibility and take accountability supports them to own tasks and problems and allows them to be significantly more involved. This creates true engagement in the work. Table 15.1 summarizes the comparisons between accountability and responsibility. This broader view suggests that every person is accountable for not only personal results but also group/team results for which they are not 100% in control. Thus they view themselves as accountable for the ultimate results of the organizational goals.

In the Workplace Accountability Study[8] researchers identified that 82% of respondents believed that their leaders had no ability to hold others accountable, yet more than 90% of these respondents ranked accountability as a top developmental need in their organization. These respondents believed their peers should be held accountable when they fail to meet job requirements, just as they feel they should receive recognition for good work and for meeting the expectations of their jobs. On the other hand, 11% of managers identified that 50% of their employees avoid taking responsibility for mistakes in their jobs or taking accountability for their actions or the consequences. This disconnect between how accountability is needed and how managers hold others accountable is a major concern. If we can convert formal leadership behavior to one of supporting accountability for all and transition that change in a just manner, we could dramatically improve care. Think of the informal leaders in

TABLE 15.2 Skousen's Accountability Traits

1. Discovering other people's perspective about a problem or issue. Asking others what they think or what perspective they have from their experience.
2. Communicating openly not just with teammates but with anyone who might have ideas about how to further a project or goal.
3. Asking for and offering supportive feedback.
4. Hearing and saying things that may be difficult for others to hear in a way that supports the process rather than making these same observations in destructive ways.
5. Being personally invested in discovering what creates success.
6. Focusing on learning from both successes and failures, or discovering what didn't work.
7. Ensuring each person's work is aligned with the key outcomes.
8. Acting on feedback provided to make changes and attempt approaches that work better.
9. Having an attitude of constantly asking, "What else can I do?"
10. Collaborating across functional boundaries, including other teams and departments.
11. Dealing creatively with obstacles, including brainstorming sessions to generate ideas.
12. Taking necessary risks to experiment and innovate and to create new approaches.
13. Doing what you say you will do (DWYSYWD), or if a problem arises, letting others know as soon as possible.
14. Refusing to blame others when problems or issues or failure arises.
15. Tracking progress (or the lack thereof) with proactive transparent reporting and identifying when help is needed.
16. Building an environment of trust.

Adapted from Skousen T. Choose accountability. 2016. Available at: https://www.partnersinleadership.com/insights-publications/responsibility-vs-accountability/. Accessed March 7, 2019

an organization who speak up separately about a concern. They can be perceived as "complainers" rather than as an advanced warning system. Leaders attend to this advanced warning system. They listen and support appropriate changes. They believe they are accountable for these actions and for facilitating appropriate changes.

REFLECTION Consider how the "complainers" behave in your organization. Are they merely being disruptive, or are they acting as an early warning system? How can you support these individuals to be effective in their alerts?

POSITIVE ACCOUNTABILITY

Both terms, *accountability* and *responsibility*, appear magically when a designated result has not been achieved. Tracey Skousen suggests that the terms have been used in a more negative perspective and that accountability should be viewed as a positive. She suggests that accountability plays a role in overcoming most challenges faced by leaders.[6]

Something more positive might be defined as a personal choice to demonstrate ownership, to achieve the desired organizational results and outcomes even if it requires exceeding one's job description or other circumstances. Skousen describes 16 accountability traits that she believes are the essence of striving for accountability individually, as teams, and as organizations. These traits are presented in Table 15.2.

REFLECTION Use the 16 items in Table 15.2 as a checklist to conduct a personal appraisal. Consider what you can do to exhibit all 16 traits consistently. Which traits do you want to strengthen? How will you plan to do so?

This list contains behaviors that are not easy to incorporate, to teach, or to role model. Becoming effective in these 16 behaviors is hard work *and* it is a choice. When these 16 behaviors are addressed at each level of the organization, positive accountability is created, and an entirely different culture evolves.

LL ALERT

- Do not blame others for problems and issues.
- Don't merely be responsible.

SUMMARY

Accountability is both a personal and a professional behavior that is demonstrated (or not) by every leader. Accountability is not the same as responsibility, although both are essential to leaders. Accountability can be seen as a positive way to move a team or an organization forward. Leaders hold themselves and others accountable for outcomes.

LL LINEUP

- Leaders refrain from using accountability and responsibility interchangeably.
- Leaders maintain clarity regarding the accountability for outcomes both in terms of quality patient care and working constructively with others.

REFLECTION Think about a time when you did not follow through on a promise or agreement. Did you apologize to the person or group? Did you inform them that you couldn't meet the timeline? Did you ignore the situation or person(s) and act as though you had not made the promise? What did you do to make amends? If you believe you held yourself accountable, what did that entail?

16

Agility

Today's health care world has been described in shorthand as VUCA—volatile, uncertain, complex, and ambiguous. (Actually, that is true of most aspects of the world, but we are concerned with health care, and it certainly is apt there!) Another way of looking at today's world is to use the acronym RUPT—rapid, unpredictable, paradoxical, and tangled. We would add an "I" to each word to represent intensity! Either acronym means we live in a very complex and confusing world that is rapidly changing and sometimes makes no sense. This statement reflects how many people viewed the 2020 pandemic–it made no sense! This view means we have to be agile if we want to survive, let alone thrive. Agility is defined as having the ability to move with quick and easy grace. Note that moving quickly isn't sufficient—agility includes ease and grace. We also may know agility by the term *nimbleness*.

PERSONAL AGILITY

Remember when you thought you were busy because you had maybe 10 tasks to accomplish in a day? We remember those days with fondness because now the tasks are multiplied, the time frame is shortened, and expectations are higher. We readily see the effects at work, but we may not think about what is happening to us. We must process information more rapidly; consider more factors; and apply research about the practice, the people, organizations, and numerous other factors. Then, to make matters worse, answers aren't always forthcoming or clear. This situation is known as a *fog of uncertainty*.[1] The term seems appropriate if you have ever driven in fog. You sort of know where the edge of the road is and you hope the vehicle in front of you has visible taillights, but you aren't really sure. You are "flying blind" and hoping you are doing the right things to stay on course. "We need inner agility, but our brain instinctively seeks stasis."[1] This uncertainty is taxing on our mental and emotional reserves.

We see this stress played out in making quick decisions that may not be the most logical if we took more time. We also see this stress played out in never getting to a decision (paralysis of analysis) because we keep hoping for just one more piece of information—the piece that will bring the whole puzzle of whatever is going on into full view. That is known as *magical thinking*. Or we become very controlling in an attempt to force order onto something that does not lend itself to order. The more forward thinking and proactive we can be, the more likely we will be able to make a decision and move forward. Notice that in the earlier possible responses, the common element is simplification— "quick, make the issue go away," "wait till the answer comes," and "just control the variables." None of these works because what is needed is to be agile.

How do we become more agile? Five practices can help us be more agile.[1] These appear in Table 16.1. In challenging situations, our normal tendency might be to respond quickly. What works better is to pause to think clearly. When we respond quickly, we typically use actions that have worked before. Although these may work in the new, complex environment, they also may not be the answer. Pausing allows us to think not only of the tested ideas but also the untested, different responses.

Sometimes when a situation is tense, we tend to try to forge ahead to resolve the situation. Rather than forging ahead, however, if we can admit our limitations, we can garner ideas from others. When we admit our limitations, we expose our vulnerability, and as Brene Brown says, that opens a different relationship in a group.[2] Embracing our ignorance allows us to garner all those ideas from others, who are also looking for solutions.

As we already discussed in the chapter on framing, we benefit when we think of something in a different way. We are always trying to see a different view to generate new ways to approach a situation. The potential in reframing is that we get to a different level of a problem. When we do that, we then create the possibility of having a broader impact as we address the original issue.

We love the next idea because so much in life is about the journey and not the destination. So thinking of setting a direction rather than a destination makes sense. This practice almost demands a purpose or vision to guide the next activities. When we are purpose driven, we have a

TABLE 16.1 Five Practices to Agility

- Pause to move faster.
- Embrace your ignorance.
- Reframe the questions radically.
- Set direction, not destination.
- Test your solutions—and yourself.

From Bourton S, Lavoie J, Vogel T. Leading with inner agility. McKinsey & Company. 2018. Available at: https://www.mckinsey.com/business-functions/organization/our-insights/leading-with-inner-agility. Accessed March 29, 2018.

TABLE 16.2 Strategies to Develop Emotional Agility

1. Find the patterns.
2. Label the patterns.
3. Accept the patterns.
4. Act on your values.

From David S, Congleton C. Emotional agility. 2013. Available at: https://hbr.org/2013/11/emotional-agility?autocomplete5true. Accessed March 6, 2019.

general direction we need to take. Dr. Susan David, who writes about emotional agility in her email service, points out the world today demands agility, and part of the success of developing personal agility and buying into an organization's purpose is to allow individuals to discuss how their personal values relate to the organization's values.[3] The point here is that individuals need to be able to see how their values are valued and how they relate to the bigger picture.

Finally, the idea of testing solutions and self is reflective of health care's approach of small tests of change. Some people call that perpetual evolution. As Dr. Beverly Malone, CEO of the National League for Nursing, says in tough meetings: "It's a cinch by the inch, but hard by the yard." Inching along allows us to gain a sense of our direction rather than plunging ahead and ending up some place we don't want to be. If we fail, we won't create fatal damage. We may be bruised, but we aren't so badly hurt that we have to relinquish our involvement. Again, leaders are vulnerable at this point because we may have declared what we planned to test and we get immediate feedback that indicates that was not a smart strategy. Although we all are disappointed whenever we feel we wasted time, this was a mere test of a small step that allows us to refocus on a different aspect. The intensity of testing care standards in the early stages of patients with COVID-19 created havoc for many. The "rules" of care were often changed by the day because we were learning in real time.

REFLECTION Consider what is going on in your life right now. It may be at work or at home or in a volunteer situation. What quick adaptations have you had to make? How did you feel as you became more engrained in those changes? Did you gain any insights into what to do with what you learned from that (those) experience(s)? Did you pause or just jump right in? Did you embrace your ignorance or try to dazzle others with your "brilliance"? Did you use reframing? Did you get a sense of where you were headed? What can you carry forward?

Now, so no one goes away with the perspective that being agile is the absolutely best thing ever, we need to consider what happens when we are consumed with being agile. Susan David and Christina Congleton offer four strategies to get unhooked from our emotions when we need to.[4] Table 16.2 lists those strategies.

First, find the patterns. For example, when we are constantly bombarded with change, which is how it feels sometimes, we may give ourselves negative messages, such as "I can't do this anymore." That little voice in our heads keeps iterating that message, and we begin to believe it. Our ability to recognize such patterns sets us on a different road—one of fixing these emotional drainers.

Second, David and Congleton say, label them. Are they thoughts or emotions? Both can be transient pieces of data if we can recognize them for what they are and move on. We need to consciously decide whether we are feeling something or thinking something. If we are thinking something, we can consider what information we are missing, if any, to reaffirm or disaffirm our thinking. If we are responding emotionally, we need to ask ourselves what precipitated that sensation and if that feeling is based on fact or leads to harm. If the feeling has no basis in fact and it doesn't suggest impending doom, we might try acknowledging the feeling to move ahead.

Third, accept the patterns we have just named. We don't have to accept them as in internalizing them. If we accept them as patterns, we can examine them and not let them rule us. Here we might examine them in more detail and determine answers to questions such as: Do I always respond to that person in that manner? Am I afraid of embarrassing myself? What can I do to recoup if I err? Could I let this go?

Fourth, act on your values. Assuming you developed a clear set of values as you moved through the Legacy *Leaders-*Ship Trajectory, you can use those to refocus what you really want and need to do to move past the current feeling.

ON BEING A SCRUM MASTER

The term *scrum* refers to a process framework for dealing with complex issues to adapt to producing high value. It is a perfect fit for today's world! Although it is most commonly used in business, especially those related to technology where changes occur very rapidly, scrum has meaning for individuals and can be used with groups, even in nonwork settings. The point of using this approach is that scrum focuses on improvements in small steps. In health care, we might call this process small tests of change or the plan–do–study–act (PDSA) cycle advocated by the Institute for Healthcare Improvement.[5]

"Knowledge comes from experience *and* making decisions based on what is known. Scrum employs an iterative, incremental approach to optimize predictability and control risk."[6] In a sense, scrum is another example of Dr. Beverly Malone's quote: "It's a cinch by the inch but hard by the yard." Inching along allows us to make small errors and gains as opposed to completing some work only to find it isn't what was needed. Because scrum is incremental work, and if we constantly have been adapting, we are more likely to demonstrate agility in a new situation than if we had not been making these ongoing adaptations. Although true scrum work requires a team, the process of scrum work makes sense for individuals: plan, scrum, review, and retrospective (or, as we would call it, reflection).

The plan starts with a goal in mind and a time frame, typically 1 month or less, and focuses on two questions: What needs to be done? How will it get done? Are those not the questions relevant for us to remain agile in our work? What do we need to be able to do differently in the ever-changing world, and how will we be able to do whatever those changes require?

In a real scrum, the team gets together for 15 minutes each day to plan what will happen in the next 24 hours. Again, this makes sense in being agile. We need to stop and think what the next thing is we need to consider or test. And every day this work starts with what we accomplished yesterday (review). We should be asking ourselves if we feel better able to handle change or if we are feeling overwhelmed by what is happening. This is descriptive of reflection—stopping to think about something specific. Admittedly, we all have days when we would declare: "OVERWHELMED!" If this happens regularly, however, something isn't working for us.

The retrospective in scrum work focuses on people, relationships, process, and tools. Although we often don't include tools in our ongoing assessments of how things went, we easily could because the lack of tools may prevent us from doing our best. However, the real focus for us should be on (1) others around us—have we inspired them to adapt to changes?, (2) relationships—have we maintained relationships to the extent we get critical information and have influence with the people with whom we relate?, and (3) process—have we figured out a safe, quality-oriented process? Our concluding questions might relate to whether or not we are on track or if we need to make minor or major adjustments and what we need to do differently to stay on our timeline. In health care (and other fields), work often is sequential, and a delay at point 1 can throw a whole process into turmoil. Doing the right thing and doing it promptly are equally important.

When we take charge of ourselves and recognize—and yes, embrace—change, we can be agile. Otherwise, we become more resistant to change, feel overwhelmed more often, become less valuable to an organization and our peers, and feel less confident about who we are and what we bring of value.

BALANCING AGILITY WITH CONSISTENCY

Being agile is critical as we have already pointed out. However, constant change probably makes all of us anxious. If we think about it, we value consistency. Consistency brings us wonderful things like a feeling of competence (because we don't have to figure out what we are going to do). Consistency makes us feel safe. (If I tell my boss X, I know she will say Y and then ask me to do Z. I won't be afraid to tell her this.) Consistency also produces efficiency (because I didn't have to stop and think about what was happening, I just responded).

John Coleman proposed a 2-by-2 matrix composed of two axes: consistency and agility and ranging from high to low on both axes.[7] When consistency and agility are both high, we are functioning on a strategic level. That is what every organization hopes every leader (and employee) is doing every day! When both consistency and agility are low, we are both unreliable and uninspired—in essence, a disaster! When consistency is high and agility is low, we are rigid. Although we aren't a disaster, no one wants to be on our team! When consistency is low and agility is high, we are unfocused. We may be able to adapt, but members of a team may not trust us.

REFLECTION In which quadrant would you place yourself? Are you often in more than one quadrant? What happens in these circumstances?

TEAM AGILITY

As we alluded to in the area devoted to scrums, agility typically is applied to teams. As with anything else, if only one member exhibits an ability and the rest don't, major movement is unlikely. Leaders (formal or informal) can help others be more agile by doing some specific things. Darrell Rigby and his team suggest that to be agile, we need to be focused on small groups and ones that have diversity.[8]

(They say multidisciplinary, but we want to expand that idea because it isn't just about the disciplines represented.) They suggest using rapid prototyping and tight feedback loops, two characteristics inherent in scrums and in rapid-cycle change (small tests of change). What is important in our view is placing more value on change and adaptation than sticking to the plan. This means that leaders need to give a team permission to break rules that aren't in place to protect safety or to ensure legality. If a senior leader doesn't convey this, any member of the team should raise the issue. The role of senior leaders at that point is to be out of the way! Agile teams need to be self-governing. As long as the timeline and the expected outcomes are clear, the teams should do their work as they see fit.

When one of us worked for a particular organization, she worked with three powerhouse groups:

"They fed on an idea, and instead of having one idea, they would generate many more, all of which brought value to the organization. To accomplish one group's important and relevant work quickly (an appropriate and accurate assessment in my view), the group met at the convenience of several members—on the weekend and in a different city. As it turned out, that behavior was not part of the work culture where I worked! I was told: others always come to us and we never work on the weekend. Fortunately, that group never needed another such meeting so I didn't have to convey that message to them. Why would we want to stop the generation of new ideas—ones critical to the success of the organization?"

BECOMING MORE AGILE

Leadership agility is the ability to deal with VUCA and RUPT, to make and implement decisions quickly, to adapt and think on your feet, and to lead with confidence. The way to develop this skill is: improv! Yes, as strange as that may sound, participating in improv sessions helps us improve our ability to be agile—and that is critical for leaders to have![9] For example, one of us had participated in a couple of such sessions in a national leadership learning activity.

"Fortunately, I had learned a lot because after those sessions, the member of the team who normally did this portion of the 3-day experience was unable to participate, so I 'inherited' this time. I have to confess, I was a little anxious because my predecessor was not only a nurse but also a former actor and someone who had participated in improv for years! How could I match that? I essentially used improvisation to help the group learn about improvisation, and it went well because I adapted the session to relevant nursing examples. I came away from that experience with an even deeper appreciation for the value of improv."

If you have ever watched improv, you know that the gist of this work is to operate in real time. No one has a script, and yet one person is expected to interact with another one or two people when given a hypothetical situation. An example of comedic improvisation is the Drew Carey–hosted television show *Whose Line Is it Anyway?*, which can be downloaded online. To be successful at improvising, each participant has to exercise the ability to listen because the words out of the second person's mouth have to relate to whatever the first person says and so forth. Each person has to be aware of the others involved in the improvisation because, as in real life, words don't convey a whole message. Our facial expressions, our gestures, our stance, and so on all contribute to the message. As with being mindful, we have to pay attention and be in the moment to be relevant. Improvisation helps with clarity of communication and promotes confidence to respond instinctively or spontaneously.

Going to an improv performance or watching one on television or YouTube isn't sufficient. You have to participate. This is not a vicarious experience. You have to be in the midst of the action. If you don't have access to a place where you can learn improv, assemble a group of people, probably at least a dozen. Form a rather tight circle; this helps you focus on paying attention to each other. One person should be in the middle of the circle and act as the facilitator for the session. That person sets up the improv by explaining each member will take turns saying one word—whatever word a person says has to relate to what the prior person said. The facilitator is to tell a story using everyone's one-word input. The facilitator has the group continue around the circle several times so that everyone gets the sense of how actively they all have to listen to continue the story. Round one can be about anything. In round two, the facilitator can present a nursing example or something with a greater intensity. For example, offering the first word as "disasters" creates a very different type of tone and content than if the first word were "summertime."

After several rounds, the facilitator can have people pair off to respond to a scenario. Each pair is given a scenario. After reading that information, the pairs are invited to participate in an exchange for several minutes to experience what the dialog (based on the scenario) might be like. The facilitator can then help everyone debrief by discussing the various responses each pair had to the scenario, describing what words or statements they used and how they felt, and considering how they might use this learning in real life. If the scenario is based on a common problem most participants experience (or will likely experience) in their roles, they now have the experience of not only how they responded but also how several others did, too.

LL ALERT

- Don't become so agile that you have given up consistency.
- Don't forget to use one or more of the practices of agility.

SUMMARY

Agility seems to be the current answer to keeping up with change and being prepared for what's ahead. It requires being proactive, and it also requires balance. If we take on the idea of being a scrum master for ourselves, we can execute a great leadership progression plan.

LL LINEUP

- Quick, easy, and grace are three key words that must remain linked in our minds if we want agility and not chaos.
- Adopt the five practices to be more agile.

REFLECTION Consider what you think will be the next big change for you at work. What new talents will you need to be successful? What adaptations will you need to make? What is your plan for being agile enough to thrive?

17

Attitudes

So, what is an attitude? No doubt, each of us could identify a negative attitude when we see it. We have all encountered others who begin an encounter with a "woe is me" story of something negative that happened to them since you last spoke to them. Hopefully, we can also identify the person who is almost always upbeat and positive, someone who tells you a happy story about a great weekend trip, or a wonderful concert, or an inspiring church sermon or sees humor in their "woe is me" story. Attitude is a way of thinking or feeling about someone or something, typically one that is reflected in a person's behavior.[1] As Charles Swindoll[2] says:

The longer I live, the more I realize the impact of attitude on life.

Attitude, to me, is more important than facts. It is more important than the past, than education, than money, than circumstances, than failures, than successes, than what other people think or say or do. It is more important than appearance, giftedness or skill. It will make or break a company...a church...a home.

The remarkable thing is we have a choice every day regarding the attitude we will embrace for that day. We cannot change our past...we cannot change the fact that people will act in a certain way. We cannot change the inevitable. The only thing we can do is play on the one string we have, and that is our attitude...I am convinced that life is 10% what happens to me and 90% how I react to it.

And so it is with you...we are in charge of our attitudes.

We see people's attitudes in what stories or events they choose to share and in what their reaction is to an event we choose to share. One of us worked where all team meetings begin with the question, "Are you able to be fully present for this meeting?" This is another way of asking if any negative or stressful situations are bothering anyone and preventing them from being 100% present and participating in the important work of the team or if they are so ecstatic about something they can't focus. One team member might share how terrible the traffic was, including being cut off by an angry driver and nearly causing an accident with another car. Another team member might share how sick her dog is and she was up much of the night with the animal. Such events trigger emotions and make it difficult to see positives and be attentive to important aspects of work. Often just sharing or talking about such events enables problem solving and a more upbeat positive approach to the situation. This sharing supports leaders to refocus and attend to the purpose of the meeting. Additionally, we all know how to filter information. For example, having been cut off in traffic might explain a special sensitivity to being cut off in our group conversation. The same distraction occurs with pleasant events. Think, for example, if you just learned you won the lottery. You probably are not fully engaged with the business of the meeting!

GENERAL OBSERVATIONS ABOUT ATTITUDE

The power of attitude, as described by many authors, is depicted as "attitude is everything." The general thinking is attitude constitutes 90% of one's success in life, and other aspects such as IQ, knowledge, and skills constitute the other 10%.[2] Would you rather be around someone who is upbeat and positive or someone who is critical of themselves and others and fills time with stories of how terrible everything is? We should surround ourselves with people and colleagues who expect more from us than we expect from ourselves. These people who expect more of us serve as a stimulus to take risks, be innovative, and, if the result is failure, attempt a different approach. This constitutes a positive mindset regarding our work, a mindset that focuses on what is possible. A positive attitude is a necessary approach to achieving positive results, innovation, and overcoming setbacks. As one author states, "Your attitude controls your life. But the good news is, you control your attitude."[3]

When we get up every day, we decide whether this will be a great day, or we might say "three negative things have already happened, I haven't left the house yet and therefore this is clearly going to be a bad day." We also could say, "I'm glad the bad is out of the way so the rest of the day can be great." At any point we can choose a good or bad day.

As some say, it isn't what happens to you but how you *choose* to respond that determines the quality of your life.[4] Salena Tully and Hong Tao conducted the first study in the United States to look at positive attitudes and stress among nurses in acute care.[5] Their work shows a strong correlation between perceived stress and using positive thinking. This is good news, because generally stress is associated with negative attitudes and thinking. Think of the attitudes the frontline nurses must have had as their workplaces filled with patients with COVID-19. They kept going back, even when their basic safety was at risk.

> **REFLECTION:** Consider how you would describe your attitude.

STRESS AND NEGATIVE ATTITUDES

Does this theme sound familiar? Negative attitudes come from repeatedly thinking negative thoughts until they become a habit, a ritual. Sometimes we are challenged to judge our negative attitudes because we have had them for such a long time. We come to expect failure and disaster. This vicious cycle, in which we expect the worst, is a self-fulfilling prophecy. Some would say "Bad situations are just a reality," a justification for negative thinking. Situations are a reality. They do show up, *and* our attitude makes a situation positive or negative. One of us learned early from her mother that the negative will pass.

"My mother would say something like: something better is in store. As a result, I have always said to others I wish for what is best for them, not necessarily what they were saying they want."

Another one of us always sees the humor in the everyday challenges we experience. Because she typically shares this view, many of us who might be ready to take on the "woe is me" attitude begin laughing, and yes, our attitudes change.

Human beings control how they think and feel. For example, rather than focus on an event such as employee satisfaction scores less than the Magnet® hospital national benchmark from a negative perspective, a more positive approach would be to discover what can be learned from these results and then develop a plan for improving the scores. Taking control of our attitudes, our states of mind, and the outcome allows us to control the results. We can create positive results with a positive attitude.

PSYCHOLOGICAL ASPECTS OF ATTITUDE AND BEHAVIORS

Psychologists identify attitudes as a learned tendency and an approach to evaluate people, issues, events, or objects in a certain way, which can be either positive or negative. Occasionally these evaluations are mixed because both positive and negative aspects can be identified. Forming attitudes can be found in a person's experiences. Some of these experiences are personal or life events that have influenced our attitudes toward situations and life roles. For example, you may recall the story about Dr. Ingeborg Mauksch from the chapter on mentoring.

"Instead of seeking a 'piece of paper/master's diploma,' I began to study in earnest, to learn about leadership, to seek out and create innovative approaches for the delivery of obstetrical care. My entire attitude about graduate school shifted."

DEVELOPMENT OF ATTITUDES

Some attitudes are acquired from observation of people we admire, such as a valued and important leader we strive to emulate. In a first director position, one of us was fortunate to have a chief nursing officer (CNO) who had amazing listening skills and asked great questions.

"She met with each director twice a month, and our little group did team-building workshops that focused on personal growth as well as the team growth. The focus was on positives, on growing and learning, and on problem solving. I watched closely all these efforts, and as I grew into other positions, I modeled my leadership behavior after what I had seen her do. My attitude was positive toward all these efforts, and I learned them from this CNO. She also insisted we all join the American Organization of Nurse Executives [AONE, now known as the American Organization for Nursing Leadership] as active members. Active membership in an organization, such as AONE, focuses on learning and taking action. These are positive actions rooted in a positive attitude."

This example is repeated across numerous organizations around the world. The role model might be the CNO, a colleague, a member of the housekeeping staff, or our patients. Think, for example, of how Christopher Reeve, who portrayed Superman and then, due to an accident, was paralyzed for years, changed our thinking about paralysis. His breakthrough attitude and funding from his foundation supported a more assertive approach to rehabilitation.

Attitudes can also be adopted from social factors, as exemplified in social roles or how people are expected to behave, and in social norms or rules for appropriate behavior. In nursing school, we learned the expected role of a nurse, especially as it related to the specific unit or care specialty. We learned about the change-of-shift report, how to perform assessments, how to create an organized workflow, or how to relate to family members. We learned how we were supposed to dress. We learned nursing care plans and the delivery of medications on the appropriate schedules. We adapted our attitude by learning the professional or nursing routine.

Attitudes can also evolve from learned behavior, such as the classical conditioning we might see in advertising where a fun time at a party is associated with a product such as a specific beverage. Learning might also come from operant conditioning in which a person suffers ridicule from family and friends for "driving under the influence" and decides to always have a designated driver.

Attitudes and behavior don't always align. For example, some people support a political party or candidate but do not follow through to actually vote. Often the behavioral alignment depends on the strength of the attitude. Behavior tends to match attitudes when we have an impactful personal experience. As an example, look at the Miracle on the Hudson, where Captain Chesley "Sully" Sullenberger landed a plane on the Hudson River in New York and everyone survived! The survivors committed to meet on a regular basis to celebrate their miracle. The commitment to show up (behavior) derives from the attitude (a miracle).

Behavior also might match the alignment when a person is very knowledgeable about a subject. When we expect a favorable outcome, the alignment is much closer. When attitudes are repeated often, behavior is more aligned. When rewards are high and what can be won is important, the behavior is much closer to the attitude.

Kendra Cherry[6] discusses the ABCs of attitudes as the affective component, the behavioral component, and the cognitive component. The affective aspects concern the feelings we may have about a person, object, or event. For example, we may have had a series of interactions with a person, none of which went well despite all our efforts. This type of interaction can easily result in negative feelings about this individual. The behavioral aspects of attitude focus on how the person, object, or event influences our behavior. For many of us an object like a wedding ring serves as a symbol of not just a relationship but also a set of promises made to another human being. A married colleague once shared an event where a man flirted with her and asked her out. Her response was, "Thank you for the compliment but I have a wonderful relationship with my husband. I hope we can be friends."

The cognitive aspect is focused on our thoughts and beliefs about the subject. For example, we have strong beliefs about "acknowledge in public, correct in private." While making patient rounds one day, one of us encountered an experienced, irate charge nurse correcting a new graduate nurse in a hallway with families and other health care professionals walking by:

"Unfortunately, I dealt with the charge nurse in private but not in a constructive/supportive way. This experience affected the relationship with her for the entire time I was at that facility. I kept attempting to 'fix' her. At that time in my career, I was totally unaware about the cognitive aspect of attitude and the impact my thoughts and judgments had on this nurse."

Cherry also identifies both the implicit (unconscious) aspects of attitude and explores the explicit (consciously aware) aspects of attitude.[6] Many leaders are totally unaware (unconscious) of their cognitive attitudes that influence their behavior. In the process of growth in addressing attitude, leaders seek to become consciously aware of both positive and negative attitudes and strive to reframe the negative perspective:

"For example, at this point in my career, I would be conscious of an employee's behavior and wouldn't be in reaction to the team leader castigating the new graduate. I would be more curious about what motivated her behavior and ask her to identify what was affecting her approach to the new nurse. I wouldn't be in reaction and, instead, attempt to create a teaching moment, perhaps by saying, 'How else could you have talked with the new nurse about her actions?' 'Where else might you have had that conversation?' She would have been more likely to integrate the feedback and be able to adapt her behavior."

REFLECTION Think back and reflect on a time when you may have been unaware of your own attitudes and the impact they had on the people around you. How are you different today? Is there additional work you would like to do regarding your attitude and how it affects others?

MINDSET

Carol Dweck describes a slightly different perspective about attitude. She refines attitudes into what she calls mindset, which can either be fixed or focused on growth.[7] Some others correlated this to a negative or positive attitude. For a person, even a really smart one, with a fixed mindset, this indicates that person is unchangeable. In comparison, a growth mindset is focused on embracing challenges. These people believe they can always learn something new. Growth mindset people may not have as high an IQ as fixed mindset individuals, and because they are focused on growth and learning, they often exceed expectations and are more successful than people with a fixed mindset. Growth mindset leaders like challenges because they simply work harder to master them. They find obstacles exciting because they can learn what works and what doesn't. They can go over, around, or through the obstacle and view effort and hard work as the path to mastery. They request critique or feedback of their performance because they learn from it. For example, one of us came home one day, and her husband announced he intended to close his business:

"That seemed to be a rash decision! He had been pushed to the wall about his building lease. What the property owner didn't know was that my husband took nothing off the table as a possible solution—including ceasing a successful business and moving out of the state. He wasn't giving up; he created new possibilities. After we talked, I could see his viewpoint and supported his intent."

Comparatively, fixed mindset people avoid challenges because the challenges may reveal that they are not perfect. When confronted with an obstacle, they are likely to give up easily because they may be perceived as not good enough to overcome the obstacle. They see exerting effort or working hard as too difficult; after all, they are good the way they are. Criticism is difficult for them because they cannot incorporate the implication that they are less than perfect. Common sense would suggest that being smart and capable inspires confidence, which is true until the going gets tough. What identifies the difference between the fixed mindset and the growth mindset is how each responds to challenges and setbacks/failures.

For those with a growth mindset, failure is information.[7] The response to failure is: Plan A didn't work and as a problem solver, a growth mindset person with a positive attitude will move to Plan B. In the example earlier, the husband (above) had moved through A, B, and C. Successful people have experienced multiple failures. These include Walt Disney, who was fired from a newspaper because he lacked imagination; Henry Ford, who had two failed car companies before Ford; and Steven Spielberg, who was rejected by the University of Southern California's film school several times.[3] These people knew they needed to be willing to fail hard and bounce back. They were resilient. They learned a lot from attempts that failed. They were passionate about their goals; they acted on their passion; they went the extra mile; and they were flexible and expected results. They grew and learned from each experience. The growth mindset can be likened to a positive attitude.

REFLECTION Think about a time when you thought you had done everything you could and you quit. What would have happened if your attitude was one of growth: "I'm learning a lot and I can go to Plan D." What would you have done differently?

GRIT

Who is successful and why? That is the question asked by Angela Duckworth.[8] She studied West Point students, National Spelling Bee contestants, and rookie teachers in rough neighborhoods only to discover that grit is not about IQ or social intelligence. Grit is about passion and perseverance for long-term goals. It is about stamina. People with grit understand that life is a marathon and not a sprint. Another way to think about grit is comparing talent and effort. She sees talent as important, but only when connected to effort. She believes talent counts once and effort counts twice.

Talent times effort = skill.
Effort times skill = achievement.
Grit = sustained effort toward long-term goals.

Although she is still in discovery about how grit is created in human beings, she believes it begins with developing a fascination with something. An example would be Ingeborg exposing one of us to leadership and the subsequent pursuit of leadership experiences. A fascination ensued. The second aspect is to improve daily, to reflect on what we have done and how it worked, and to strive for improvement. Next, Duckworth believes that leaders with grit are working toward a greater purpose. It isn't just about what brings pleasure and enjoyment; it's about passion and a burning desire to reach a long-term goal. And finally, she believes the approach is one of a growth mindset, or a positive attitude, whereas a fixed mindset is actually a negative or constricted view of self, a justification that I am who I am and I will never be smarter or more capable. Successful leaders believe that the ability to learn is continuous. We are always learning, and failure is not a permanent condition but rather an opportunity to learn and improve. We can mold our brains through this learning, and as an adult, IQ can increase. This is the epitome of a positive attitude.

REFRAMING NEGATIVE TO POSITIVE

To reframe is to view or think about beliefs, ideas, and relationships in a new or different way; it changes the way we look at something.[9] Reframing can change a really bad day into a low point in an overall wonderful week or a negative

TABLE 17.1 How Reframing Works

Attributes	Actions
1. Learn about thinking patterns	Educate yourself about negative thinking patterns that increase your stress levels (e.g., all-or-nothing thinking, overgeneralization, mental filters, jumping to conclusions, discounting positives).
2. Notice your thoughts	Catch yourself when you are slipping into overly negative patterns, become more mindful of your thoughts, and observe yourself.
3. Challenge your thoughts	Examine the truth and accuracy of your thoughts: Are the things you tell yourself even true? Can you shift to a more positive perspective of the thought?
4. Replace your thoughts with more positive thinking	Asking patients about discomfort rather than pain is reframing—using different words. Change your self-talk to less negative words and emotions.

Adapted from Scott E. 4 steps to shift perspective and change everything: how to reframe situations so they create less stress. 2018. Available at: https://www.verywellmind.com/cognitive-reframing-for-stress-management-3144872. Accessed February 10, 2019.

event into a learning experience. Reframing is a way we can create a more positive self-view before any actual changes in life circumstances. Reframing to the positive supports us to counteract negative thoughts. We can schedule daily positive activities and reframe disappointment as normal which can lead to more success.[10]

Being able to reframe an event optimistically is about resiliency, which helps leaders overcome adversity in achieving their objectives. We likely remember the old metaphor "Some people see the glass as half-full while others see it as half-empty." This is a perfect example of how the same event can be viewed in a positive or negative light by different people. One of us had such an experience early in her career:

"I attended a particularly tense national meeting with my boss. She came away with a negative attitude and stirred up the rest of my group upon returning home. I saw the turmoil at the national meeting as bad strategy but the intent as exceedingly positive—I was too intimidated to pose an alternative view by saying something like, "On the other hand," a strategy I now use frequently. I have learned that positive reframing translates as viewing events positively, and it is a powerful way to transform thinking."

Elizabeth Scott believes four approaches help leaders rethink how to approach reframing experiences[11] (Table 17.1). First she suggests that leaders focus on educating themselves and understanding negative thinking patterns, such as the way negative thinkers view life experiences. Self-education lays a groundwork for understanding and then creating change. Next, she suggests that we focus and catch ourselves when we are responding to a situation in a negative way. Challenging our own negativity begins with awareness and attending to identified negative behavior.

Journaling could support being mindful of the attitude and the surrounding thoughts. We could then examine these thoughts from a different perspective and, as an observer, notice what contributes to the thoughts rather than being stuck in them. Following these observations, we can challenge our thinking by examining the truth or accuracy of the negative thinking and then seek optional ways to view the events that precipitated the negative thoughts.[11] Finally, replacing these thoughts with more positive thoughts is important. For example, we often begin conversations with "you" messages: "You forgot to chart the urine output on patient A." This is a negative way to address the issue. A more positive approach would be to simply ask, "What was the urine output on Patient A?" Replacing the "you" with a different approach changes the way the message is received.

Table 17.2 identifies approaches for reframing with seven specific strategies to address changing an attitude.[10] These seven approaches can reinforce our efforts to be more positive and spend less time castigating ourselves for any missteps or getting stuck in negative self-talk.

MOTIVATION TO REFLECT ON NEGATIVISM?

Some people would say they "lack the motivation" to carefully examine the attitude they project. Motivation is the general desire or willingness to do something; it's the reason for acting or behaving in a particular way. What do we know about motivation? James Clear writes extensively about motivation and notes that sometimes we are highly motivated and enthusiastic about a project and can work for hours, not even noticing how much time has passed.[12] At other times, we seem stuck in procrastination and unable to extricate ourselves from this downward spiral. What

TABLE 17.2 Approaches to Reframing

Negative Thinking	Reframing Thinking to Improve the Mental Outlook
1. Counteract negative thoughts	Write down negative thoughts so you can examine them more closely and check for evidence supporting or negating your thinking.
2. Brainstorm	Write down your biggest problem, for example, finances. Identify as many solutions as possible. You could use mind mapping with money. Write down every possible solution, such as winning the lottery, finding a better-paying job, going back to school, getting certified (with an increase in salary), getting a loan, finding a second job, and so forth. Write down everything that comes to mind and have fun. Consider every possibility.
3. Conduct experiments in both thought and behavior	Test your thinking. Which thoughts seem most reasonable? If an option is returning to school (increase your salary), test this possibility by checking a couple of programs and assessing costs and requirements, and the difference between part-time and full-time study. What are some creative ways you could finance school? Does your employer have tuition reimbursement? Are scholarships or loan forgiveness programs available? These are all tests to determine how you might establish this goal and actualize it rather than adhering to the negative message, "It takes too much time" or "I can't afford it."
4. Use visualization	Visualize positive outcomes. Before getting out of bed in the morning, picture a very good day. Think of positive outcomes for the day. Imagine your colleagues smiling when you come to work and ask them about their weekend. Visualize your boss saying yes to the proposal you are developing. Before going to sleep, reflect on any positive events of the day. If something negative occurred, reframe it as a learning experience, identifying what was learned. Use this as a method of instilling hope and opening yourself to possibilities.
5. Practice positive thinking	When practicing, expect success; look for good aspects in everything. Adopt the attitude that there is no failure, only results or outcomes. Instead of looking outside at the 12 inches of snow and declaring the weather is awful, think of five positive things about the snow, such as the water being stored in the ground for the summer, the exercise you will get from shoveling, making snowmen with the neighborhood kids, completing an indoor project, or connecting with someone who is significant in your life.
6. Scheduling daily positive activities	Schedule a brief 20 minutes of positive activity, such as practicing meditation, playing favorite music, watching a favorite YouTube video or TED Talk, or reading a journal article. Such activity can help you "recharge" and create good feelings. You could look forward to this time each day, which helps create positive pathways and relieves stress.
7. Reframe disappointment as normal	Reframe disappointment as a normal part of life. You can feel disappointment and realize that everyone experiences this feeling. Focus on the learning that comes when something didn't work as well as you had hoped. Differentiate between what you had control over and what you didn't. Look objectively at each event.

Adapted from McGauran D. 7 Cognitive behavioral techniques to help reframe your thinking. 2016. Available at: https://www.activebeat.com/your-health/7-cognitive-behavioral-techniques-to-help-reframe-your-thinking/?streamview=all. Accessed February 10, 2019.

moves us out of this stuck place? The writings of Steven Pressfield described the way in which the pain of not doing the project, the manuscript, or the difficult feedback becomes greater than the pain of doing the work or taking the risks.[13] Clear believes the pain of not doing the project to be the essence of motivation. Each of these choices has a price, but when motivated, we more easily tolerate the anxiety of taking action than to remain inactive. Clear[12] believes this is a mental threshold, and consequently, the pain of not doing the work in the face of deadlines and procrastination becomes greater than the pain of doing the work.

However, the good news is processes exist that help us cross the threshold and overcome the inertia or lack of motivation. One of the misconceptions about motivation is that we must be motivated before beginning the work. Actually, the opposite is true; motivation is the result of taking action. Beginning a project can be a form of inspiration that produces momentum. In other words, once a task is begun, it is easier to continue moving it forward. The key seems to be how we make it easier to start.

Clear also suggests that getting started is about automating the early stages of the process.[14] Automating the process simply means developing some structure around the activity. For example, if the goal is to work out 5 days per week and we have no structure about the time in which we work out, each day we are wondering and hoping to find a time to work out today. With this approach, we easily fail to find the "time" to work out. This thinking likely was considered in wrist watches that remind us to breathe deeply, stand, and move.

In comparison, setting a schedule puts decision making on autopilot. In the workout example, if we get up at 5 a.m. and work out either at home or at the gym, we form a habit. The same schedule puts structure in what we do. Likewise, if we are focused on a writing project, we waste time and energy deciding when and where to do the work. Rather than waiting for inspiration and motivation to "strike," a schedule and structure make it possible to take action in an organized way. This is about ritual and turning structure into ritual. Amateurs wait for inspiration to strike; professionals and leaders set a schedule and keep it.

LL ALERT

- Don't make a habit of being negative.
- Don't surround yourself with people who are negative.

SUMMARY

The attitudes leaders project are critical to others. Attitudes of leaders are reflected in the culture and the people. So little research has focused on those who follow, yet we can surmise attitudes are reciprocal. If we think of attitude as a contagious condition, we know we can all spread the condition. A positive attitude is paramount. A positive attitude or mindset focuses on growth and learning. Our whole lives are about growth and learning. No one is perfect and has nothing further to learn. Role modeling a positive attitude is one key to legacy building. Because attitude and how it is conveyed are personal attributes, it appears in the "Personal triangle" of the model, affecting the trajectory toward the *Leaders*-Ship Legacy. Part of the admiration and respect we have for leaders is due to their attitude and positivity, acting as though nothing is impossible. A leader can always grow both as a person and a leader by enhancing this positive attitude.

LL LINEUP

- Practice reframing to strengthen positive attitudes.
- Align your behavior with your attitude, especially when the attitude is positive.

REFLECTION For 1 week, keep an attitude diary. If necessary, set an alarm for every few hours to force yourself to record attitudes. Begin at the start of the day by using a few words to describe how you feel. Throughout the day, note events that trigger positive or negative attitudes. Be certain you enter your assessment whenever your alarm sounds. At the end of each day, summarize how your attitude changed throughout the day and look for patterns. Do you need to be more positive? If so, what will you do to change?

18

Authenticity

Have you ever thought that you would really like to be *just* like a leader whom you admire? Most of us have had that thought on occasion and perhaps have even tried to mimic the behaviors of that person. While "trying to be *just* like" is a natural impulse, it is not an effective strategy for a leader. Certainly, we may be attracted to some aspect of a respected colleague's behavior and determine to improve our own behavior in that area. For example, one of us admires those who think before they speak, and she has worked to develop the habit of taking a breath before she gives her opinion. As she says, "I can incorporate this habit into my own behavior, but I remain who I am, even as I improve myself."

According to Bill George and his colleagues, over the last 50 years, more than 1000 studies have been conducted with the goal of determining the specific styles, characteristics, or personality traits of great leaders.[1] Not surprisingly, the research did not identify one or two characteristics that define great leaders; instead, a wide range in leadership behaviors seemed to be effective. This makes perfect sense; think of all the leaders you have known. We would hazard a guess that they represent many different personalities and characteristics.

In *True North*, Bill George described his team's groundbreaking work on being authentic as a leader.[2] North's team extensively interviewed 125 leaders, from 23 to 93 years old, who were considered to be authentic leaders. The purpose of the interview was to determine how the respondents became and remained authentic in their leadership activities. These interviews highlighted the leaders' stories, focusing on how they realized their potential and shared their life stories, personal struggles, failures, and triumphs. These stories demonstrated that those interviewed used their real-world experiences to discover their purpose in leadership. They found that being their authentic self made them more effective leaders. So how do we lead from a place of authenticity? Read on.

WHAT DOES AUTHENTICITY IN LEADERSHIP LOOK LIKE?

Bill George and his team first defined authentic leaders as genuine people who are true to themselves and to what they believe.[2] They bring people together around a shared purpose and empower them to also step up and lead authentically to create value for all stakeholders. Similarly, Bruce Avolio,[3] early in his exploration of authentic leadership, characterized such leaders as individuals who are deeply aware of how they think and behave and how they are perceived by others. They consider their knowledge and strengths and the context in which they are operating when determining their leadership strategies. In their interactions with others, they are confident, hopeful, optimistic, resilient, and high on moral character. Most authors suggest four components of authenticity are inherent in a leader: balanced processing, moral and ethical perspective, transparency, and self-awareness. Table 18.1 gives us a look at the definitions of each of these components of authenticity.

Those sound like characteristics that we would all like to have. The question is how do we become more authentic, particularly in our leadership roles?

EMBRACE YOUR STORY

Our past influences our future. The people and experiences in our early life that had a great impact on us; the values that are important to us; and those individuals, events, or goals that motivate us all influence our authentic or true self. Understanding our own story can help us determine what qualities we bring to leadership and what characteristics we would like to cultivate. For example, in what way does our story affect our current world? What have we consistently been passionate about? What values remain important to us? Are our values consistent with our behavior?

TABLE 18.1 Definitions of Components of Authenticity

Component	Definition
1. Balanced processing	Analyzing objectively all relevant information and seeking the opinion of others before making decisions.
2. Moral and ethical perspective	Involves behaviors of leaders who are more guided by internal norms and moral values than external pressures from their peers, organization, or society.
3. Transparency	Making personal disclosures, such as sharing information and openly expressing one's truths, thoughts, feelings, and moral values with colleagues.
4. Self-awareness	Having confidence in one's own motivations and desires, as well as recognition of strengths and weaknesses.

Does our heart, as well as our head, guide our decisions? How important are personal and professional relationships to us? Are we sufficiently disciplined to accomplish our goals?

To be an authentic leader, we must reflect on our own story. This is very much like peeling back an onion (Fig. 18.1). The first layer is the way we present ourselves to the world—our facial expressions, our attire, and the way we express ourselves verbally and nonverbally. The next layer of the onion exposes our strengths, weaknesses, and what we hope for from our lives. Recognizing the characteristics in this second level leads us to an exploration of our values and the ways in which various experiences may put our values in conflict and, finally, to what motivates us. We must also explore our blind spots and vulnerabilities. The result of this introspection is to find our authentic or true selves.[2] Recognizing—and accepting—our own stories increases our self-awareness. This awareness prepares us to act in a manner that is consistent with our own true selves.

AUTHENTICITY AS A JOURNEY

As our self-awareness grows through reflection and introspection, we must move forward toward new action. We must not depend on our current behavior patterns. These new experiences and their outcomes, whether they are positive or negative, will help us make sense of our journey thus far and allow us to make changes as we go.[4] To make this plunge requires the willingness to take risks, recognizing that some may bring failure. Although failure is really just that necessary struggle called *learning*, exposing ourselves to the potential of failure also requires courage. However, these new experiences, regardless of the outcomes, broaden and deepen our leadership capabilities.

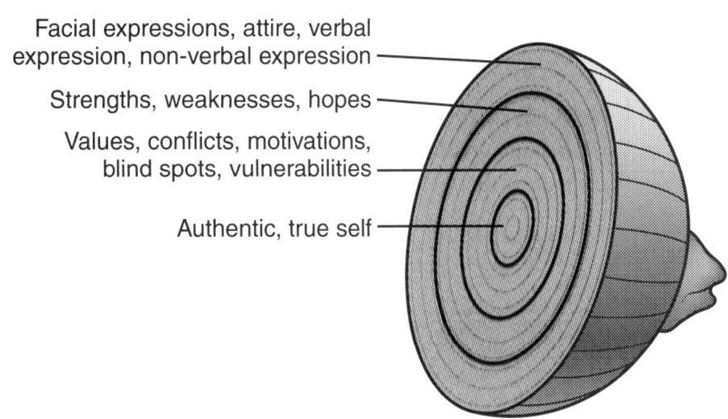

Fig. 18.1 Authentic leadership.

This focus on action can be described as "adaptively authentic." Most of us believe that in general, consideration of the possibilities comes before action. However, in times of transition or uncertainty, action should come before thinking and introspection. Action changes who we are and what we believe is worth doing. In these circumstances rather than thinking that we are working on ourselves (that sounds hard!), we can frame these activities as "trying on possible selves."[4]

It may seem counterintuitive that while we are trying to be authentic, we are also trying on new roles. However, this paradox provides necessary experience for a leader.[5] Authentic leadership requires learning to adapt to the context—identifying the skills that are best in a particular context. Making these adjustments does not mean that the leader is putting on an act. It means that they are able to identify the personality traits that should be revealed, as well as to whom and when they should be revealed. We might choose not to divulge many aspects of who we are because the environment doesn't support such revelation in a positive way. It is possible that revealing your personality profile might be used against you rather than being something on which you can capitalize for your personal growth and development.

Despite this ability to adapt, authentic leaders do not lose their identities in the process. Instead, they rely, in part, on intuition developed as a result of past, often painful, experiences to understand the expectations and concerns of their colleagues. Their actions are derived from their authentic or true self, but they know how to work within the culture they find themselves.[5]

"Earlier in my career, I was the administrator of a public, not-for-profit hospital for the seriously and persistently mentally ill. The governing body was the local mental health authority that had not operated an inpatient facility in the past. Because of an exception in state law governing medical practice, the physicians were employees of the agency, accountable to the administrator (me). We were successful in instituting shared-governance practices in this facility, in large part because of the collaborative team approach already present in other community programs of the mental health authority. Some years later, I became the administrator of inpatient and outpatient mental health services of an established regional health care system. The attending physicians were independent contractors with private practices and very different schedules. The organization had a more formal and traditional culture compared with the public hospital where I had previously worked. When we began the process of introducing shared governance and I used some of the same strategies with which I had had previous success, we met serious roadblocks. Context does matter, and our leadership actions must adjust to that context!"

REFLECTION Think about leaders you have known. Have you observed them adapting their behavior to the circumstances? Did these changes in behavior affect the outcomes of the team's work? Did they affect your perception of the leader?

ESTABLISHING ENDURING RELATIONSHIPS

Our authenticity is confirmed by what other people see in us, and what they see affects the extent to which they are eager to engage with us. Because leaders cannot be effective without the support of others, developing relationships and teams is critical to effective leadership. All of us have worked with leaders who make us feel as if we are an integral part of the group. These leaders give us the impression that what we do—and who we are—is very important. They demonstrate their passion for the team's goals and care about the part we play in achieving those goals, providing relevant feedback that improves our work. In short, these authentic leaders empower others to lead.

Maintaining authenticity—not losing our way—is critical to effective leadership in the long run. Developing and maintaining relationships, at work and in our personal lives, is an important strategy to maintaining authenticity. Being in groups that provide professional or personal support is effective to keep one grounded. Having a friend or colleague who will be honest with you is also powerful. Emma Seppala[6] describes one Stanford study that found that chief executive officers (CEOs) were looking for more advice and counsel, but two-thirds of them don't get it. She suggests that this isolation can skew the perspectives of the leader, resulting in potentially disadvantageous leadership choices. We need others who have our best interest at heart and who will be willing to tell it as they see it.

VULNERABILITY AS A PART OF AUTHENTICITY

George and Sims[2] suggest that when authentic leaders reveal their vulnerabilities, they develop trusting human connections with others that motivate and empower those they engage. However, vulnerability suggests the possibility of being attacked or harmed either physically or emotionally—not necessarily a position we want to experience, particularly when we are in a leadership role. The question then becomes how can we reveal our vulnerabilities in a way that promotes growth rather than harm? Brene Brown, an expert on vulnerability, suggests that "to feel is to be vulnerable. Believing that vulnerability is weakness is to believe that feeling is weakness."[7] However, she suggests that leaders should always be clear about what our intentions are when sharing our vulnerabilities. Is the sharing related to our leadership responsibilities? Are there other more personal or spontaneous reasons that we share? We must set boundaries to be sure that expressing our vulnerability is related to the needs of the group. As Dr. Brown says, "Vulnerability without boundaries, is not vulnerability; it is confession, manipulation, desperation, or shock and awe. It is oversharing, indiscriminate disclosure."[7]

REFLECTION Where are you in your journey toward authenticity? Have you used your own story to "peel the onion" of your life? Consider the components of an authentic leader: balanced processing, moral and ethical perspective, transparency, and self-awareness. In what ways do you integrate these characteristics into your leadership roles? What areas do you want to work on going forward?

AUTHENTICITY IN HEALTH CARE

The complexity of today's health care environment, as well as the diversity of patient needs, the impact of technology, and the burden of increased regulation and reporting make it difficult to maintain a healthy work environment for health care personnel. Recognizing this challenge, a number of organizations are focusing on improving health care work environments. For example, the American Nurses Association has a Healthy Work Environment initiative that addresses nursing staffing, incivility, and a variety of other health care issues.[8] In addition, the American Association of Critical-Care Nurses (AACN) established six standards for a healthy work environment in health care. They are (1) skilled communication, which results in equal proficiency in communication and clinical skills; (2) true collaboration; (3) effective decision-making, where valued and committed partners lead organizational operations; (4) appropriate staffing, which matches patient needs and nurse competencies; (5) meaningful recognition, including authentic acknowledgment of the value each person brings to the work; and importantly for our discussion, (6) authentic leadership.

The AACN Standards for Establishing and Sustaining Healthy Work Environments[9] illustrate the potential of authentic leadership within the health care workplace. For the last 10 years, a limited number of published nursing research studies explored the impact of this type of leadership on nurses, patients, and other health care workers. For example, Wong and colleagues[10] tested a theoretical model that linked authentic leadership with staff nurses' trust in their manager, work engagement, voice behavior, and perceived unit care quality. The findings suggested that authentic leadership and trust in the manager play a role in fostering trust, creating a positive work environment, establishing an affirming voice behavior, and increasing quality of care among staff nurses.

Lisa Giallonardo and colleagues[11] examined the relationships between new graduate nurses' perceptions, their preceptor's authentic leadership, work engagement, and job satisfaction. They found that new graduate nurses who were paired with preceptors who demonstrate high levels of authentic leadership felt more engaged and were more satisfied than those who did not have such a preceptor. Similarly, Heather Laschinger and her colleagues[12] also tested a model linking authentic leadership, areas of work life, occupational coping, self-efficacy, burnout, and mental health among new graduate nurses. The findings suggested that authentic leadership plays an important role in creating working conditions that optimize the match between new graduate nurses' expectations and the reality of the work environment and strengthen new nurses' confidence in their abilities to cope with the demands of their jobs. This interaction with leaders who are authentic appears to protect them from burnout development and poor mental health. Although the research in nursing and health care is relatively sparse, for those of us who are in nursing, it appears likely that developing authenticity will prepare us for the future of health care.

LL ALERT

We are likely *not* being an authentic leader when we:

- Don't indiscriminately share feelings with your team.
- Don't avoid giving negative feedback for fear of harming staff morale.
- Don't transfer programs or policies from one organization to another without considering the organization's context.

SUMMARY

The work about authenticity is still developing. Yet we know the concept is an important one because few, if any, of us would choose to work with someone who is not authentic. We might behave differently at a formal event than we would at a family event, but our underlying "true" selves remain the same. Being an authentic leader requires that we embrace the story of our lives, reflect on our behaviors, and engage with others throughout our leadership trajectory. This requires work, yet the results pay significant dividends to the leader and team.

LL LINEUP

- Peel back your own onion in a thoughtful way.
- Keep ethics in mind.
- Continue to be self-aware.

REFLECTION Think about your own work environment. How healthy do you believe your workplace to be? Can you identify leaders in your environment that you believe have the characteristics of an authentic leader? If so, can you describe their impact on those with whom they work? Can you compare their impact with other leaders in the workplace who use other leadership styles?

19

Capacity

Most of us have looked at the leadership trajectory of colleagues and thought, "Wow! I could never accomplish what they are doing." When faced with a leadership challenge, we may have also said, "I simply don't have the time, competence, and/or energy to move through this problem." In both cases, our reticence may stem from our fear that we don't have the *capacity* to lead in increasingly unknown or complex situations. In those of us who aspire to leadership, this common fear occurs on occasion throughout our careers. However, if we don't experience some anxiety, we may not be pushing ourselves beyond our comfort zone. However common, this fear can slow (or stop) us from achieving the Legacy *Leaders*-Ship outcomes that meet our particular hopes and dreams. How can we build our leadership capacity as a strategy to achieving those things we are not sure we can do?

WHAT IS CAPACITY?

Merriam Webster gives us a variety of definitions of capacity.[1] The following are samples:

- An individual's mental or physical abilities
- The potential for experiencing or appreciating
- The power to produce, perform, or deploy

Each of these definitions provides a component of important characteristics required for a leader. We must have not only theoretical knowledge of leadership but also a number of mental skills, such as the ability to think quickly, assess the context, and make effective decisions. A leader must also have emotional intelligence, including the ability to recognize and appreciate the "said" and "unsaid" messages coming from the environment and act upon these as appropriate. Finally, the leader must have the internal drive and external power to work with all stakeholders to accomplish a goal while maintaining hope in the face of a negative turn of events. Taken together, these leadership characteristics can result in what Warren Bennis and Robert Thomas describe as "adaptive capacity."[2] These well-known authors on leadership define adaptive capacity as the ability to change action plans based upon the context of events. This has never been more evident in our lifetimes than in the early months of 2020 as health care workers made life adaptations to provide care.

Throughout this book, we discuss various concepts that make up the Legacy *Leaders*-Ship Trajectory model. Much overlap can be found among the definition of capacity provided earlier and many of the other concepts we have identified. Capacity in our discussion of Legacy *Leaders*-Ship requires that we *recognize* the strengths and weaknesses that we have and then decide to act to harden our strengths or address our weaknesses. If we don't recognize what we have and don't have in our "leadership box" and then take action to get a "bigger box," we cannot expand our capacity.

> **REFLECTION** Are you aware of what your capacity for leadership is? Do you think your leadership capability might be lacking and unable to prepare you for some future opportunities? If so, what might you do to increase your capacity?

LEADERSHIP CAPACITIES

Jeff Boss, a principal and senior advisor at N2 Growth, says:

"Leadership isn't a title and it's not a position. *It's not tenure and it's not rank. Leadership is about capacity—being the type of person, who is able and willing to learn, be courageous, tackle difficulty and question the status quo."*[3]

Boss suggests three leadership characteristics—courage, clarity, and curiosity—build our leadership capacity.[3] Courage is defined as the ability to control fear in order to be willing to deal with something that is dangerous, difficult, or unpleasant (according to the Cambridge Dictionary). We can all tell stories of times when it took courage to step forward for an opportunity where the outcome was uncertain. One of us accepted a job to develop the structures and processes for an inpatient psychiatric hospital without actually ever having worked in an in-patient mental health facility.

*"Okay, I had worked in an outpatient clinic for patients with seriously and persistent mental illness, but that hardly counted. Of course, I was scared to death, but I knew I could depend on my listening skills and the assistance from supportive colleagues who had the kind of experience that I didn't have to complete the project. Courage and my sense that I **did** know how to develop health-related programs, which really was the goal, helped me to take the leap. Ultimately, this leap expanded my capacity for leadership in other situations."*

Another one of us moved from Colorado to Texas to help start a school of nursing *after* the governor line-item vetoed the funding. This experience led to a greater willingness to risk other strategies that developed leadership skills.

Boss defines clarity as being clear about what is important to us and why.[3] This reduces the need to second-guess, wondering if we are making the right decision. We can focus on the work, because we are clear about the image of success. In the situation described earlier, *"perhaps I was not clear about the specifics of the program development, but I did have a framework of program development and knew that I could support a group of experts to meet the goal of developing a program."* The second example showed faith that funding would follow.

Boss also believes that curiosity fosters questions that can lead to clarity.[3] He suggests questions like, "What do you think?" "How might we…?" and "What do you think would be the best way to achieve…?" can be a successful way to learn *and* lead. We (the authors) would all certainly agree.

> **REFLECTION** Evaluate your own professional development. When have courage, clarity, and/or curiosity been necessary to help you move forward? Did you use these attributes to decide what actions to take? Why or why not? What was the outcome of the situation(s)? What would you do differently if you had this to do over?

DEVELOPMENT OF COGNITIVE FITNESS

Roderick Gilkey and Clint Kilts, in the *Harvard Business Review*'s articles on mental toughness, describe the relationship between cognitive fitness and our ability to improve our leadership capacity. They suggest that the first step to cognitive fitness is to understand how experience makes the brain grow. It turns out we have a biological impact when we have new experiences. Neuroscientists have identified "mirror" neuron systems in our brains that represent objects, people, and actions in our environment. Stimulation of these systems within the brain allows us to internally reflect on our physical and social experiences through direct and indirect experiences and observations. For example, the authors suggest that leaders spending time talking to colleagues and stakeholders is not just a good leadership strategy; it is also a sound form of cognitive exercise.[4] They also suggest several other strategies that affect the structure and function of the brain and thus cognitive fitness. Table 19.1 outlines these strategies.

HAVE YOU NOTICED?

Let's consider each of these suggestions from Roderick Gilkey and Clint Kilts.[4] When we think about our leadership capabilities, we often think that enhancing our capability means we must work more! Yet how often have you been asked to deal with a leadership challenge, and you have ruminated endlessly over the possible approach. Finally you give up in despair and go to exercise, have coffee with a friend, or even go to a movie.

- Have you noticed how a plausible answer to your problem seems to "pop" into your head after you played?
- Have you noticed that after a vacation where you see new things and talk to new people you return to work refreshed, better able to solve problems that seemed insurmountable before you left?
- Have you noticed that listening to new viewpoints, often those that you may not agree with, and analyzing them can often expand your understanding of a situation?
- Have you noticed that learning new things—things that may not necessarily pertain to your leadership role—can often give you new ideas that *do* apply to your role?

When you have had such "a-ha" moments, you realize that developing your leadership capabilities is not necessarily improving the specific work that you do. Instead, it is enhancing who you are. Let us repeat that: leadership development isn't necessarily about the work—it is about the person!

DEVELOPING LEADERSHIP CAPACITY IN TEAMS AND ORGANIZATIONS

As our leadership capabilities expand, the scope of our leadership may also increase. This will likely allow us to be instrumental in increasing the leadership capacity in the teams and organizations within our sphere of influence. As Bill Hogg, a leadership consultant, says: "There is a commonality between successful organizations and leadership

TABLE 19.1 Strategies That Influence Cognitive Fitness

Strategies	Neural Changes
Work hard at play.	Play engages the prefrontal cortex, nourishing the part of our brains related to incentive and reward processing, goal and skill representation, mental imagery, self-knowledge, and memory, all of which are necessary for improving our leadership capacity.
Search for patterns often by: Challenging your own existing mind-set Listening and reflecting on different viewpoints Visiting different places with learning goals in mind	The left hemisphere of the brain is the source of routine tasks that get us through the day. This includes pattern recognition (the ability to scan the environment, quickly assessing a situation so that appropriate action can be taken accurately and quickly). Pattern recognition is critical for determining action in a complex situation.
Seek novelty and innovation in order to find out what you are not learning. On a regular basis, use this to identify new things to learn.	The right hemisphere deals with novelty, including less linear and structured experiences and data. This skill allows us to increase our own capacity to innovate.

Adapted from Gilkey R, Kilts C. Cognitive fitness. On mental toughness. HBR's 10 must reads. *Harv Bus Rev.* 2018:37-52.

capacity. Successful leaders understand the importance of harnessing leadership talent in others and taking the time to develop it."[5]

Examples of strategies that companies use to prioritize leadership development may include:

- Encouraging employees to take "stretch assignments" that give them leadership opportunities
- Using hiring practices that ensure internal candidates have equal opportunities for positions
- Conducting leadership assessments of selected employees with ongoing feedback as they progress
- Providing coaching opportunities and mentoring programs
- Ensuring opportunities for cross-training and job shadowing
- Developing formal leadership training programs
- Devising special opportunities that allow employees to observe effective leadership
- Holding periodic forums (formal or informal) that cover core aspects of leadership
- Forming developmental councils composed of senior leaders who meet regularly to discuss the development of promising employees (adapted from Hogg[5] and Dotiwala and Unni[6]).

Faridun Dotiwala and Naveen Unni (2013),[6] leaders in a prominent consultant company, McKinsey & Company, suggest that "a small group of excellent leaders is not sufficient to steer an ambitious business, a fact that is especially relevant to businesses that have grown rapidly. A critical mass of excellent leaders is required to trigger and sustain corporate growth." We believe that this principle is not only true in rapidly growing for-profit businesses but also in all organizations, large and small.

LL ALERT

- Don't send yourself messages that convey the idea that something is beyond your abilities.
- Don't ignore those insights that "simply come to you."

SUMMARY

We have all observed circumstances in which employees with leadership potential do not take advantage of opportunities to expand their leadership capacity. Numerous reasons explain this behavior, including fear, negative pressure from family or friends, other time commitments, and lack of interest. Leaders who do not explore the consequences of rejecting these opportunities with such employees are missing an opportunity to help them move forward. Developing our leadership capacity is a critical element in developing our own leadership trajectory. Similarly, organizational leaders have a responsibility to help others in their sphere of influence to develop their own capacity. Developing the capacity of a number of leaders throughout the organization increases the potential success of both the individuals and the organizations.

LL LINEUP

- Remember to create opportunities for those who come behind us.
- Provide a step up to leadership opportunities to build the skills of others.

REFLECTION Think back to your leadership trajectory. Who provided a "step up" for you? How did this happen? Have you had one or more opportunities to return the favor to that colleague? Did you pay it forward? How did this work out? How did it make you feel? What will you do in the future?

20

Courage

No industry in the United States is more in need of courageous leadership than health care. Understanding how to be courageous is critical to creating any legacy. Legacies don't just happen, and they often aren't wildly endorsed upon introduction or supported throughout the organization. They require people who have the courage to take risks and to speak up and be willing to be the targets for blame if something goes wrong.

Have you ever been in a situation where a colleague was providing care in a way with which you disagreed? Perhaps it was a safety issue for the patient. Did you speak up? Perhaps it was the implementation of the policy that seems unfair for some staff. Did you speak up?

Speaking up involves a risk, perhaps being seen as wrong or different from others, upsetting colleagues and supervisors with whom you disagree, and perhaps even risking your own position. Eleanor Roosevelt once said, "You gain strength, courage and confidence by every experience in which you really stop to look fear in the face. You are able to say to yourself, 'I have lived through this horror. I can take the next thing that comes along.' You must do the thing you think you cannot do." Her wisdom highlights that speaking up requires courage. Because of the importance of courageous behavior in the workplace, we need to consider how to use courage in our professional lives, particularly when we are in a leadership role.

WHAT IS COURAGE?

Courage is defined as the ability to control fear in order to be willing to deal with something that is dangerous, difficult, or unpleasant (as defined in the Cambridge Dictionary). Because stakes are high in these situations, these actions require thoughtful deliberation. Equally important, the truly courageous person pursues a morally worthy goal or idea.[1]

Courage is an individual behavior; however, individuals often come together to act in courageous ways in a work environment or any other group endeavor. Leaders in these groups have a special obligation to act with courage because of the diversity in most organizational environments and the relationships that are a part of their leadership responsibilities. The explosion of health care technology, the growing needs of patients and their families, and the economic challenges in health care provide myriad opportunities for courageous leadership.

Courageous leadership may be defined as "the heart to step up front and transform vision into reality."[2] Courage is required for us to "step up" to lead, often in uncomfortable or risky situations, and leadership is required to move from an idea for change to implementation, particularly when there is opposition. The complexity of being courageous in a leadership position requires us to implement a number of related behaviors, including taking risks, connectivity, communication, empowerment, decisiveness, honesty, trustworthiness, self-awareness, resilience, and persistence.[2]

Courage is a personal characteristic described in the Legacy *Leaders*-Ship model. However, the environment also makes a difference in how safe we feel to act courageously. For example, a reciprocal relationship exists between courageous leadership in an organization and courageous behavior among individuals within that organization. Susan Tardanico, a contributor to *Forbes*, suggests that "demonstrating leadership courage—whether it's having an uncomfortable conversation, communicating when you don't have all the answers, or making a decision to move ahead on a new project—can be scary. Yet it's precisely the kind of behavior that fosters trust and sets a crucial example for others to follow at a [time] when they'd rather hunker down and wait for the storm to pass."[3] She suggests courageous leaders exhibit 10 traits. These are found in Table 20.1.

Courage is a term we associate with people who serve in the military. People who enlist and their leaders know that at some point they might be called on to take bold steps to confront danger. Often, however, many of us forget the less dramatic examples of courage. We can find them in almost any setting. Acts of courage typically relate to safety, both our own and that of others. Whistleblowers, some of whom might be disgruntled employees, have to have courage to report something that has not been addressed in the system.

TABLE 20.1 Ten Traits of Courageous Leaders

1. Confront reality head on. Don't avoid what is real just because it is difficult.
2. Seek feedback and listen. Be prepared to hear hard truths, often about yourself.
3. Say what needs to be said. This can be done without attacking the other person.
4. Encourage push-back. Don't be defensive when you hear something you don't agree with.
5. Take action on performance issues. Don't wait, hoping miraculously things will get better without intervention.
6. Communicate openly and frequently. Tell the truth.
7. Lead change. Recognize that avoiding change is a risk.
8. Make decisions and move forward. Don't spend too much time on regrets.
9. Give credit to others. When others do well, you do well.
10. Hold people (and yourself) accountable.

REFLECTION Use these 10 traits as a checklist for yourself. You may want to use simple responses such as yes, no, and sometimes. How many of those items would garner a yes? How many would garner a no or a sometimes? What is a logical first step you could take to strengthen one of those traits?

CATEGORIES OF COURAGE

We can categorize courage depending on the circumstances an individual or group may face. Table 20.2 outlines six possible categories and the definition of each. We use most of those types of courage in leadership work; one, however, has a major influence for us.

Moral courage is the type of courage we are most likely to need in difficult, high-stakes issues. If we are able to endure distress while managing a high-risk situation, we are drawing on moral courage. How do we deal with such a situation? Initially, we need to de-catastrophize the circumstances. We should ask ourselves: What is the worst that could happen? What would be the consequences? We may also use various calming techniques—deep breathing, meditating, exercise, or debriefing with an impartial colleague. Once we are calmer and the situation is more manageable, we should be able to decide our course of action. What is the right course of action to answer the question? One of us was involved in a highly challenging situation. *"I kept repeating to myself, 'This is unethical.' Because I felt compelled by the organization's mission, I stayed in the position and chose to speak the truth when it was distorted. My life would have been less complicated if I had left. But, as with not abandoning patients, I chose not to abandon the staff with whom I worked. They needed a buffer and I was it."*

A review of the circumstances and our own emotions in the context of our values can help us identify what the right course of action is. At this point, we can make a nonemotional assessment of the situation. For nurses, the American Nurses Association Code of Ethics for Nurses with Interpretive Statements can provide a context for analyzing the nurse's responsibility in a high-stakes situation.[4] The bottom-line question when dealing with a high-stakes situation is to ask: Should I act? In truth, not all battles should be fought. Several questions can help us decide whether we should speak up or remain silent. Is it really a high-stakes situation—for me and for others—or is the risk in my own mind? Are values, beliefs, and principles involved? Is it the right time? Has the situation escalated from prior similar situations? How much am I willing to risk?

COMPETENTLY COURAGEOUS

People who successfully negotiate high-stakes problems in the workplace are considered to be "competently

TABLE 20.2 Types Of Courage

Categories	Definition
Physical	Showing bravery at the risk of bodily harm or death. Involves physical strength, resiliency, and awareness.
Social	Involving the risk of social embarrassment or exclusion, unpopularity, or rejection.
Intellectual	Engaging with challenging ideas, to question our thinking, and the risk of making a mistake.
Moral courage	Doing the right thing, particularly when risks involve shame, opposition, or the disapproval of others. Driven by ethics, values, and ideals. "Steadfast determination to do what is right, no matter the consequences."[9]
Emotional courage	Being willing to feel the full spectrum of emotions.
Spiritual courage	Fortifying in the exploration of faith, purpose, and meaning.

courageous."[5] Competently courageous people can take several steps when dealing with workplace challenges. For example, those who spend time establishing themselves in the work environment are more likely to be successful in handling difficult situations. Their reputation tends to engender trust. Because they have demonstrated that they are invested in and excel at their job, they have developed a stock of goodwill that can be used when challenging power or norms.[5] Thus if we are new to a workplace and have some concern about a situation, we should talk to a more seasoned colleague we trust to give us advice moving forward.

When a decision is made to act in a courageous manner, focusing on three factors can help us move forward. First, we can frame the issue by evaluating the problem and identifying potential solutions. The potential solutions can then be compared with the organization's priorities or values. This allows decision makers to understand the problem and solution in the context of the organization. Second, we can use relevant data in an understandable way to describe the risks and possible solutions. Finally, we can manage our own emotions, setting an example for others who are involved in the conflict.[5]

Our emotions play a role in deciding whether or not to act; thus we must identify our own feelings as part of analyzing the situation. However, presenting the situation to the final decision makers is best done in a factual manner. In short, using moral courage appropriately means learning to express ourselves in an honest and direct manner at the right place and time. We must explain what we hope to change in a nonjudgmental behavior—simply via a statement of the desired behavior change.[4,5] For example, one of us was expected to eliminate some educational programs that were not meeting the enrollment numbers that were projected:

"One of the programs under review was a curriculum to which I felt an attachment. Part of me (the selfish part) wanted to protect this program through 'over the top' advocacy. (As the leader, I probably had enough 'clout' to convince at least some of the committee to save the program.) Instead my 'better self' prevailed and I said, 'You all know how invested I am in X program, so it is hard to be rational about potentially closing it. I suspect others have similar feelings about other programs we have to evaluate. Shall we agree that we will let the quantitative data (# of students/cohort) guide our decision?' Unfortunately for me, the quantitative data clearly demonstrated that 'my' program was the biggest loser. However, fortunately for me, I did not lose my team's confidence, because I was willing to be honest about my feelings and apply the quantitative data equally."

After relevant decisions have been made to resolve the concern, the "competently courageous" follow up with all stakeholders. If the outcome is positive from our perspective, we share credit with our colleagues. If the outcome is not what we hoped for, we recognize that learning is often disguised as failure and continue to advocate for our goals or values. We sometimes see groups claim victory and brag about their success. This action causes the "losers" to be more entrenched and potentially vengeful. If we "win," especially if it is a decisive win, we should be as gracious as possible and help those who see the outcomes as a loss to save face and declare a willingness to move forward together.

REFLECTION When in your past work environment have you demonstrated moral courage? What were the circumstances? What process did you use to determine whether you should act? What would you do differently in the future?

MANAGING RISK

Sometimes, even with the best of intentions, speaking up doesn't work out well. When we are "competently courageous," we recognize the risks that can potentially occur if things don't work out to our advantage after standing up for what we believe to be right. To compensate, we can develop strategies that will minimize any risks likely to occur. Such strategies may include maximizing our value within the organization, being aware of other employment opportunities, or minimizing our economic reliance on the employer.[5] For example, a colleague of ours was involved in a serious disagreement with the executive team to whom she reported. The disagreement involved an ethical issue about which she felt strongly. As the dialogue about the possible solution continued, she began to receive signals that to continue to push for her position would put her job at risk. She discussed the issue with a trusted colleague and ultimately decided that her position represented her core values. So as she continued to articulate her position, she also "polished" up her resume and began to look for other employment opportunities.

REFLECTION Would you describe yourself as competently courageous? If not, what strategies could you undertake to identify and then minimize risks?

APPLICATION OF COURAGEOUS LEADERSHIP

In the news and social media, we see numerous examples of organizational leaders courageously speaking on behalf of the common good, rather than the best interest of themselves or the organization's stakeholders. A well-known example of the courage of nurse leaders is the 3-year battle of two Texas nurses who reported the unsafe practices of a physician in a small, west Texas town to their hospital administrator and the state board of medical examiners. In retribution, they lost their jobs and were criminally indicted, alleging that they improperly disclosed information not public "with intent to harm" the physician. After 3 years, the matter was settled, the nurses were vindicated, the hospital administrator and a public official were charged with misconduct, and the physician ultimately lost his license to practice medicine—a positive outcome long in coming. In the interim, however, the nurses suffered significant financial and emotional harm.[6]

This example demonstrates how important it is for nurses and other health professionals to speak out against unsafe or unethical practices. It also shows the risk that those who do speak up may incur. Speaking up, or using *safety voices*, as it is sometimes called, has generated a great deal of concern in the health care environment. When do professionals speak up? What can health care leaders do to increase the likelihood that they will speak up to ensure patient safety?

Beginning with the 2005 report, *Silence Kills*, highlighting research completed by Vital Smarts, Inc., in partnership with the American Association of Critical-Care Nurses, health care began to consider how to make it safe for providers to speak up.[7] The *Silence Kills* study identified categories of conversations in health care that are especially difficult and, at the same time, especially essential for patient safety. The study showed that the quality of these crucial conversations influenced medical errors, patient safety, quality of care, staff commitment, employee satisfaction, discretionary effort, and staff turnover. The researchers grouped these concerns into seven areas, Broken Rules, Mistakes, Lack of Support, Incompetence, Poor Teamwork, Disrespect, and Micromanagement, because more than half of the health care workers surveyed had occasionally witnessed behaviors that fell into these categories. Table 20.3 outlines the extent to which the respondents of the *Silence Kills* study identified these problems.

TABLE 20.3 Silence Hurts: Percentage of Health Care Providers Who Experienced Difficult Conversations

Categories	Percentage of Health Care Providers Experiencing Difficult Conservations
Broken rules	84% of physicians and 62% of nurses and other clinical care providers observed some of their coworkers taking shortcuts that could be dangerous to patients
Mistakes	92% of physicians and 65% of nurses and other clinical care providers worked with some people who have trouble following directions 88% of physicians and 48% of nurses and other clinical care providers saw some colleagues show poor clinical judgment when making assessments, doing triage, diagnosing, suggesting treatment, or getting help
Lack of support	53% of nurses and clinical care providers reported 10% or more of colleagues are reluctant to help or refuse to answer questions
Incompetence	81% of physicians and 53% of nurses and other clinical care providers had concerns about the competency of some nurse or other clinical care provider they work with; 68% of physicians and 34% of nurses and other clinical care providers had concerns about the competency of at least one physician they work with
Poor teamwork	81% of nurses had been in a team that gossiped or were part of a clique that divided the team 55% had a teammate who tried to benefit at others' expense
Disrespect	77% of nurses and clinical care providers worked with those who are condescending or insulting 33% worked with a few who were verbally abusive—yelling, shouting, swearing, or name calling
Micromanagement	52% of nurses and other clinical care providers worked with some number of people who abused their authority—pulled rank, bullied, threatened, or forced their point of view on them

> **REFLECTION** Consider how many of the categories in Table 20.3 you have experienced. What actions did you take? Would you do something different if this happened again today?

Almost 25 years later, health care is still working to develop strategies to improve the environment for health care professionals to speak out. A literature review regarding health care professionals' speaking-up behavior for patient safety with the intent to assess the effectiveness of speaking up and of speaking-up training identified the factors that influence such behavior.[8] Table 20.4 lists the factors that were identified as influencing speaking up.

Numerous conclusions can be made from the literature review, and the resulting model, that can be helpful as courageous leaders evaluate the impact of speaking up. Evidence suggests that because the perception of the risk of negative outcomes is a prerequisite for speaking up, the courageous leader must evaluate the "harm-rating" of the situation—asking what the level of the risk of harm is in this situation. Interestingly, physicians typically ranked each risk lower than nurses did.[8] Another factor that influences the likelihood that personnel will speak up is the clarity with which the clinical situation can be described. Those who speak up report being more satisfied with their jobs than those who do not. Those who speak up also are more likely to feel confident in their abilities in such situations, particularly if they had had previously favorable experiences in similar circumstances. Current strong and visible administrative support is also an important factor in encouraging staff to speak up.[8]

TABLE 20.4 Factors That Influence "Speaking Up"

Factors	Examples
General contextual factors	Hospital policy Interdisciplinary policy making Team relationships Attitudes of leaders
Individual factors	Satisfaction with the job Responsibility toward patients Roles as professionals Confidence and previous experience Communication skills Education background
Perceived safety vs. costs	Fear of the responses of others/ conflict Concerns of appearing incompetent
Perceived efficacy vs. futility	Lack of change Personal control and impact
Outcomes for the patient	Harm rating Clinical situation
Voice: messages, tactics, targets	Collected facts Positive intent
Outcomes for the patient	Error correction

How do nurses and other health care workers speak up instead of remaining silent when patient safety is at risk? Four themes in a meta-analysis study were identified: (1) hierarchies and power dynamics negatively affected safety voice, (2) open communication was unsafe and ineffective, (3) embedded expectations affected safety voice, and (4) nurse managers exerted a powerful positive or negative affect on safety voice.[9] In short, hesitation to speak up is pervasive among nurses, often due to their lack of confidence in their communication skills or power inequity. In addition, they believe that speaking up will not make a difference in patient safety. Nurse leaders in health care organizations have the opportunity to positively alter this reality. How? We can speak up in situations that support nursing staff and/or patient care. For example, the nurse leader who asks to speak to a physician in private after the physician demeans a staff member in public establishes a precedence for others to speak up. The nurse leader who listens to the staff's concerns about a patient safety issue and provides resources to investigate the incident demonstrates that staff observations can support change in care behaviors.

Unfortunately, when we talk about the provider having the courage to speak up, the emphasis is almost always on *individuals* doing the right thing, often in the face of organization obstacles to safe care. Leadership groups at every level of the organization must also be courageous in providing a work environment that formally and informally supports the caring of staff and patients, peer support for speaking up, and an organizational commitment (codified in policy and actions) to safe, open cultures. When these behaviors can be seen at all levels of the hierarchy, the dialogue across the organization will open up and speaking up becomes the norm.

LL ALERT

- Don't avoid a difficult conversation.
- Don't ignore pertinent feedback.
- Don't punish by word or action those who disagree with you.

SUMMARY

Courage is a critical characteristic for a nurse leader in today's health care environment. Given the diverse viewpoints within the health care environment, we shouldn't be surprised that significant conflicts require courage to resolve. Nurses in all positions can enhance their success by developing courageous leadership skills.

LL LINEUP

- Act in accordance with your values and the mission of the organization.
- Be accountable for your own behaviors.
- Think through the consequences before acting on your emotions.

REFLECTION Is the leadership in the organization where you are employed courageous? Do leaders provide an environment that supports speaking up? Have you had the opportunity to speak up? Was this supported by the leadership above you? What would you have done differently? What do you do to encourage others to speak up?

21 Creativity

What is creativity? To create is to bring into existence. Creativity could be a thought or a theory or an idea, but it could also be something tangible such as a painting or an invention. Some confusion exists between creativity and innovation, and we will discuss both. The distinction between the two is creativity is the ability to have original ideas, to see a different way of doing something. In contrast, innovation is the ability to make new things actually happen. Innovation is the action side of the process, whereas creativity is the thinking, dreaming, idea creation side of the process.

> *"The creative is the place where no one else has ever been. You have to leave the city of your comfort and go into the wilderness of your intuition. What you'll discover will be wonderful. What you'll discover is yourself."*
>
> *–Alan Alda*[1]

A CREATIVITY PERSPECTIVE

One of the most important competencies for leaders of today's complex health care systems is creativity. Innovation and creativity are not necessarily an end. Rather, they are a means to an end, which is continuous improvement of patient care. Leaders don't have to be the most creative people in the organization, but they must support and facilitate creativity and innovation at all levels of nursing services. Perhaps the most important level of creativity is at the patient care level where direct care nurses and the frontline leaders make adaptations daily. Effective leaders understand they must create a culture in which nurses are unafraid to risk and try new things. These leaders embrace experimentation because they do not view unsuccessful ideas as failure; rather, the focus is on learning.[2]

Creative leaders are open-minded and inventive. They promote disruptive innovation and facilitate others to discontinue outdated approaches and take balanced risks. This approach is particularly important in engaging younger generations of nurses, as is moving from hierarchies to networks and from focusing on individuals to working in effective interprofessional teams. Perhaps we need an innovation budget that emphasizes creative and innovative options. The Magnet Recognition Program® has a focus on new knowledge and research. Such pathways support nurses at all levels of the organization to "dream" and imagine new solutions to problems. Creative, innovative leaders embrace these dreamers and support them, encouraging them to apply their creativity in ways that support improved patient care. Sometimes that encouragement comes from a leader who has budgetary support for developing an idea. Other times that encouragement comes from a colleague who takes the lead in urging a group to be a cheering squad for testing an idea.

LEVELS OF CREATIVITY

Daniel Burrus suggested that three levels of creativity exist: discovery, invention, and creation.[3] These distinctions are helpful to consider as leaders strive to facilitate more creativity and innovation in their organizations. Thinking about creativity in this manner, as levels, makes it easier to enter the process at the lower level—one of becoming aware of problems. Most all of us are aware of problems, and this framework gives us a constructive way to approach these problems using creativity and innovation.

Discovery is the lower level of creativity. When we become aware of a problem or issue, we have discovered it. For example, when the Colorado Center for Nursing Excellence (the Center) began to receive phone calls from advanced practice registered nurse (APRN) graduates concerning the inability to find jobs in the state, we "discovered" a problem. This is called *discovered art*, and much creativity begins with discovered art.

> **REFLECTION** What is a major problem you can identify at work?

The next higher level of creativity is *invention*. For example, the Wright brothers have credit for inventing a flying machine. You might ask, "Would a flying machine have been invented without the Wright brothers?" Yes, multiple inventors were working on flying machines, and another team would have been successful. Although invention is higher than discovery, the inventions will happen eventually. Invention is a matter of time.

> **REFLECTION** What hasn't been tried to resolve the problem you identified earlier?

Creation is the highest level of creativity. For example, Andrew Lloyd Webber, a composer, is credited with reinventing musical theater. Musical theater would still be a part of Broadway, but we most likely would not have had *Phantom of the Opera, Jesus Christ Superstar, Evita,* or *Cats* without Andrew Lloyd Webber. No one else would have written these musicals, which ran on Broadway for more than 10 years each. Organizations can create things that are as individualistic as these musicals. We simply must discover what those are.

> **REFLECTION** If you were "in charge," what would you actually do to address the problem related to APRNs noted earlier?

"Once the Center discovered the state was losing 60% of its new APRN graduates because physicians and clinics would not provide oversight for prescriptive authority, we wanted to discover how to resolve this problem. The work began with changing the legislation. New graduates were required to have 3600 hours of physician supervision to obtain prescriptive authority. An 18-month endeavor resulted in changing the law to 1000 hours of supervision by either a physician or a qualified nurse practitioner with prescriptive authority."

This example used the discovery level of creativity to address a problem. While at a conference we might discover a tool, a technology, or a process that we didn't know before. We bring the tool back to our organizations, and the discovery of the new tool helps everyone work better. After some time, that discovery may also spur a creative idea of how to apply the discovery. We may then use that creative idea as an inspiration that yields something never seen before, something created by our organizations that helps us and others. That's how the three levels of creativity can work together. In the APRN example, the effort was collaborative with other state organizations interested in access to care for rural and underserved people. First, we discovered the problem and then we created an innovative solution: change the law. Someone else would have eventually come to the same realization. A similar example occurred in Texas when planning a new school of nursing:

"When funding was denied, I developed an accredited continuing nursing education program while the 'dean' mapped out the curriculum for an undergraduate program. By doing these—and many other—things, the school could admit students immediately after the next legislative session when the funding for the school was approved."

The highest level of creativity related to the APRN issue occurred when we asked the question: What else can the Center do to increase access to care for the rural and underserved population? Funding had been available from both state and federal sources for physician loan forgiveness if they served 2 years in rural areas of the state. Many physicians took advantage of these programs, worked in rural areas of the state for 2 years, and then went back to the city. This is an inadequate solution. Consequently, the Center team came up with the "Grow Your Own" program (the creative idea) in which the leader of this effort toured the rural areas of the state and recruited nurses, rooted in those communities, to return to school for their nurse practitioner education with the support of scholarship funds acquired by the Center. The Center now has over 100 APRN students and graduates who will (or did) return to their communities to provide primary care (action on the creative idea is an example of innovation). Many of the communities matched the scholarship funding for their nurses.[4] Other organizations might not have devised such a plan.

Because the levels of creativity are much clearer, strategies to support the development of creativity and innovation are explored in Table 21.1. Notice that some structure and support can facilitate creativity and innovation. Leaders can exercise these strategies and share them with others. For example, a journal club could focus on journals and magazines outside of health care, and people could discuss creative possibilities learned from exploring proposals and projects from business, futurist thinking, or training and how these might be applied to health care.

ADDITIONAL THOUGHTS ABOUT CREATIVITY AND INNOVATION

The late Clayton Christianson, author of *The Innovator's Dilemma: When New Technologies Cause Great Firms to Fail*, is famous for the work he did on disruptive innovation, which described new industries that usurped famous and supposedly

TABLE 21.1 Increasing Your Creativity and Innovation Through 10 Strategies

Strategy	Description
1. Observe and use all of your senses	Fine-tune the use of your senses, including your intuition; use observational skills to see what is going on across your sector and what you are hearing in the community.
2. Expand knowledge	Because innovation is based on knowledge, continually expand your knowledge and read articles and books not in health care (i.e., *Fast Company, Forbes, Harvard Business Review, Future,* etc.)
3. Defer judgments	Perceptions can limit your thinking and reasoning. Be careful about perceptions and bias. Be open.
4. Practice guided imagery	Visualization and guided imagery are helpful in "seeing" a concept or possible project materialize. Practice visualizing the goal or end product.
5. Facilitate incubation	Take breaks from the thinking process. Take a walk or run, cook something, or whatever allows your brain to shift into another place. When you return, you will be more creative.
6. Seek new experiences	Try new things that you haven't done before. Teach a new class, find a new hobby or activity, visit someplace you've never seen before. These activities broaden you and stimulate new ideas.
7. Develop new patterns	Structured patterns can be a problem—seeing and doing the same thing. Something as simple as creating a different way to drive to work establishes a new pattern. This can stimulate different thinking.
8. Redefine the problem	All problems have solutions. Frequently, the problem is defined incorrectly. Go back to the beginning and redefine the problem, because if you are truly "stuck," another problem underneath the "stuck" problem is what needs to be addressed.
9. Look in different places	"Look where others aren't looking." Some of the most important discoveries came from outside of the businesses they influenced.
10. Come up with creative ideas	Structure the creative time with an endpoint. Then focus on innovation, which is the action segment. Implement some of the ideas rather than continuing to create more ideas.

Adapted from Burrus D. Creativity and innovation: Your keys to a successful organization. 2017. Available at: https://www.huffingtonpost.com/daniel-burrus/creativity-and-innovation_b_4149993.html. Accessed March 24, 2019.

solid corporations. One example is Kodak, which disappeared in a couple of years as digital cameras, such as those in your cell phones, completely disrupted the photography business. Kodak was unable to respond quickly enough.[5]

Ideas resulting in innovations in health care are apparent in the creative use of APRNs.[6] Many grocery stores and pharmacies have ambulatory clinics that are provided by nurse practitioners (APRNs). Primary care practices have been affected by these clinics. Patients use these clinics when they go shopping. Many ambulatory problems, such as urinary tract or respiratory infections, are easily managed in these clinics. Patients can receive immunizations, sports physicals, and so on easily. Some of these clinics have collaborative agreements with physician groups. These groups send their chronic care patients to grocery store/pharmacy clinics, and these clinics send any complicated patients to the physician groups. This is a disruptive innovation in health care.[6]

Weberg and Davidson have addressed the challenges of leading with creativity and innovation.[7] Traditional leadership behaviors in leading teams are inadequate to facilitate creativity and innovation today. Practices, such as linear thinking, poor readiness for innovation, and leader centricity, or doing what members think the leader wants, cannot result in creative ideas and innovation. These are 20th century approaches and won't work today. What is needed to facilitate creative ideas and innovation are behaviors such as boundary spanning, risk taking, visioning, leveraging opportunity, adaptation, and coordination of information flow. We can learn any of these skills. We simply need more practice or experience working with them. "Trial and error" is great. It encourages team members to also experiment with creative idea generation and the resulting innovative behaviors. We saw how innovative people and organizations can be as many groups converted their usual business to be part of the response to the 2020 pandemic.

INCREASING YOUR CREATIVITY AND INNOVATION

How do we increase creativity and innovation in our organizations? Table 21.1 reviews strategies that support the development and expansion of creativity and innovation. Expediting both creativity and innovation has been recognized as an excellent pathway to success, both in patient care and nonpatient care areas. Costs can be reduced while patient care is improved. Encouraging new nurses to think differently, including assuring necessary resources, as well as asking critical questions to support the development of innovative ideas, is the responsibility of the leader. Supporting creativity improves the process of problem solving by clinical nurses at the bedside and gives a competitive edge to the organization. This approach also respects patients who can be involved in discovering what can improve care. Creative ideas and innovative strategies can be helped through open dialogue and an exchange of ideas with all who function in the organization.[8]

BRAINSWARMING

In contrast to the recommended strategies in Table 21.1, most of us have been involved in brainstorming sessions to hopefully create new ideas and strategies. Brainstorming can occur when a team spontaneously shares ideas while withholding judgment about the suggestions offered. Brainstorming has been around since the 1950s, but many have questioned its effectiveness.[9] It relies on the storming metaphor, which swirls in, raises a lot of dust and dirt, and passes on. And frequently, a lot of discussion ensues among a few group members, which can lead to all storm and no brain.[10] Research has not demonstrated that it works any better than team members working alone and then coming together to share their ideas and expand on them. This traditional method can encounter some challenges, such as strong personalities dominating the discussion, leaving some team members quiet and introverted; some ideas being discounted as unworkable or missing the theme; and the process being time-consuming, especially when the group is large.[11]

For these reasons, some have suggested an alternative strategy: brainswarming. In this approach, a single problem or goal is placed at the top of a flip chart or whiteboard (Fig. 21.1). A few known available resources are identified at the bottom. As team members make written suggestions,

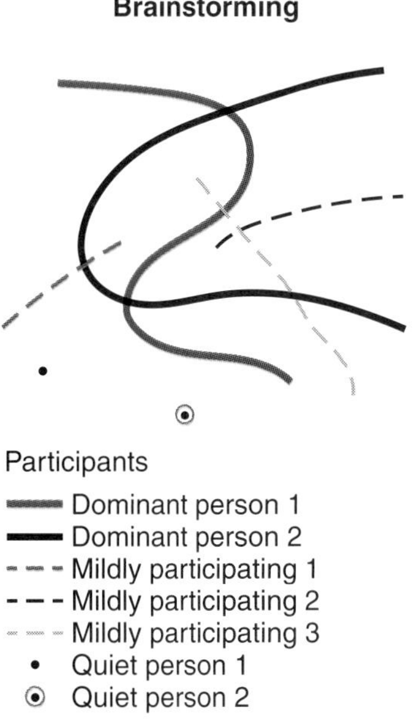

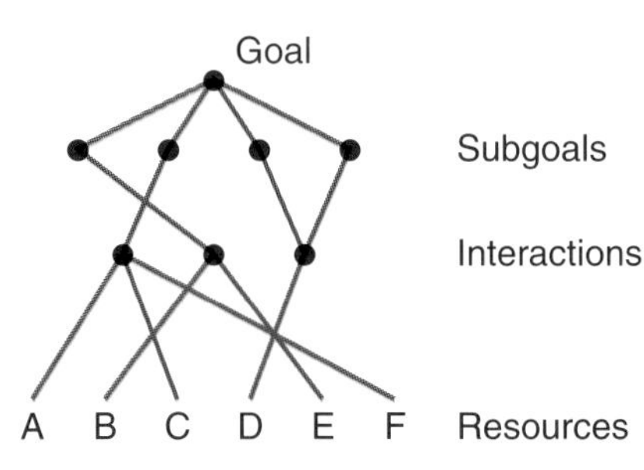

Fig. 21.1 Brainstorming vs. brainswarming. The figure on the left shows how a brainstorming session among different personality types might progress. The figure on the right shows a major goal as it might be written at the top of a whiteboard, and available resources are listed at the bottom. Participants identify subgoals, shown on the level below the major goal. Interactions (which can include discussions and/or suggestions) connect the subgoals to the available resources.

the main problem expands with "subgoals," or subsections of the problem/goal. The big thinkers tend to gravitate to the top of the flip chart, whereas those who tend to be more detail oriented frequently focus at the bottom. Thus more resources are added at the bottom as they are identified. Lines are used to connect resources to the activities that derive from the goal or problem. With these connections, potential solutions materialize. Some studies show that over 100 ideas can be generated in approximately 15 minutes.[12] It seems that switching from talking to writing improves the overall effectiveness of the activity.

> **REFLECTION** How would you set up a brainswarming session? Experiment with a problem identified by the team and see what happens.

LL ALERT

- Don't do things the way you have always done them.
- Don't jump on the first idea offered as a solution.

SUMMARY

Leaders plan for what strategies to use to stimulate teams. We need to develop exercises or activities to stimulate thinking and implementation of an innovation. If we want others to be creative, we have to convey that it is safe to think in new ways and to create projects to test their ideas. National specialty conferences are great places to exchange new ideas and receive stimulation to think about creative ideas and their application in your own facility—an innovation. Creative leaders are open-minded and employ strategies that encourage people to think differently and to experiment with possibilities. They know and use disruptive innovation and encourage others to experiment with different approaches to achieving goals or solving problems. They are not afraid of mistakes or failure and promote experimentation.

LL LINEUP

- Be creative in devising ways to stimulate thinking.
- Establish and maintain an environment in which diverse thinking and input are supported.

> **REFLECTION** Would you describe yourself as creative or innovative? What do you need to become skilled in each? What problem could you begin to tackle in a new way tomorrow?

22

Integrity

We look for integrity in our leaders, but what does integrity mean? Integrity is being honest, consistent, and uncompromising as it relates to our stated moral and ethical principles and values. Or, as C. S. Lewis said, "Integrity is doing the right thing, even when no one is watching."[1]

In ethics, integrity is regarded as the honesty and truthfulness or accuracy of one's actions. Integrity can also relate to internal consistency and the importance of resolving internal conflicting values. We demonstrate integrity when we act in alignment with our stated values, beliefs, and principles.[2,3] Integrity isn't easy. It requires courage to be in integrity on an ongoing basis. And almost every one of us can experience diminished integrity at some point in our week.

COURAGE AND INTEGRITY

Integrity is easy when no stress or pressure exists and life is good. When the going is tough and stressful and includes personal assaults, it is much more difficult to be in integrity. When we think about what it takes to maintain integrity during tough times, such as difficulty with children or a spouse, with coworkers or supervisors, or with a public health crisis, the word *courage* comes to mind. Courage is the willingness to uphold your beliefs and values, despite the possible costs, when it would be easier to "stretch the truth" or to tell a little "white lie" or blame others. When you know that the truth will be upsetting and cause a scene, yet you tell the truth regardless of the upset and cope with the "scene," you demonstrate courage.[4]

We were thinking of the true story depicted in the movie and book, *Hacksaw Ridge,* in which the World War II hero was a conscientious objector due to his faith. He insisted on joining the army even though he refused to carry a weapon. He served as a medic, and on Hacksaw Ridge in the South Pacific, he rescued 75 wounded Americans under heavy enemy gunfire during the night. He worked tirelessly to lower each of the wounded down a tall cliff, even when the enemy overran the American position. Before that event, the troops hadn't trusted him and they made fun of him (and his faith) because he refused to carry a weapon. He maintained his integrity and beliefs, even under nearly unbearable stress and persecution. For his actions, he received the undying respect of his fellow soldiers and the Congressional Medal of Honor.

WHAT DOES INTEGRITY LOOK LIKE IN OUR PERSONAL LIVES?

Both in our personal lives and the workplace, we could choose to treat others the way we (or, as some say, *they*) would like to be treated. Friends and associates would also like to be treated well. This translates into "Do what you say you will do." Promises made to others should be honored. For example, if we promise to take children or grandchildren to a special event, we cannot cancel or back out on the commitment. If we do, what family members learn is that work or other priorities are more important than they are. This is an integrity problem when you break your word, or as Don Miguel Ruiz conveys, "Be impeccable with your word. Speak with integrity. Say only what you mean. Avoid using the word to speak against yourself or to gossip about others. Use the power of your word in the direction of truth and love."[5] Honesty and trust are at the core of integrity.

HOW TO DEVELOP INTEGRITY

"The supreme quality for leadership is unquestionably integrity. Without it, no real success is possible, no matter whether it is on a section gang, a football field, in an army, or in an office."[6] What an interesting perspective on what it means to live with integrity. So how do we develop personal integrity in our lives, and how can we apply this to our professional lives? Table 22.1 describes 10 suggested strategies for increasing integrity.

We (the authors) want to emphasize the importance of assessing where we are in relationship to being successful leaders and positive human beings. A concerted effort is needed to not only exercise a self-assessment but also monitor where we are on an ongoing basis. Once we identify areas we would like to work on, we need to monitor

TABLE 22.1 Strategies for Developing Personal Integrity

Strategies	Description
1. Perform a self-assessment	A better understanding of who you are, including your strengths and weaknesses, helps you understand how to develop or expand your integrity. Do you procrastinate? Are you open to constructive feedback? Several tools are available to assist (see the chapter on intelligence).
2. Keep your word	Honoring your word is integral to integrity. Remember Don Miguel Ruiz. When you dishonor yourself by lying to someone, it destroys trust and it is very difficult to regain trust.
3. Don't overpromise	In your professional life, a promised outcome that is not delivered will cause loss of respect in your organization. It is best to underpromise and overdeliver.
4. Learn from masters	Find a role model of professional and personal integrity to learn from. Find a role model in an associated field (such as leadership). Focus on learning and be teachable.
5. Practice doing for others what you would want done for you	Be consciously aware of how you treat others. They should be treated the way you want them to treat you.
6. Giving leads to multiplication	Research reveals that charitable work literally makes the heart grow stronger. It helps your health. When you give, you are opening yourself up to selflessness and blessings, and it adds to your integrity.
7. Face your weaknesses	Whatever your self-assessment reveals, expand your strengths and work on your weaknesses. Face whatever flaws you may have and work on lessening the negatives that result from them, using self-discipline to counteract their effects.
8. Surround yourself with positive people	You need to surround yourself with encouraging and successful people. Find someone who has advanced further than you and who can help you get to the place you want to be. That someone needs to be a person whom you respect and who will keep confidences.
9. Review your growth	Establish a timeline for your efforts in improving your integrity. Evaluate your progress. Recognize your progress and identify what will be most helpful next. Identify new goals and seek help or support as you need it.
10. Teach others to do the same	Share with others what you are learning. Teaching them is another way to solidify your own learning and continue to grow.

when we are successful and when we need more work. Consistently being in integrity is not easy until we have developed a habit.

One of us shops at a grocery store that also has a pharmacy:

"I like the convenience. The store changed the policy regarding paying for prescriptions at the checkout stand and wanted customers to pay at the pharmacy. During the transition, they were willing to have a 'runner' go to the pharmacy and pick up the prescription so that it could be paid for at the checkout stand. As I can be somewhat resistant to certain types of change, I made use of the 'runner.' In the process, I checked the receipt as I was leaving the store and discovered that the clerk had not charged me for the prescriptions (which were $40.00). I went back to the clerk, and he insisted he had charged me for the prescriptions. Could I sell my integrity for $40? I'm not sure what I would have done at 20 years old, but at this juncture of my life, I had to insist that I pay for the medications. It would be against my value of honesty to let it pass. This is an example of a decision that adds to or detracts from personal integrity."

The good news is we increase or detract from our integrity each and every day with each decision we make, as in the example of the clerk's error. Adhering to personal integrity is decided with each choice. No one forces us to live one way or the other. And often, advantages for failing to adhere to our stated values exist. However, when we live a life of integrity, life is often filled with personal happiness and achievement. In addition, we sleep better at night.

> **REFLECTION** Consider an everyday situation where "cheating" would have been easy and likely successful. What did you do? Consider what motivated you to do what you did.

WHAT IS INTEGRITY IN THE WORKPLACE?

People who adhere to integrity tend to attract other people to them, and nowhere is this more important than in the workplace. These people tend to be principled, and we know we can count on them—for example, when a formal leader is making rounds and talking with staff and says she or he will check into an issue or a problem. People with integrity have a priority to circle back with information about the issue.

Another example is when leaders keep others informed and involved with issues, such as nurse-sensitive indicators and infection rates. Consequently, no surprises occur, and the nurses can address the issues with support from the leaders. Thus financial problems resulting from nonpayment due to failure to meet benchmarks can be addressed together. We are all smart and understand that financial difficulties could result. These problems can be avoided with creative solutions and hard work. When leaders are truthful and open about issues, others are more apt to trust and be willing to problem-solve with the leader. When crises occur, such as a flood or pandemic, it is even more important to be truthful and open because of how rapidly conditions change.

Integrity issues can be big, as in the outcome measures affecting the bottom line, or they can be small and look like consideration for others. If we are in a public place and see liquid on the floor, we can either notify someone, who can clean the area and post a warning sign or attempt to clean it ourselves. This is about treating others the way we ourselves would like to be treated. We don't want to risk slipping on the liquid, and we don't wish that for someone else.

What happens when we walk into a room and hear two people discussing a third person who is not present? They are gossiping and complaining about the third person's performance and behavior. What do we do? Hopefully, we ask the two if they have talked with the third person. Our tendency, of course, is to hear the latest issues about the third person. That doesn't help that person, and our listening only adds to the "juiciness" of the discussion. If we don't have the courage to help the two people stop the discussion, we can leave or we can say we aren't participating in this discussion unless that person is present.

In another example, a colleague might come to us to discuss a situation with a physician who is believed to be demonstrating "bullying behavior." After listening to this person, we agree that additional discussion is needed. We can support the colleague to speak to the physician with us as support or to report the concern through the appropriate channels. The key is that we don't merely listen to reinforce our view of this person, nor do we simply leave our colleague without support.

Leaders are responsible for maintaining certain standards, and doing so is a demonstration of integrity. Others may request that we bend standards for them, but they really want standards to be maintained equally and fairly across the system. These examples demonstrate leadership integrity.

WHEN INTEGRITY IS MISSING

Lapses in integrity in the workplace matter because of the impact on the workplace culture. Regardless of employee handbooks regarding codes of conduct, mission, and values, lack of integrity and ethics can be rampant. These violations are not about misconduct of the chief executive officer (CEO)—they can occur anywhere in an organization. Often, human resources (HR) policies are responses to situations where misbehavior of employees necessitated a restrictive policy.[7] It could be about unfair treatment, discrimination, favoritism, or what is known as "a hostile work environment."

Behaviors demonstrate values, beliefs, and character each day in the workplace; they demonstrate people's integrity. Some examples of everyday occurrences that are out of integrity include calling in sick because it is a beautiful day. This is the reason many facilities replaced sick time and vacation time with the concept of paid time off (PTO). Or a clinical unit sponsors events such as picnics or lunches or holiday parties. People sign up to go and then don't. Integrity of your word is at risk.

Another common example is taking office supplies from work for other purposes. This seems like a small thing, but when one of our values is honesty, we are out of integrity. What about hoarding certain supplies in lockers so we have them when we need them? Where does that leave others who also need those supplies? What about passing on juicy gossip about a colleague? Is that a demonstration of integrity? What happens when we claim credit for work done by someone else or we are told the correct information to include in a document but ignore it? All of these are examples of being out of integrity.

> **REFLECTION** What other decisions could you make where integrity isn't maintained?

HOW DO WE RECOUP FROM MISTAKES WITH INTEGRITY?

What do we do when we know we have violated our stated beliefs and values? One approach is to begin afresh each day with a renewed desire to live a life of integrity. We must not allow our own misgivings or negative self-talk to stop us from doing better each day.[8] First, we must guard our words. Choose them with great thought. Don't just talk without thinking. Consider responses carefully before answering questions. We can speak without regard to how truthfully we are speaking. For example, exaggerating stories is easy when we are attempting to impress others. Are we conveying the truth? We also must be sure our words are like beautiful gemstones—that they are viewed as valuable and trustworthy.

Another example is returning phone calls and emails. This is highly disrespectful to others when we do not. We in essence are conveying how unimportant the other people are to us and how much more important we are than they are. By consistently responding to calls and emails, we build trust and demonstrate our integrity and respect for the others. Being timely is equally important. Being late demonstrates disrespect for others' time. One of us worked in an organization where everyone said meetings and appointments started late, which translated to 10 minutes after the scheduled time. On the other hand, being early (perhaps 15 minutes before the scheduled time) shows respect for others. If we are going to be late, we need to let others know. We might ask about rescheduling if we need to be at the meeting. We can't deceive ourselves into thinking that late behavior is okay. If the culture believes that being late is okay, be on time anyway. People will notice, and their timeliness might increase.

> **REFLECTION** Consider some group gathering—a meeting, a webinar, a change of shift report, or a conference. Did the gathering start on time? (You likely won't remember if it was close to the designated time.) What happened next? Were you distracted by people entering the gathering? How did the leader manage these interruptions, if they occurred? Can you recall what happened to your mental expectations of the meeting? What were they?

To be effective, however, the person in charge has to start the meeting and not stop the meeting to bring late arrivals up to date. If starting on time is an agreed-to expectation, bringing late arrivals up to date disrespects those who were on time. We have to assess which is more important—keeping those who are committed and engaged actively committed and engaged or accommodating people who are "violating" the standards. We all can be late; however, some of us could easily name the chronic abusers of time.

We also need to remember to express gratitude. Being grateful is a demonstration of our personal integrity. By focusing on connecting requests to please and responding to what we are given with "thank you," we can add integrity to the culture. The words "please" and "thank you" show tremendous respect and honor to the people with whom we interact. Additionally, showing gratitude has demonstrated a relationship to other positive aspects of life.

Showing gratitude is equivalent to having personal integrity. Simply by making requests with the inclusion of please and receiving a gift with words of thanks can add integrity to the very atmosphere. Probably the most important aspect of resurrecting our integrity is owning our failures. Blaming others all the time is inaccurate and a problem. We live in a society of blaming. It is unhealthy to consistently never own responsibility for what doesn't work. We all make mistakes; it is a part of being human. If we make a mistake (and we all do), just own it and offer a sincere, authentic apology. Follow the apology with a period. Do not add a *however* or *but,* which negates the apology. Simply say, "I'm sorry." This simple heartfelt response can be a freeing experience. The ability to acknowledge our failures is critical to reestablishing our integrity.

The process of regaining or reinventing integrity is accomplished one event at a time. Integrity is not rebuilt easily or quickly. In a society where integrity is collapsing and the focus is on money and power at any cost, leaders need to commit to rebuilding and reinventing integrity in our lives. Be persistent in applying these suggestions in Table 22.1. Over time, integrity will become consistent in your life.

> **REFLECTION** How often are you late to meetings or appointments? Do you speak before you think? What are the negatives of your self-assessment?

LL ALERT

- Don't assume no one is watching when you are tempted to be out of integrity.
- Don't break promises.
- Don't break simple social graces, such as timeliness and showing gratitude.

SUMMARY

Leaders have the opportunity to exhibit integrity every day. Others look to leaders to set the behavioral expectations. When leaders slip in those behaviors, they lose trust and respect. Integrity is important because we do not need to spend time and energy questioning ourselves or berating ourselves when we violate our values, beliefs, or principles. When we listen to our hearts and do the right thing, life becomes simple and straightforward. We don't have anything to hide and can be open with our thoughts, spoken word, and actions.

LL LINEUP

- Remember that leaders set behavioral expectations.
- Promise only what you know you can deliver.

REFLECTION Look back. When in your life have you been out of integrity? What did you learn? Could you or did you forgive yourself? If you have held onto it, what was the benefit of not practicing self-forgiveness?

23

Intelligence

How many of you took an intelligence quotient (IQ) test in high school. Perhaps you thought, "Well, I'm stuck with an average IQ and probably won't do much with my life." Or maybe you thought, "I need to figure out a way to get around this!" That's because 50 years ago, intelligence was simple. It was measured by our IQ, and when we were tested in high school, we knew we were stuck with that number for the rest of our lives. Thankfully, things change. Today, intelligence has expanded to include intellectual, appreciative, emotional, and visual measures. Each of these realms is important to be an effective leader; and if we don't possess the related skills, we can develop them.

GENERAL (INTELLECTUAL) INTELLIGENCE

General intelligence is defined as the ability to acquire and apply knowledge and skills.[1] This definition is foundational and just the beginning of how we think about intelligence today. Currently, we define intelligence as the capacity for logic, understanding, self-awareness, learning, emotional knowledge, reasoning, creativity, and the ability to perceive information and retain it. We take this knowledge and apply it to behaviors as they relate to a specific context.[2] An example of how thinking changes regarding intelligence is apparent in considering artificial intelligence (machines or software capable of exhibiting intelligent activity). Undoubtedly, our thinking will continue to change.

Writing different content with each hand at the same time, playing classical piano well, and speaking multiple languages well may be different skill sets, but each is thought to be an indicator of general intelligence. The IQ typically measures a wide variety of verbal and spatial skills and is the most widely used measure to assess intelligence.

The general public believes that a high IQ score equates with success, and many people have attempted to determine whether the level is a characteristic acquired at birth, which remains the same throughout one's life, or if it changes in any way. Psychological research has repeatedly demonstrated that contrary to common beliefs, IQ can change dramatically, with the greatest changes in childhood and adolescence.[3] IQ seems to stabilize with age and perhaps decrease in old age.[4]

In the 1980s, Howard Gardner of Harvard University was the first to offer the concept of multiple intelligences and identified seven intelligences comprising language, logical-mathematical analysis, spatial representation, musical thinking, use of the body to solve problems, an understanding of other individuals, and an understanding of ourselves. Human beings differ in the strengths of these various intelligences and how they are combined or interrelated to solve problems and perform tasks.[5] From this work comes such concepts as visual, auditory, and kinesthetic learning and, of course, such concepts as emotional intelligence (EI).

APPRECIATIVE INTELLIGENCE

The definition of appreciative intelligence is the ability to perceive the positive generative potential in a given situation and to act purposefully to transform the potential into outcomes.[6] It is the ability to reframe a situation in a way that recognizes the positive possibilities within situations that are not apparent to the untrained person. According to Tojo Thatchenkery and Carol Metzker, we are not talking about simple optimism. People with appreciative intelligence are realistic and action oriented. They have the ability to identify positive potential and to devise a course of action that uses this positive potential to obtain a specific goal or outcome. Three components of appreciative intelligence were identified: reframing, appreciating the positive, and seeing how the future unfolds from the present,[6] utilizing reframing and appreciation.

One of us, as the head nurse of the labor and delivery unit (L&D) in a university hospital, followed a small group of patients antenatally and then provided nursing care in L&D on an "on-call" basis[7]:

"One of my patients was a dear friend, a psychiatric nurse, who had published her qualitative research on a small group of patients experiencing stillborn infants. As she approached her due date, she began to experience decreased fetal movement. She was admitted in early labor with no fetal heart tones. I provided her

nursing care all night and, when she delivered, supported her husband to be with her in the delivery room (even though this was not standard practice at the time). Because I had read her research, I asked her if she wanted to hold her baby girl (this was not standard practice at the time). Of course, she did and held and touched the baby everywhere and said, 'She's so warm; why doesn't she breathe?'

"Because of this nurse/patient and her research, we changed all our policies relative to care for patients with stillborn births and became one of the first university obstetric services to show stillborn infants and allow parents to complete the process of saying goodbye in whatever way they needed.[8] *I saw the need for this patient/friend and perceived the positive generative potential of supporting the bereavement process in this critical life event for parents. Traditionally, stillborn infants were whisked away to the morgue before the mother recovered from general anesthesia. Fathers were not in the delivery room, so neither parent saw the infant. We showed all infants if the parents wanted, even those with physical abnormalities. Outcomes for parents changed, and they could actively begin the bereavement process with support rather than being stuck in denial. We reframed the experience and developed an appreciation for facilitating a positive psychological bereavement process."*

Those leaders with high levels of appreciative intelligence often have four key qualities: persistence, the conviction that their actions make a difference, a high tolerance for uncertainty, and irrepressible resilience.

> **REFLECTION** Look at the last paragraph again. Which of those components and qualities would likely describe you? How might you deliberately enhance one that is missing or that you are less likely to see as an immediate quality?

Leaders easily see the power of adopting a positive generative approach to especially difficult situations and thus to effect potential outcomes in a more positive way. Leaders are realistic and action oriented to accomplish specified goals and to harness the positive potential not just in ourselves but also in others. Without persistence and conviction, we would be challenged to move a team forward. Inevitably, obstacles appear, and we must demonstrate resilience when we don't overcome them during the initial effort.

EMOTIONAL INTELLIGENCE

The concept of EI was popularized by the New York Times bestselling book, *Emotional Intelligence: Why It Can Matter More Than IQ*, by Daniel Goleman.[9] Although the scientific community has criticized his analysis, it has been useful in the business community. EI refers to the ability of leaders to identify and manage personal emotions, as well as to identify and manage the emotions of others. Although questions exist from the research about the validity of the model, clearly, leaders who are sensitive to the emotions of others and their social environment can make a stronger, more powerful impact. And the good news is, these are learned skills. Those leaders who can manage their own emotions and influence those around them are more effective leaders.

Goleman describes the five components of EI as follows:

- **Self-awareness** is the ability to recognize and understand one's own personal moods and emotions, including strengths, weaknesses, drives, values, and their effect on others. Some attributes of this understanding include self-confidence, realistic self-assessment, and a self-deprecating sense of humor.
- **Self-regulation** is the ability to control or redirect disruptive impulses and moods, to suspend judgment, and to think before acting. Attributes that denote this behavior include trustworthiness and integrity, as well as being open to change and comfortable with ambiguity.
- **Internal motivation** emphasizes a passion to work for internal reasons beyond money and status, such as an inner vision, a joy in the work, and a curiosity for learning. Attributes include a growth mindset that leads to pursuing goals with energy, persistence, and optimism in the face of failure and organizational commitment.
- **Empathy** focuses on understanding the emotional aspects of other people. Attributes include successfully building and retaining talented people, being sensitive to cultural issues, and focusing on service to patients and clients and their families.
- **Social skills** refers to a focus on managing relationships and building networks, seeking common ground, and building rapport. Attributes include leading change and an extensive skill set in persuasiveness.

These concepts are represented in Table 23.1. Goleman's idea that the ability to understand and manage emotions significantly increases our chances of success has influenced all areas of business. For leaders to understand what constitutes the demonstrably high levels of EI, Justin Bariso has identified everyday behaviors that he believes are evidence of EI in action.[10] People with high levels of EI can recognize the impact of emotions on themselves and on others. They can reflect and respond to questions such as: What are my strengths and weaknesses? How does my mood affect my thoughts and decision-making? What thoughts and emotions influence other peoples' language choices and behavior? The answers to these questions can lead to valuable insights about ourselves and others.

TABLE 23.1 Goleman's Representation of Emotional Intelligence

	Self	Others
Awareness	**Self-awareness:** Knowing one's internal state, preferences, resources, and intuitions accurately, leading to self-confidence	**Social awareness:** Awareness of others' feelings, needs, and concerns and employing empathy for others An organizational orientation such as service to others
Management	**Self-management:** Managing one's internal state, impulses, and resources; self-control; transparent and adaptable Taking initiative Demonstrating achievement and drive	**Relationship management:** Adeptness at inducing desirable outcomes Understanding responses in others, developing others, influencing others, managing conflict, building relationships, creating teamwork and collaboration Serving as a catalyst for change

Adapted from Goleman's work as represented in https://web.sonoma.edu/users/s/swijtink/teaching/philosophy_101/paper1/goleman.htm. Updated February 1, 2009.

REFLECTION Use Table 23.1 to identify behaviors reflecting how you perceive yourself. What did you conclude?

Another action that could demonstrate high-level EI is for the leader to pause and think before speaking. The task is to think about the situation and our response. At the same time, we exert some control over our thoughts. By focusing on our thoughts, we can slow down emotional reactions, or as Bariso says, "You can't prevent a bird from landing on your head, but you can keep it from building a nest."[10]

Although few people enjoy negative or constructive feedback, it does provide leaders with an opportunity to learn. Even when we feel it is unfounded, the feedback provides information about how the other person thinks, which is also valuable. Rather than being defensive (getting emotional about it), we can ask ourselves what about the situation can make us better leaders. The toughest part of entering a feedback situation is remaining authentic—authentically interested in the interaction and authentically listening to the feedback. Utilizing our principles and values can support us in stressful situations. We can be authentic about valuing interactions, and that attests to our ability to manage ourselves.

Sometimes the person giving the negative feedback is more uncomfortable than we are. In this case, we can be empathetic, understanding how awkward or difficult the situation is for the person. Remember, empathy doesn't mean we agree with the other person—it means we are seeking to understand the other person. When leaders give feedback, they reframe messages as constructive, as coaching, and as an opportunity that coincides with the other person's stated goals. One of our favorite questions to ask a new group of learners—for example, students in a clinical rotation or leaders attending a conference—is "How many of you want to be a mediocre nurse/leader?" Clearly no one raises a hand. We might also ask if they want to be the best possible version of themselves, and, of course, no one denies that statement. The point is this: all of our discussions, interactions, and feedback will be focused on the goal of supporting learning so they can be the best nurse or leader possible. The feedback is designed to make the good great.

By "setting up" a group of people to recall that sometimes as we move through situations, we might be uncomfortable, we help them know we are supportive—that we are there to support them on their journey to be their best. As Don Miguel Ruiz says: "Always do your best."[11] That is true of us as leaders facilitating someone else's development and of others as they do the work of developing.

Acknowledgment, including praise, is an important part of leadership, and the ease with which we do this in an authentic manner can be invaluable. As a leadership skill, praise can result in an amazing response from those receiving praise because it meets the need people have for acknowledgment. All human beings crave appreciation, and some even believe that's why people come to work every day. Focus on the good in other human beings and acknowledge it.

When we make mistakes (and we all do sometimes), simply apologize. Saying you're sorry demonstrates courage and humility. The ability to apologize means valuing the relationship we have with others more than protecting our egos. If someone makes a mistake, simply forgive and forget. Move on. Hanging onto a misstep, an error, or a slight is like leaving a sponge or instrument in a patient: the wound festers. We are unable to heal, to move on with our lives. Meanwhile, the other person has no idea that we are holding on to the event and they go about living their lives. We can't afford to let others rule our lives without even knowing it. Instead, let go of such issues and reach for dreams and goals.

One of the most important actions for a leader is to keep commitments. If something happens such that a commitment or promise must be broken, let the other party know as soon as possible. When we keep our word in situations like an evening at the movies with a friend or being timely with a business deadline, we demonstrate reliability and trust. When we consistently fail to keep our word by breaking commitments or being late, we are distrusted.

Volunteer to help others. Asking what we can do for them positively affects them. Help can be as simple as listening or as complex as discovering data and information they need for a project. Or it could be working with someone. One of us once had a chief executive officer (CEO) who shadowed a nurse for 4 hours on each unit. It was a significant dedication of time and interest in what nurses were doing with patients. The way he enrolled staff with just that activity was amazing. Even better is the example from a colleague who took another CEO to the clinical area. At about 10:30, the CEO thanked the CNO and decided to take a coffee break. The CNO placed a hand on the CEOs arm and pointed out that the shift wasn't even half over yet! The CNO had booked the CEO for the full shift to appreciate the full impact of what it means to be on the front lines for the duration and not just a visit.

REFLECTION When was the last time you worked alongside someone else just as a demonstration? What value was it to the other person? What value was it to you?

VISUAL INTELLIGENCE

The concept of visual intelligence is somewhat new and is defined as the ability to see what's there that others don't see and to realize what's not there that should be. In other words, the visually intelligent see the positives and the negatives.[12] Amy Herman believes we find more things competing for our attention than ever before in human history. The bite-sized interactions that exemplify our daily lives are a detriment to concentration, focus, and productivity. As an example, when many meetings, as well as people's jobs, went online in 2020, we talked about the increased intensity of following what was happening in meetings. More importantly, this environment can endanger our personal safety and impinge on our functioning intelligence. A BBC report describes a 2005 study at King's College, which found that distracted workers (from excessive environmental stimuli) can experience a 10- to 15-point IQ loss.[14] This decrease is greater than what occurs when smoking marijuana. When the brain is inundated with too much information or is made to switch focus too quickly, it simply slows down as much as 40%, as demonstrated in a study of students working on complicated math problems while being bombarded with distractions. Herman believes sharpening our visual attention skills greatly enhances our effectiveness in our jobs. Visual intelligence is critically important to being able to both see and understand the details in any of the well-constructed plans or efforts and then be able to recognize any details that can disrupt the well-thought-out plan. We can incorporate visual, emotional and appreciative intelligence in our efforts to be successful.

LL ALERT

- Don't immediately discount emotional, appreciative, or visual intelligence.
- Don't decide someone is "smart" based solely on an intellectual basis.

SUMMARY

Multiple types of intelligence exist, and we are not tied only to the basic concept of IQ. To be successful, additional types of intelligence can be explored and implemented to enhance our leadership skills.

LL LINEUP

- Notice how well influential leaders get along with peers, subordinates, and superiors.
- Observe how they deal with difficult situations.
- Notice the various types of intelligence they use.
- Learn more about these types of intelligence during your leadership journey.

REFLECTION Think about the last time you noticed details about another person, about the surrounding environment. What was gained by noticing those details? Think about the last time you launched a project or a new idea: Were you positive and upbeat? Did you enroll your people? Is there one person who challenges you? How do you relate to that person?

24 Mindfulness

Have you ever headed off to work in your car or on the bus or train and suddenly looked around and wondered where you were? That is an example of not being mindful. We weren't "in the moment," nor were we attending to the "now." Our minds were somewhere else and suddenly for some reason we returned to the present. We had been moving all the time, but we were somewhere else mentally, so we were confused about where we were until we found a familiar landmark that snapped our minds back to where we were physically. So, if that is not mindfulness, what is?

WHAT IS MINDFULNESS?

Even if we had never heard of this concept before, we could guess its meaning by the word itself. Fullness of mind is a big clue. In the opening paragraph we probably recalled our own fullness-of-mind example—it's just that the mind wasn't focused on what was going on around us! Because mindfulness, or *intentionality* as it is also known, is about being in the moment, it requires our full attention to wherever we are and whatever is happening around us. Mindfulness is defined as a deliberative, active process of focusing on the here and now. It requires actively attending to the environs and the persons. It allows us to be introspective in examining a situation by thinking through how we responded and how that response may have shaped subsequent events. If we are focused on the present, we can't be running our memory tapes about comparable situations, and we can't be planning what our responses will be. Mindfulness is a powerful tool *any one* of us can use. Don't we all feel special when we think someone is paying full attention to what we are saying? Part of the point of practicing mindfulness is so we are focused. What we focus on precipitates the actions we take, which according to Al Kleiner, Jeffrey Schwartz, and Josie Thomson, happens in the brain and determines what we will be like as leaders.[1] When we focus on positive behaviors, we are training the brain to respond differently than if we focus on the negative.

REFLECTION Think back to yesterday when you woke up. Can you list what you did and in the exact sequence? Now think of the last discussion you had with one or two other people. What were they wearing? Did they have on jewelry? If so, what did the jewelry look like? What kind of shoes did they have on? What did their facial expressions convey—happiness, sadness, frustration, anger? Did they engage in any physical activities such as standing or pacing or jiggling their feet? Can you quote or paraphrase anything they said? Based on your responses, how mindful do you think you were?

PRACTICAL USES OF MINDFULNESS

In addition to the benefits others who experience our undivided attention receive, we benefit by gaining much more information about a person, a problem, or a situation. Consider how much time we can save by not having to do additional follow-up work because we didn't engage the first time. Mindfulness is important, and it's one of the 16 critical competencies for health care executives.[2] Before we talk about the mindfulness competencies, let's look at that model developed by Carson Dye and Andrew Garman. Four major areas comprise the model: well-cultivated self-awareness, compelling vision, masterful execution, and a real way with people. These four areas and the 16 competencies use different words than the Legacy *Leaders*-Ship Trajectory, but the content is the same. Note, however, that we believe these competencies are about leadership in any position at any level and are not distinctive to any particular title.

The thirteenth competency for health care executives is mindful decision-making. In essence, mindfulness is combined with reflection to make us aware of how to make decisions. The authors refer to this as the lessons-learned step. Information about how we make decisions is highly useful to any leader because if we are seen as leaders, others want our input (and sometimes decision). If we need to exhibit some consistency, we should have a framework reflective of how we approach decision-making. The intentionality of how to make decisions is something that can be learned. Specifically, Carson Dye and Andrew Garman say, "The best decision makers decide how to decide,"[2] and that can only happen if we have reflected on our past decisions. They also identify two qualities that set apart highly skilled decision-makers from others. The first quality is selecting from a broad array of options. The second is explaining why leaders made the decision they did.

Most of us are accustomed to generating options, but fewer of us think to share how we decided on the option we selected. Think how powerful that one step is for the development of others. First, we need to be mindful about how we make decisions, so we are making more good decisions than bad ones. Then we can reflect on the process we used, the data we considered, and the opinions we sought—first, so we know how we are making decisions and second, so others know why we chose what we did. Consider how addressing a "because" statement helps others understand our thinking. Instead of merely telling a colleague we expect him or her to report an occurrence to our supervisor, let's add a rationale such as "because this situation from our experience can escalate into a major issue." That addition helps our colleagues see we aren't whimsical, we paid attention, and we used our wisdom to offer support for a positive outcome.

Another strategy to consider is thinking aloud. When we do this, we help others see our line of reasoning from beginning to end. Unfortunately, speaking what we think slows down the action process, so this is not always the best strategy. However, for less time-sensitive decisions, thinking aloud helps anyone who listens hear how various data points are pulled together to make a tapestry of decision making.

As we thought about speaking aloud our rationale, we couldn't help but wonder how many rumors could be stopped by such action, because in the absence of information, people fill in the blanks. When one of us was a senior in high school, she was identified as the source for a rumor that two teachers were involved in an affair:

"I was stunned! Not only had I not started the rumor, I hadn't even heard it before. I immediately went to one of the teachers, who was also my summer swim coach, and told her what the rumor was. That person helped me realize I knew both of the targets of the rumor in a more detailed way than the average student (I was also in the band and orchestra, and the other teacher was involved with both of those activities). She pointed out that when people have incomplete pieces of information about a story, they may freely (and falsely) fill in blanks. The two teachers had been seen in the parking lot talking together and that apparently triggered the idea of affairs. She also pointed out that people who spread rumors want them to be believable, so they attach a key name (in this case mine!) to add credibility. After all, I knew them both in ways that few others would."

If people fill in the blanks, isn't sharing how we reach a decision (thinking aloud, if you will) a great strategy to make sure people can agree or disagree with the outcome or the process? The rationale becomes a damper to thwart rumors. Simultaneously, by thinking aloud, we are helping to develop the thinking of other leaders.

Mindfulness can also help us determine which risks to take. If we look at the model for creating innovation in nursing, we could overlay the concept of mindfulness. This overlay can illustrate we must be mindful in gathering information. What we gather shapes our decision to take a risk or to do so in a considered manner (mindful manner). This deliberative process prevents really irrational actions or a reticence to act.

REFLECTION When, if ever, was the last time you shared your rationale for some action or a direction to someone else as a part of the decision statement? If you have not tried this approach, find at least one opportunity in the next 2 days to state your rationale openly. If you have used this approach, consider what types of reactions from others you have received. Were some situations more conducive to using this approach than others? What were those situations like?

MEDITATION AND MINDFULNESS

Mindfulness and meditation are concepts often considered together in the literature. Common benefits of meditation for leaders are identified in Table 24.1. Additionally, meditation seems to increase one's capacity for compassion.[3] Other benefits exist, but these all relate to how leaders can feel calmer, more in control, and more energized while leading. Meditation can be as simple as focusing in the

TABLE 24.1 **Benefits of Meditation for Leaders**
↑ sleep
↓ stress
↓ anxiety
↑ attention
↓ job burnout

moment, accepting one's self, and breathing. When we jokingly have said, "breathe" when something dramatic happened, even if we didn't know the related research about breathing, we were giving good advice. The practices of meditation include walking, standing, sitting, and lying down. In essence, we can meditate almost anywhere without any special clothing or equipment. This also means no one has an excuse for not practicing meditation! (Yes, we know many people who have to have the "right clothes" before they can jog, or bike or lift weights or…!) Meditation is really an inexpensive way to contribute to our health, effectiveness and leadership.

> **REFLECTION** Even if you have tried meditation, stop what you are doing and devote 5 minutes to the process. If you need a quick guide, go to: https://www.mayoclinic.org/healthy-lifestyle/consumer-health/in-depth/mindfulness-exercises/art-20046356.

When one of us first moved to a new state, she lived next door to the parents of a local, famous songwriter. His lyrics come to mind whenever she thinks about the force of self:

You can go too near;
You can go too far.
But wherever you go,
There you are!

–Andy Wilkinson

Leadership is about being you and using your strengths for the greater good wherever you are. Meditation helps us be in touch with our real selves. No matter what type of meditation you might engage in, the key is to be quiet, slow, and thoughtful. Being aware of slow, deep breathing; moving slowly; or wearing noise-canceling headphones all enhance our focus and work.

> **REFLECTION** Stop reading for a minute. Focus on you and your breathing. Choose to inhale as research supports our doing: 5-2-7. Inhale for 5 seconds, hold your breath for 2 seconds, then exhale for 7 seconds. Repeat for 2 minutes. This approach helps us feel less stressed, and as a result, we make better decisions.[4]

A final thought about mindfulness: although studies have shown mindfulness practices have positive effects, considerable limitations have been identified.[4] For example, mindfulness has no formal, universal definition. Outcomes are difficult to measure because they are self-reports about perceptions. As a result, we should consider the quality of the findings thus far and know that practicing mindfulness will cause no harm. Likewise, justifying specific decisions based on mindfulness only could be challenging. One major exception comes from work by Benjamin Shapero and Gaelle Desbordes, who studied brain changes associated with meditation and is included in a review on mindfulness and meditation.[5–7] As additional research evolves, we will know how much we can rely on meditation to enhance effective decision-making.[6]

LL ALERT

- Don't become addicted to being mindful.
- Don't avoid sharing what you are thinking.

SUMMARY

Mindfulness has been studied from numerous perspectives, almost always with positive results—decreasing negative effects and increasing positive ones. It is low cost, minimally invasive in terms of time and place, and habit forming. Leaders who use a mindful approach to decision-making and share their thinking with others are seen as more effective than those who do not. Mindfulness is a powerful tool immediately available to anyone anywhere.

LL LINEUP

- Practice mindfulness.
- Tell others how you reach decisions.

> **REFLECTION** If you are journaling, use a symbol to indicate entries related to a decision you made. Then, review all of those entries. Can you find a pattern regarding how you make decisions? If you are not journaling, start making a summary statement with each decision you make to help with determining a pattern. Include a statement you could use to tell others your rationale for any decision you made. This might include something so basic as "I already had something scheduled then" or as complex as a detailed statement with a rationale for how you make decisions and what was particularly compelling. Practice telling your colleagues your "because" statement.

25

Presence

Presence. That is a powerful word. We know someone who has presence and yet we aren't sure what it is that makes us say this person has it or seems influential or powerful. The research is clear, however. If we don't have it, we better get it if we want to be considered a leader!

WHAT IS PRESENCE?

Known also as executive presence (even when the person is not an executive), presence can be explained simply: it is the interaction of appearance (A), behavior (B), and communication (C) (A + B + C = presence). Presence creates a sense of power, confidence, and trust about who a person is. Paying attention to only one of these factors is insufficient, but if you must focus, choose behavior because it is seen as acting out your values and evidence of who you really are.

In a study about registered nurse (RN) satisfaction that focused on the characteristics of nurse directors (NDs), a specific group of leaders, the authors found four themes related to RNs. One of the four RN themes is especially relevant to presence: Visibility Promotes Interpersonal Connections and a Safe and Caring Environment.[1] In other words, leaders (in this case NDs) must be seen or their presence must be "felt." The ND themes identified three of the four themes related to behavior. They were: (1) Authentic Presence Allows NDs the Ability to Come to Know Staff; (2) Visibility Fosters Staff Accountability, Autonomy, and Responsiveness; and (3) In Role Modeling Professional Behaviors, NDs Set Clear Standards and Expectations for All Staff. (The fourth theme was NDs Empower RNs by Balancing Autonomy and Support/Advocacy.) Behavior, in part, includes visibility, physical presence, and role modeling. If presence (the overarching concept) can contribute to a safe and caring environment and positive interpersonal connections, as well as foster accountability, autonomy, and responsiveness, we need to attend to what our presence conveys!

The combination of poise, confidence, authenticity, communication, and social awareness is how Sylvia Hewlett[2] defines the concept of presence, and Kristi Hedges[3] (both leading authorities on presence) says it is about "creating an impression on others." If others see us as leaders (formally or informally), they are watching us. We want them to see us at our best because our best makes a difference.

> **REFLECTION** Have you ever had someone say a message to you that conveyed they remembered your encouraging words or that you reached out to them when they needed to have someone care? Did you remember those words or that act? How did you feel when the person conveyed how much your actions meant?

Presence also fits with the model Jim Kouzes and Barry Posner created.[4] Presence is reflective of their concept of modeling the way. How leaders act, how they appear, what they do, how they communicate—and more—are seen as cues to others regarding how they, too, should act, appear, do, communicate, and so forth. Perhaps John Maxwell says it best in his video chat on presence: "When you see it, you feel it."[5] And he says presence is based on competence. When we think about that for a moment, it is hard to envision people who are competent not acting as if they knew what they were doing. Yes, some competent people are hurried or may even seem distracted, but those whose presence fills the room convey they are competent in whatever the task is that is before them.

THE ABCs OF PRESENCE

Appearance, behavior (gravitas), and communication comprise presence. Table 25.1 summarizes what each element contributes. Each element has relevance to the overall perception of presence, but it may not be what we expect.

TABLE 25.1 The ABCs of Presence and Leadership Elements

ABCs of Presence	Examples	Leadership Elements
Appearance	Professional attire and comportment	Confident: Belief in your own abilities
Behavior/Gravitas	Acting with integrity to one's values when no one is watching	Character: the core of who you are
	Following through on promises made or decisions to act	Commitment: a promise or a pledge
Communication	Intentionally seeking to be with and getting to know others	Connectedness: being in a relationship with others
	Demonstrating empathy through listening genuinely to another	Compassion: an openness to feelings

Developing presence, as is true of every other element in the Legacy *Leaders*-Ship Trajectory personal triangle, contributes to a new way of thinking. As an example, women have often been excluded from the meeting before the meeting and in the actual meeting speak hesitantly or present ideas in a hypothetical manner rather than offering "the plan."[6] Another example might be when new leaders (in a formal position) fail to communicate regularly with the people with whom they work, aren't available (for example, feeling secure in the office and not venturing out to be with people), lack consistency in decisions, or are demanding of others. A final example is from research about questioning. Rather than talking about ourselves, if we ask frequent, probing questions, we are perceived as more responsive and are better liked.[7] Asking questions, as it turns out, is even more powerful than we first thought.

> **REFLECTION** Think of at least three questions that would precipitate responses to help you know someone else better. Remember they don't have to be personal. Asking something about a current event can precipitate insights. Over the next week, test those questions on at least three people. What did you learn you didn't know before?

In 2015, the *Wall Street Journal* carried an article with three graphics.

1. Behaviors people use to try to look smart
2. Behaviors people use that actually make them look smart
3. Behaviors others look for when judging who's smart

Rather than focusing on the first or the third lists, we are sharing the four strategies that seem to make a difference. They are looking at others when speaking, standing or sitting up straight, using a middle initial, and wearing glasses.[8] Although we may not want to wear glasses if we don't need them, the other strategies are easy to adopt if they aren't already a part of who we are.

When study participants were asked to rate candidates for leadership roles, they were given specific criteria. These individuals were the final decision makers in a formalized process. Appearance accounted for 5% of the influence on selecting a given candidate.[2] Initially, that might surprise us; however, another way to think about this finding is that those with inappropriate appearance had likely been eliminated from the interview process before they reached the final decision-makers. We like to think of appearance as the "ticket" to entry into whatever activity you wish to pursue.

The best part about appearance is this: we don't have to grow several inches, lose a lot of weight, change our gender, or buy expensive clothes. The aspect of appearance that seemed to have the greatest influence was being clean, neat, polished, and groomed—something we all can achieve. A second aspect is to look like the position we are seeking. In other words, in a rural community, wearing jeans and boots to work might be acceptable, whereas that style likely would not fit in at a large health care organization's executive headquarters in a major metropolitan area.

Looking like, acting like, and talking like are all ways to influence others to see that we are a perfect fit for a position. In other words, we need to be clothed in a manner reflective of the current organizational culture, our behaviors need to be seen as positive if they blend in with how people in the organization currently behave, and our language needs to be appropriate to the organization. Just to be clear, all of this assumes the person has the basic skills and competencies for a particular position. The ABCs can be the influencing factors when all other factors are equal.

In this same study, behavior at the micro and macro level was the most important aspect of the decisions made by the subjects. The micro level is something we are generally familiar with—body language, how we act, how we move, and even how we eat. We need to consider if we are sitting and standing up straight, if we make eye contact with others, and if we shake hands in a firm manner—if shaking hands is appropriate. Many leadership positions often involve dining experiences. Any general etiquette book helps with the basic expectations of how to function in such situations. As if the art of eating wasn't important enough, couple the art of carrying on a conversation with eating, and we readily see a challenge if we aren't prepared for it. One of our colleagues shared a story about going to his first board luncheon, piling up his plate with food, and beginning to eat when he realized no one else had really taken much food. Those who did were mostly "pushing" the food around on the plate. They were all engaged in conversation, however. Figuring out what the cultural norm is for meetings we have not previously attended is important prework. If we don't have a trusted colleague to ask, we need to be especially alert to how a group appears, behaves, and converses so we can blend in with the standard. If our intent is to be disruptive, however, we likely need to be more focused on the risks we are taking in being so.

The macro level is reflected by how well we live by our values and goals (or purpose). For example, if leaders say they believe nurses must be involved with a community effort but nothing about doing volunteer work for a community activity, board, or committee appears on their schedules or in their evaluations, no match exists, and the leaders are then less believable. Of the study participants, 67% said behavior was important. In other words, we can look great, but if we don't have that combination of micro and macro behavior, we likely will not be successful candidates for positions we seek. When micro and macro are combined, Hewlett calls this gravitas.[2]

One of us once interviewed for a key leadership position. This position included accountability for all of nursing and fundraising for the department.

"I spent the first day with several key people who were interesting and informative. Two events were very discouraging, however. First, when meeting with the current, interim occupant of the position (who had been portrayed as a noncandidate), I asked what deterred her from applying for the position. Imagine my surprise when she said, 'Oh, I am a candidate!' Competing with an internal candidate wasn't a problem—lack of truthfulness from the recruiting source was. The following morning I met at breakfast with the person who would be my immediate boss. As we were talking (about fundraising no less!), he put his finger in his mouth and scraped something off the roof of his mouth. Imagine asking people for major donations while being distracted by this physical behavior!"

We share this story to remind us all that interviews are two-way streets and what applies to applicants also applies to interviewers. This person was obviously brilliant, but the microbehavior was off-putting!

Communication accounted for 28% of the decisions made by the study subjects mentioned earlier. Superior speaking skills, the ability to command the room, and forcefulness and assertiveness were the factors comprising communication. Superior speaking skills for leaders at every level are important because we influence others through what we say and how we deliver the message. Commanding the room is suggestive of the old E. F. Hutton advertisement. The punchline of the ad was "when E. F. Hutton speaks, people listen." This statement was always delivered where a group of people was present and noise was evident. When investment words were uttered, everyone stopped speaking to listen. Although we may not want people to "hang on our every word," if we are seen as powerful (having presence), they do attend to what we say and do.

Vikram Chib of Johns Hopkins and his colleagues found that having people watch us actually might increase the quality of our performance.[9] "Speaking up proactively, not allowing the conversation to become an argument, and stating clearly what is needed/what the outcomes are to be/what actions we must take are examples of being forceful and assertive."[10] Being watched—or even thinking we are—might enhance our potential to be better at executing a positive presence.

REFLECTION Think back on the last major organizational event you attended. That event may have been a fundraiser, a summer picnic, or a board meeting. Who sticks out in your memory? Some of those outstanding people may be in your memory because they were dressed inappropriately or behaved poorly or were ineffective in communicating with others. Others of those outstanding people likely are remembered because the person looked like an ad for the event, behaved appropriately, and held others' attention when speaking. Which person do you wish to be?

INCREASING OUR PRESENCE

As Cuddy says, "Presence isn't about pretending to be competent; it's about believing in and revealing the abilities you truly have."[11] Five key practices can increase our ability to have presence. These appear in Table 25.2.

Being present requires mindfulness to be fully engaged in the moment. Focusing on the present conveys to others we are interested in them *and*, more importantly, leads to better responses. What we are doing, in a sense, is creating a more memorable experience.

TABLE 25.2 **Key Strategies for Enhancing Presence**
1. Be present: You must be known to others. To be effective, you must also be vulnerable.
2. Value trust: Trust is the most important element of creating teams.
3. Be real: Insincerity is evident, and so is sincerity.
4. Practice: Determine what you need to do to enhance your appearance, behavior, and communication.
5. Reflect: Evaluate what you have done and determine what you need to work on.

Valuing trust creates a situation where others feel free to be honest because we exhibit trust and trustworthiness. Trust relies on the bidirectional process of trusting and being trustworthy. Perhaps some of us have experiences where we misread another person or thought we could trust somebody and then were betrayed. In addition to no longer trusting that person, we become more hesitant to open up to anyone else because this situation is what we anticipate when we trust others.

Being real involves being yourself and not adopting false behaviors or mannerisms. That doesn't mean we shouldn't try to improve ourselves. Rather, we need to adopt what fits with our purpose and values. For example, if we really don't want to drink alcoholic beverages, just because the group gets together after work doesn't mean we have to drink when joining the group. If we really don't support the idea of alcohol consumption, we can politely decline the invitation while knowing (1) that act may limit our potential connections and (2) we are true to our values.

Practicing refers to anything about the ABCs that isn't fully developed and seems natural to us. We need to practice these skills just as we would practice any critical skill in our profession. If we are really concerned about how we appear, act, or communicate, we can ask a trusted colleague to video us (even on a smartphone) so that we can experience for ourselves what others do.

The last practice is reflecting. Just as we need to reflect on our functioning in general, we also need to practice on specific skills we are trying to develop. To do that, we need to reflect on our ABC skills progression.

LL ALERT

- Don't ever think "no one will notice!" *Everyone* watches a leader.
- Don't assume you can just sneak into work! Someone will see you and likely judge your appearance and behavior, even from afar.

SUMMARY

Presence is an essential part of leading effectively. Although appearance is important, being neat and polished—not necessarily fashionable—is what contributes to presence. In other words, anyone has the potential to meet this expectation. Behavior exhibits people's purposes and values. If a mismatch exists, behavior is believed over communication or appearance. Communication in leadership demands a high level of performance. All of these areas require that each of us devote energy to improving ourselves.

LL LINEUP

- Attend to both micro and macro behaviors.
- Critique the ABCs of other leaders to gain insight about being influential.

REFLECTION Consider recording a self-made video. Be your best critic. If you were meeting with your boss, evaluate your own appearance. How are your micro behaviors exhibited? Are they hinderances or helpers? What about your communication? Do you sound convincing? Are you hesitating? Based on your assessment, what is your plan to gain more presence and fully develop your ABCs?

26

Resilience

We know we have said each element of the total model is important. And yet we are going to tell you this one is critical. If you cannot be resilient, you will have the energy to do very little, and leading is tough, energy-consuming work. The Human Performance Institute defines resilience as "the ability to regularly recover, adapt and grow from stress."[1] Resiliency has also been referred to as a characteristic, skill, or process designed to reduce stress and burnout.[2] If we fail to recover, adapt, and grow, we are likely to experience disengagement, acute and chronic fatigue, and burnout. How we manage our energy levels determines how effective we can be as a leader. And if all we do is "bounce back," we are returning to where we were before. That is not a condition sustainable for leadership, which is all about advancing and being and doing better than before. The most important consideration about resiliency, however, is that it promotes personal and professional growth—in other words, it takes us beyond just bouncing back. Who among us doesn't want to be better able to adapt to life's challenges?

In an interview by Adam Grant for *FastCompany*, Doris Kearns Goodwin, the historian and political scientist who has studied presidents, said a leadership quality commonly overlooked is replenishing their energy and creativity.[3] That ability to replenish energy to accomplish major goals is what allows us to be resilient. It is akin to the "secret sauce" of leadership.

The importance of resiliency is evident in considering clinician and patient health, as seen in the National Academy of Medicine's conceptual model: Factors Affecting Clinician Well-Being and Resilience. This model illustrates the complexity of elements that affect those two aspects of health.[4] Our well-being affects our relationship with patients, which affects their well-being. Because we operate in complex environments burdened with rules and regulations, overwhelming structures, and numerous demands, our well-being can be fragile.

In a study about fatigue in nurse managers and administrators, the researchers found different themes that contributed to fatigue.[5] Managers identified their sources of fatigue as 24/7 accountability, visibility and responsiveness to staff, and interruptions in work flow. Nurse executives, on the other hand, identified meetings, long work days, leadership responsibility, and age and decreased stamina. The constancy of "being on" can lead to fatigue and the need to reenergize.

HOW RESILIENCY WORKS

Although a lot has been written about resiliency, Angela Prestia suggests that we move from the incident to the postcrisis to transformational resiliency.[6] Integrating the work of Judith Rodin[7] and Brene Brown,[8] she first detailed what happens in the incident phase where we deal with readiness, reckoning, rumble, and responsiveness (words from the work of Rodin and Brown). During the postcrisis, we deal with revitalization and revolution. Assuming we were successful in each of those phases, we experience a strengthening of our ability to deal with the next issue.

The phrase "tough old bird" probably was used to describe someone who was resilient before we really knew about the concept or the research. That phrase didn't really refer to someone who was particularly tough, in the physical sense, or old. It was a phrase designed to say the person rose up when knocked down and went on to the next challenge. If you remember, framing is a valuable strategy for leadership development. So, let's reframe challenges to growth opportunities (GOs). That reframing allows us to distance ourselves a bit from the intensity that some GOs precipitate. Our challenge now is not to survive this challenge, but to capitalize on the GO.

REFLECTION How resilient do you feel? What do you use as strategies to recover? Think back to a recent frustration at work. What precipitated it? Was it an ongoing issue or a new one? Identify who else was involved in the frustration and if a policy and/or system issue was involved. Using the idea of GO, what would it now be called?

To be ready to deal with GOs, we again need to have solid self-insight into our ability to deal with the situation. We might ask ourselves if we have the necessary skills to address the various aspects of the situation. We likely should start with a pause to consider our emotions so we don't act on those alone. The postcrisis stage involves learning that leads to better ways to adapt in the next situation, which is also the rationale for the reframing of GOs.

What makes us more resilient is probably something we all need to know, and it's especially useful information for people pursuing leadership opportunities. A study of nurse managers provides what we think is very useful information. Two questions were asked in this descriptive, cross-sectional survey: What is the level of resilience at work among first-line nurse managers? and Are years of experience in that role, years of experience as a registered nurse, and other profile characteristics related?[9] Using the Resilience at Work scale, 48 nurse managers responded to this study. The highest mean score was scored on "living authentically," a score reflective of high resilience. This was followed by "interacting cooperatively," which suggests openness to feedback, and "finding one's calling," which suggests connection of purpose at work with personal values and beliefs. That is all good news. The less good news is that "maintaining perspective" had the lowest mean score, which suggests that these nurse managers tended to worry about the problems at work as opposed to feeling they could find solutions.

HOW TO BECOME MORE RESILIENT

Several activities can help each of us be more resilient. Table 26.1 provides a list of suggestions. In the postcrisis stage mentioned earlier, we know learning occurs and that leads to better ways to adapt in the next situation. Additionally, Noreen Bernard provides a toolkit appropriate for leading self to leading organizations (and students).[10]

As with many other areas of experiences, keeping a journal is highly valuable because it allows us to review entries to determine patterns. As an example, we know a nurse (let's call him Carl) who worked with a colleague (and we'll call her Jo) who frequently had personal crises. Tracking these crises, which always affected Carl, allowed us to see a pattern. That pattern was that about every 2 months, Jo would call in sick at the last minute. Eventually we determined that timing coincided with a meeting involving a third party who was verbally aggressive. We learned this by first figuring out the pattern of the absences and then figuring out a particular meeting was scheduled and then who the players were. By pointing out this pattern to Jo, Carl could challenge the core issue of verbal abuse. Rather than intervening on behalf of Jo, however, Carl worked with Jo to build courage to challenge the behavior and the lack of anyone addressing the behavior.

TABLE 26.1 **Suggestions for Increasing Resilience**
• Adhere to policies designed to prevent and correct workplace violence, harassment, and other inappropriate behaviors.
• Keep a journal.
• Reinforce a just culture.
• Document suboptimal staffing.
• Sleep.
• Create a task force to analyze work flow to decrease load and increase productivity.
• Share your values and purpose.
• Provide individually appropriate responses to others.
• Tackle system-related issues of inefficiencies.
• Create a culture of autonomy.
• Devise meaningful recognition programs and activities.
• Take a break!
• See the potential.
• Balance your energy.
• Write a letter to someone to tell them why you admire and value them.
• Remember that our greatest learning opportunities often derive from failure.
• Identify what needs to change in our organizations to support some of these suggestions.

From Human Performance Institute. Available at: https://www.jnj.com/innovation/resilience-in-the-workplace-training-human-performance-institute. Accessed March 8, 2019.

Additionally, Press Ganey's white paper on burnout and resiliency suggests that leadership must be engaged in solving the issues clinicians identify as those that lead to burnout.[11] In general, the common stress physicians experience is comparable to that of nurses—the burden of documentation, managing the electronic health record, experiencing suboptimal staffing, excessive workloads, demands for increased productivity, inefficiencies, and limited autonomy. Examples of what seems to work for both groups are intradepartmental teamwork and recognition. Both decompression (disconnecting from work) and activation (engagement with work) seem to be important in determining who will be successful in being resilient. Additionally, being able to create contexts where clinicians can reinforce each other and their pride in care seems to be an emerging critical aspect. Perhaps what is most concerning is that younger nurses are less engaged and less able to decompress and feel activated in their roles. This has major implications for the support we provide these people, who will be the leaders of the profession in the future. Additionally, we can reduce our exposure to job stressors.[12] Of course, that is what was happening with the Carl and Jo story presented earlier! It is also the point about why we must all be vigilant about violence, harassment, and other inappropriate behaviors in the workplace.

THE IMPACT OF PERSONAL ON PROFESSIONAL

As dramatic as some workplace issues can be, they usually can be topped by personal issues. If we are stressed one place, we are likely to be stressed, or at least restrained in our ability to be resilient, in the other. We always talk about personal and professional as if we could divide ourselves or our day into those two categories. The reality, however, is that we lead integrated lives where our two views of us blend, merge, separate, reintegrate, and evolve. When one of our daughters worked for a world-famous consulting firm, she called one day, clearly exhausted. She said, "I'm making all this money but don't have time to spend any of it. I barely have time to change clothes!" That is an example of when one of our roles in life has almost been subsumed by another.

REFLECTION Consider what you did last week. When you were at work, what personal work/thoughts occurred? When you were at home, what professional work/thoughts occurred? Is it even important to separate personal and professional fully unless one has totally consumed the other?

In a *Harvard Business Review* interview, Sheryl Sandberg identified how she got to the new book, *Option B: Facing Adversity, Building Resilience, and Finding Joy*, coauthored with Adam Grant.[13] You may recall that Sheryl Sandberg lost her husband suddenly due to a cardiac condition. Now she needed someone to help her son at a father–son event. When a friend volunteered, Sandberg said she really wanted her husband to be able to do this. The friend pointed out Option A (Dave, her husband) was not an option, so Option B had to become the wow factor. "When you suffer a tragedy, the secondary loss of having it bleed into other areas of your life is so real."[14] And because we deal with loss differently, the one-size-fits-all typical policy regarding bereavement leave doesn't fit with the needs people experience. Some need to distract themselves with work; others struggle to get to work.

This discussion focuses on grief, but Adam Grant, in the same interview, points out that it really is about adversity. Maybe that is another way for us to reframe the situations we face at work. They are about situations or people who are trying to suck the life out of us. Our opportunity is to triumph over such adversity.

RESILIENCY AND WOMEN

Because the profession of nursing is still dominated by women, we felt compelled to include some thoughts of two researchers from the United Kingdom. Rosalind Gill and Shani Orgad identify that middle-class women (which is what most nurses would identify themselves as being) "possess the substance that helps them to defy the obstacles set by adversity and precarity."[15] Think about the way in which nurses persist in overcoming organizational policies, lack of supplies, bureaucratic hierarchies, incivility, and the instability of assured scheduling and care load. Even the public became aware of how nurses overcome such obstacles as story after story appeared in the media during the 2020 pandemic. We seem to thrive sometimes in figuring the best "workaround" of the day. Actually, that is a sad statement because we should have been able to identify an issue, report it to some person who has the authority to change the policy, secure the supplies, and so forth.

Many of the insights that Gill and Orgad provide are comparable to content in this book. To be clear, we are not providing information about strategies such as journaling, reframing, "run to the lion," and so forth as ways to tolerate what might be poor workplace practices. (Those are but some of the examples the authors provide from their study.) Rather, we have provided those strategies because they help us maintain forward momentum in bringing about needed changes in spite of poor workplace practices. Being firm and being tactful, as an example, are strategies that frequently work in our society. We certainly don't want to cave on a topic of great importance, nor do we gain anything by not being tactful.

The idea of resiliency, or bouncing back as it is often called, is even an expectation of female employees. Perhaps those of us who are female are too good at being resilient because others rely on us to be the flexible element. For example, what other services are available throughout a hospital 24/7? What other profession "fills the void" in numerous ways? In part, we do so because what we typically fill in relates to quality patient care. How many other departments in a hospital have "flex" staff who come in or stay home on short notice? It isn't that other areas don't have these same commitments; rather, our numbers make the point a dramatic one. Our resiliency has supported these practices. Maybe some need to remain, but maybe some need to be examined to be certain we aren't being detrimental to our health in our attempt to be flexible. Several of the founding faculty at Texas Tech University Health Sciences Center called ourselves willows. Like a willow tree, we would gracefully move from one position to another and "go with the flow" as the new school developed. We had to in order to implement the new program. This is analogous to any totally new venture. Even extremely well-developed plans are seldom comprehensive in implementation. Resiliency is a key factor in new endeavors.

LL ALERT

- Don't engage in "bad habits" to tolerate issues that are stressful rather than learning to become more resilient.
- Don't allow one aspect of your life to overtake your entire being.

SUMMARY

Resiliency is a critical consideration for anyone interested in advancing their leadership. Being able to motivate ourselves, knowing how to navigate tough situations, and becoming more resilient help people have the ability to go back into the same situation with enthusiasm for change.

LL LINEUP

- Live authentically.
- Solve problems that are described as leading to burnout.

REFLECTION Imagine for a moment that you experienced a significant personal loss. How much time are you able to take away from work to reorganize your life? Will your position be protected? Is the time allocated too much or insufficient? What resources will you draw on to thrive during this period? Now repeat that process assuming you experienced a significant professional loss. How much time can you take away from family to reorganize your life? Will your family life be "protected?"

27

Risking

Taking a risk, whether small or monumental, can be unnerving—even scary—for the risk-taker.

"Years ago, I had two simultaneous job opportunities. One of these offered slightly more responsibility than I had in previous assignments but in an environment that was similar to my previous roles. The second opportunity was in a role in which I had little practical experience but offered exciting professional opportunities, to say nothing of significantly more reimbursement. What to do? One job offered very little risk. The other had the potential for excitement and challenge; however, the risk of failure was much higher.

"I sought counsel from a wise mentor. He gave me one of the best pieces of advice I have ever received. He suggested that I sit quietly and review each offer. He recommended that I not think of the money offered or the security provided. Instead, he suggested that I decide which opportunity made me most excited to do the work. I did what he suggested and realized that the opportunity that offered excitement and challenge—and more risk—was the position I should accept.

"How did this decision turn out? Well, it was a 3-year journey of excitement, challenge, learning, and stress. Although I ended up being downsized in a time when the organization was retrenching and letting go of many employees, I have never regretted my decision. Despite the stress, anxiety, and some very difficult moments, this risk was one of the greatest intellectual and emotional learning opportunities of my life. I am most grateful for the opportunity to accept this risk."

REFLECTION Have you taken a risk that did not turn out well? Was there anything you could have done to reduce the risk potential of this situation? What did you learn from this situation?

TAKING RISKS

Risking is a key component of leadership. The Oxford English Dictionary defines *risk* as exposure to loss, injury, or other adverse or unwelcome circumstance.[1] Despite this negative connotation, taking a risk also implies that if the loss, injury, or other adverse circumstances can be overcome, the rewards may be substantial. In fact, the possibility of a reward is frequently the motivating factor for taking a risk. A *risk factor* is defined as the probability of something happening multiplied by the resulting cost or benefit if it does. Fig. 27.1 illustrates this definition.

As T. S. Elliott once said, "Only those who will risk going too far can possibly find out how far it is possible to go."[2] Let's explore the type of person who is likely to take risks and factors that often stop us from taking that step toward risking.

Deborah Piscione suggests that riskers, usually individuals with an innovative spirit, "refuse to accept the status quo." They are in touch with a much greater purpose in life and focus on ideas that emphasize value creation above all else. In short, they are creators, not observers, perhaps because they are incredibly curious about why things are the way they are. They believe that anything is possible. They value talented people and understand how and when to collaborate with them. Because of this they are able to effectively execute an innovative idea, at times because they can do it themselves or they can delegate it to others.[3]

This description sets a high bar, and many of us may think that it certainly does not describe our behaviors. Why in the world should we put ourselves in such a scary and uncertain position? Yet it is true that being risk-averse also

$$\text{Risk factor} = \frac{\text{Probability of occurrence}}{\text{Cost or benefit}}$$

Fig. 27.1 Risk factor formula.

TABLE 27.1 Steps to Improve Willingness to Take Risks

Steps	Suggestions
Step 1: Listen to your intuition.	Sit quietly and consider what actions best fit with your values.
Step 2: Don't become paralyzed in the assessment process	In making a decision, rarely are the timing and situation perfect—at some point you have to "step off the ledge."
Step 3: Don't let what you know guide all of your actions.	Sometimes what worked before will never work again. Sometimes what has not been tried will actually work. This step is particularly helpful in response to those who say, "We tried that before and it didn't work."
Step 4: Start with baby steps.	For example, starting by implementing a pilot study can give you the courage (and data) to take a bigger step.

Adapted from Tull M. How taking risks evokes leadership success. Huff Post Blog. December 6, 2017. Available at: https://www.huffingtonpost.com/megan-tull/how-taking-risks-evokes-l_b_10843744.html. Accessed February 2019.

carries risk. Often risk-adverse people see themselves as deliberate, cautious, and thoughtful. Unfortunately, these characteristics can also be seen as lacking in courage and confidence, traits that may limit our professional trajectory.[4]

GENDER DIFFERENCES IN RISK-TAKING

In both individual and group decisions, women seem to be more risk-averse than men. However, women's tendency to take fewer risks than men is much less rooted in nature than it is in the way women are nurtured.[5,6] This has considerable impact on the limitations in innovation in nursing. Fortunately, we can all improve our ability to take considered risks by examining the positive and negative aspects of our own behavior.

> **REFLECTION** Does your experience suggest that gender differences in risk-taking exist? Provide some examples of your observations that validate your observations.

IMPROVING YOUR RISK-TAKING SKILLS

Fear is at the core of the inability to take risks: Fear of failure, fear of success; fear of looking like a fool, fear of seeming stupid or too aggressive. Becoming a competent risk-taker means that we must confront these fears and gather the courage to move. To help us move past this fear, we need to realize that failure is simply an opportunity to learn from our mistakes. The very real discomfort we feel when we fail can motivate us to analyze our actions and make corrections. Through failure, we learn about our own strengths, talents, and resilience, all of which improve our chances of getting it right the next time. The feedback we receive after a failure is often the critical difference in ultimate success. In addition, the confidence we develop from acting, failing, and then moving forward toward success will stimulate us to take risks more often. Megan Tull,[8] a columnist for Huffington Post, suggests four steps to improve our willingness to consider taking a risk. See Table 27.1.

Tull[7] also suggests several other ideas that can support us as we try to "step out of our comfort zone." We must be willing to think big and have a vision of where we want to go. Limiting our thinking contributes to being risk-averse. Renaming the behavior of risk-taking can often help us to take the risk. For example, we can think of risk-taking as innovation—that sounds much more positive—and appealing—than taking a risk. In addition, focusing on the outcomes and the rewards rather than the possible negative consequences of our action can motivate us to act.

"When I was 'moaning' about the possibility of failing in a particular situation, a dear friend said to me, 'Well, you will certainly fail if you don't try.'"

> **REFLECTION** Consider the last time you "stepped out of your comfort zone." What was the result? What did you learn? Is there anything you plan to do differently the next time you take a risk?

CONSIDERED RISK-TAKING

Despite the importance of embracing risk as the path to success, we must not be impulsive in our risk-taking. Crenshaw and Yoder-Wise[8] call a measured approach to

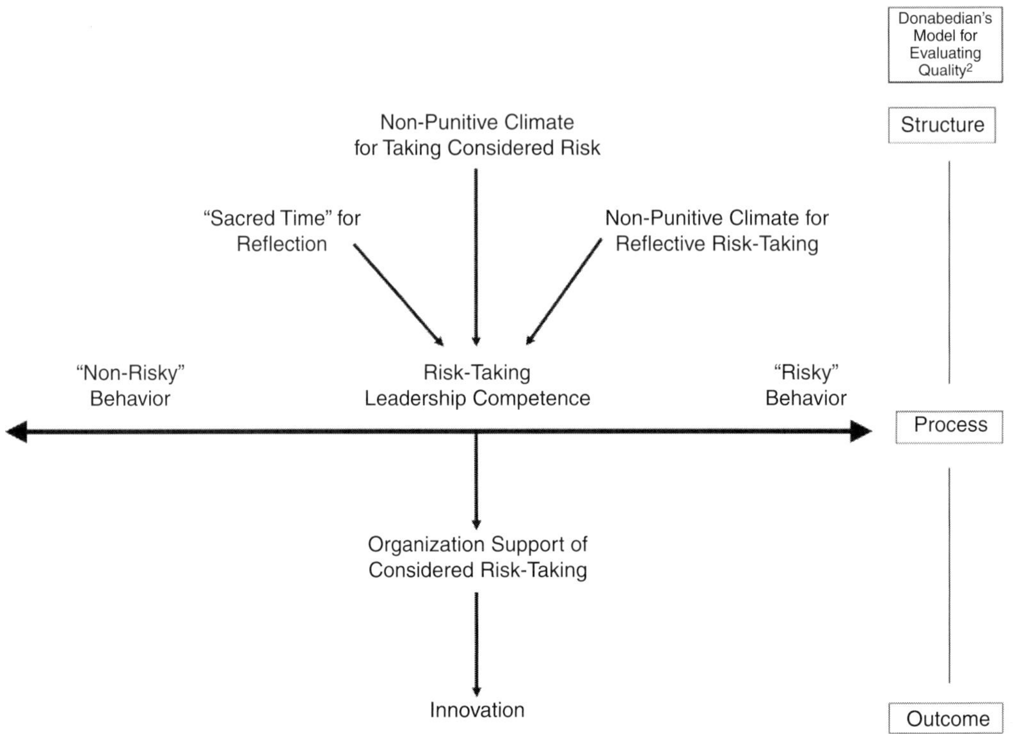

Fig. 27.2 Risk-taking model.

risking "considered risk-taking." They suggest that risk-taking can be thought of as a continuum from nonrisky behavior on one end to risky behavior on the other. Considered risk-takers' position is typically located in the middle of the continuum. This position requires the risk-taker to assess the environmental structure and processes, as well as the evidence associated with the possible action. The evidence must be compared with the innovation (risk) being considered. Taking time to reflect on the risks and benefits in order to balance the innovation with the evidence is critical to remaining in the center of the risk-taking continuum.[8] Fig. 27.2 illustrates the continuum.

An additional component of the conceptual model of considered risk-taking is the extent to which the organization supports the risk. The organization must allow time for reflection for the risk-taker and colleagues involved in the innovation—often a change from the action orientation of many organizations today.[8] In addition, the organization must create a culture where failure is embraced and seen as an opportunity to grow. Nurse leaders within the organization can serve as role models in this regard by valuing and supporting the mistakes of those with whom they work. They can also acknowledge their own mistakes.

"This approach is in direct opposition to an experience I had when I was 'pitching' an innovative idea to my boss. She said, 'I really support taking risks, as long as they are successful.' Imagine the pressure to succeed in this sort of environment.

"On the other hand, I have" had many examples of support for innovation in my career. Some years ago, my university received a grant to institute a collaborative community simulation center for the university's Bachelor's of Science in Nursing (BSN) and allied health programs, an Associate's degree in nursing (ADN) program from another college, and a regional hospital. One of the innovations of the program was to use BSN-prepared registered nurses (RNs) as staff for the simulation lab, under the supervision of a Master's of Science in Nursing (MSN)–prepared director. In a geographic area where MSN-prepared faculty was at a premium, this approach allowed us to increase the number of students we could serve, ultimately addressing the shortage of nurses in the area.

"At that time, using BSN nurses to teach health assessment for RN students was not permitted in the state board of

nursing (BON) rules and regulations. Faculty members who taught health assessment were required to hold at least an MSN. Fortunately, the state BON was very supportive of this innovation in staffing of a simulation center. So in the absence of specific evidence that a clinical simulation experience is ineffective without an all-MSN staff and with a strong evaluation process in place, we were given permission to proceed. This risk resulted in successful education for an increased number of BSN and ADN prelicensure students, as well as ongoing competency evaluations of a host of hospital staff. This ultimately increased the number of graduates available to practice in the area. In addition, as an added benefit, each of the BSN simulation coordinators ultimately earned a MSN and became full-time faculty members. This was a considered risk that worked out well."

LL ALERT

- Don't let fear stop you from taking a risk.
- Don't implement an innovation impulsively.
- Don't berate a colleague or employee for making a mistake.

SUMMARY

Considered risk-taking is a leadership competence.[8] Risking is a necessary personal characteristic for effective leaders who are charged with leading change in a team or organization. Since the future is unknowable, no amount of planning can guarantee that a plan for change will result in positive outcomes. A leader must be able to choose strategies that have the greatest chance for success, while planning for potential negative consequences—and then take the necessary risk.

LL LINEUP

- Approach risks from a standpoint of considered risk-taking.
- Test risk-taking to make some progress.

REFLECTION Consider a situation where you took a risk. What strategies did you use to prepare for taking a considered risk? Were they effective? What did you learn as part of this process?

28

Spirituality

What is spirituality, and why would we include this concept? Some would say that "spirituality is a broad concept with room for many perspectives. In general, it includes a sense of connection to something bigger than ourselves, and it typically involves a search for meaning in life. As such, it is a universal human experience—something that touches us all. People may describe a spiritual experience as sacred or transcendent or simply a deep sense of aliveness and interconnectedness."[1] Another way to view spirituality, according to Christina Puchalski,[2] is an aspect of humanity that refers to ways people seek and express meaning and purpose and the way they are connected to the self, to other human beings, to nature, and to what is significant to them or to the sacred. Many people think of spirituality in association with significant questions, such as: What is my sense of purpose? Am I a good person? What is my connection to the world around me? Do events in life happen for a reason? What is the meaning of suffering? Or how can I live my life in the best possible way?

From another perspective, let's examine similarities and differences between spirituality and religion.[3] These two concepts can be used in similar contexts, and in reality, some overlap exists between the two. We can have a belief in organized religion that is very spiritual, yet this spiritualism may not lead to an organized religious system. And some people can be very thoughtful about spirituality but are not committed to an organized religion. Likewise, it is possible for a very "religious" person to lack a deep spiritual connection to their faith or organized religion. In other words, religious behavior can become a pattern or habit.

SPIRITUALITY AND RELIGION: HOW THEY ARE DIFFERENT

Some people think of spirituality in a religious framework, and it can incorporate aspects of religion. However, spirituality and religion are not the same. In spirituality, the focus is on where each of us as leaders finds meaning and value. From a religious perspective, the focus is on what is right or true. Some think of the two as circles slightly overlapping. In the intersection of spirituality and religion is a personal experience that affects thinking, feeling, and behavior. In this overlapping space, belief systems also exist, and these serve as a reflection on life and experiences that influence current behavior and provide comfort and reassurance in our beliefs, ethics, or moral principles. Such beliefs or principles govern behavior, activities, and "awe," which is a feeling of reverential respect mixed with fear or wonder.

SPIRITUALITY COMPARED WITH EMOTIONAL HEALTH

Spirituality has also been associated with emotional health. Practices that support spirituality are similar to those that are focused on improving emotional well-being. In Table 28.1 we have identified "12 Symptoms of Spiritual Awakening,"[4] and it becomes clear that many of these symptoms resemble those provided for improving emotional health. In expanding our spirituality, we seek meaningful connections with something bigger than ourselves, and this searching can culminate in positive emotions, such as contentment, peacefulness, gratitude, and acceptance. In this process of seeking, we can connect with other people and, perhaps, a sense of higher purpose. We can see that the linkages of emotions and spirituality can become deeply integrated, one with the other. What is needed, as Thomas Merton said, is "to know precisely what is happening, or exactly where it is all going. What you need is to recognize the possibilities and challenges offered by the present moment, and to embrace them with courage, faith and hope."[5]

WHAT MAKES SPIRITUALITY IMPORTANT?

Research is now beginning to indicate that spiritual practices are associated with better health and feelings of well-being. Some spirituality practices that support improved health include meditation, prayer, yoga, and journaling. Contemplative practices can be both practical and transformative due to developing a capacity for deep concentration. Matthieu Ricard, a neuroscientist who has lived in the Himalayans with the Dali Lama, has been involved with

TABLE 28.1 **Symptoms of a Spiritual Awakening**

Spiritual Symptoms	Emotional Well-Being
1. An increased tendency to let things happen rather than make them happen.	Avoid or curtail the desire to control most of those events or happenings around you—they are "out of your control."
2. Frequent attacks of smiling.	Research has shown that smiling releases serotonin, a neurotransmitter that produces feelings of happiness and well-being.
3. Feelings of being connected with others and nature.	Being connected to other human beings is at the core of the human experience and increases positive feelings.
4. Frequent overwhelming episodes of appreciation.	Appreciation and acknowledgment are about recognition of you or another human being, and receiving recognition usually leads to feelings of well-being.
5. A tendency to think and act spontaneously rather than from fears based on past experience.	Fear is false evidence appearing real. To allay fears and identify their false aspects can reduce fear and increase spontaneity.
6. An unmistakable ability to enjoy each moment.	Power is in the present moment. Focusing on the present moment and taking action increases well-being.
7. A loss of the ability to worry.	Worry refers to negative thoughts and emotions and can be described as a response to a moderate challenge when the person has inadequate skills. Decreasing worry increases emotional well-being.
8. A loss of interest in conflict.	Conflict is disagreement or disharmony between people, and people who are emotionally distraught can be more susceptible to creating conflict. Decreasing conflict increases emotional health.
9. A loss of interest in interpreting the actions of others.	A common practice can be to imagine motivation for the actions of others. Letting go of such imaginings increases emotional well-being.
10. A loss of interest in judging others.	Judgment of others often occurs with initial interactions and very little data or understanding. Being curious about the reasoning of others rather than judgmental increases emotional well-being
11. A loss of interest in judging self.	Who is the toughest person on you? Yourself, of course. Practicing self-forgiveness leads to increased emotional well-being.
12. Gaining the ability to love without expecting anything in return.	Think about the unconditional love of your dog or other pet. We want to love others unconditionally. Having no expectations increases emotional health and well-being.

Adapted from Anonymous. 12 Symptoms of Spiritual Awakening. Available at: https://www.bing.com/images/search?q=12+symptoms+of+spiritual+awakening&qpvt=12+symptoms+of+spiritual+awakening&FORM=IGRE

research projects in France and the United States dealing with contemplative practices and their impact on the human brain.[6] It is possible to quiet the mind in the midst of the action and distraction of everyday activities. A state of calm centeredness can serve as an aid in dealing with crisis situations, as well as serve to explore meaning, purpose, and values, particularly as they relate to the crisis. Contemplative practice can be experienced as meditation, which induces feelings of clear-headedness and calm while improving concentration. Research has shown that meditation increases brain density and reduces sensitivity to pain. In addition, the immune system is enhanced and stress can be relieved. Specifically, the research has shown improvement for patients with conditions such as depression, anxiety, cancer, and chronic pain.[6]

Contemplative practices also consist of various forms of meditation; focused thought; writing; and contemplative arts, including drawing, painting, and dance. Some devotees find activity is helpful, such as yoga or tai chi. Others prefer silent practices, like mindfulness meditation. Some people appreciate religious or cultural tradition and find them soothing to the soul. At the same time, whereas some practices are done in solitude, groups and communities can engage in practices that involve social reflection. As mentioned earlier, yoga, journaling, and prayer can also stimulate feelings of hope and compassion. Prayer is founded in a belief in a higher power that can influence our lives. This gives credence to a resulting sense of comfort, support, and healing.[7]

REFLECTION Experiment with one approach, such as meditation, reflection, yoga, or journaling. Practice your chosen approach for 2 weeks and evaluate the outcome.

Yoga, a centuries-old practice, can yield a sense of unity within a person through breathing and physical positions. For many, the regular practice of yoga can reduce inflammation, lower blood pressure, and decrease stress. It can increase the sense of well-being. Like yoga, other forms of structured physical activity such as tai chi, martial arts, and dance can also provide a sense of well-being. Journaling can help us become more aware of our inner thoughts and our inner sense of values, and it can serve to clarify thinking and issues or struggles in life. Writing about what happens, what feelings resulted, and what values were involved can help to identify specific challenges and to see ourselves and others more clearly.

Spirituality may help us make healthier choices due to some of the traditions around spiritual practices, such as avoiding unhealthy behaviors (e.g., smoking, excessive drinking, or violent behavior). At the same time, because of these rituals, we may be more likely to adhere to healthy behaviors such as exercise, participation in community activities, and giving to others. Forgiveness is taught by many of these practices, and "letting go" of negative feelings such as anger, revenge, and blaming has been shown to increase immune function, lower blood pressure, and improve general health.

DEVELOPING SPIRITUAL RESOURCES

Spirituality may be as important as exercising or building strong relationships. Finding meaning in life, as well as thinking about life's central issues of meaning and lived values, can enhance a sense of connectedness within ourselves, as well as with a greater presence. Cultivating spirituality can include a focus on empathy and compassion for ourselves and others. Empathy and compassion have a strong connection to spirituality. One of us served in the Army Nurse Corps in Vietnam in a surgical hospital not unlike the one in the television series *MASH*:

"Many of us who served in Vietnam, attempting to make sense of the death and destruction, experienced posttraumatic stress. In the ensuing spiritual struggle, I transferred many of these feelings into work in my specialty area, obstetrics. My compassion and empathy was focused on parents experiencing stillborn/newborn loss. The process began with changes in the labor and delivery policies, which focused on giving parents choices to see and hold newborns and on facilitating a positive bereavement process. To this end, a colleague and I started one of the first stillborn loss parent support groups through hospice. I researched and wrote about these processes and completed my doctoral dissertation with a qualitative study of the influence of social networks on the process of bereavement for parents. This was my effort to integrate the violence and destruction of war into something positive.

"When I became a director of maternal child services, staff would ask me to see bereaved parents. I would sit down on the bed and say to the parents, 'The staff are very concerned about you. Can you tell me about your experience?' They would talk and cry for most of an hour or more. Sitting with this kind of psychological pain and being 100% present is some of the most exhausting work I have done. Much of this work emphasized spirituality and the empathy and compassion for parents experiencing so much psychological pain and distress. In retrospect, this work allowed me to come to terms with my wartime experience."

Empathy is demonstrated by a willingness to understand another person's emotions, especially upset. When we see the upset involved with patients and families in crisis, we choose to see the behavior as fear, shock, pain, and lack of control. We choose to console or deescalate situations rather than to judge and make them wrong. Think about applying this same approach to upset coworkers.

REFLECTION When was the last time you judged yourself? Think about what you did and why. Then be your own nurse and sit in nonjudgment. How would you describe that situation in nonjudgmental terms?

Practicing empathy and compassion actually serves to increase our spirituality because it helps us relinquish self-centered ways of thinking and increase our relationships with colleagues and coworkers. Three aspects of empathy and compassion include listening deeply with a focus on prioritizing the other person's narrative above what we might like to say, considering the other person's perspective through imagining what it would be like to be in their situation, and looking for the good by actively thinking about the other person's positive attributes.

REFLECTION What are your good attributes?

Another aspect of increasing our spirituality is to identify our beliefs and values and to strive to live by these in a daily intentional way. We might ask ourselves what matters the most. What drives our actions and behavior? What do we believe is the right thing to do?

TABLE 28.2 **Nine Steps to Forgiveness**

Actions	Discussion
1. Know exactly how you feel.	Articulate what was not okay about a situation. You can share with one or two trusted friends to support you in reflection on the situation.
2. Commit to yourself to feel better.	Forgiveness is for you, not for the other person.
3. Forgiveness is not about reconciliation.	Forgiveness is not about condoning the person's actions. Rather, you are seeking peace and understanding that comes from blaming people less and taking offenses less personally.
4. Get the right perspective.	Recognize that distress is the result of hurt feelings, thoughts, and physical upset in the moment, not from the event minutes, hours, or days before.
5. Practice stress management at the time of the event.	Soothe the fight-or-flight response. Breathe deeply and consciously or take a walk outside.
6. Manage expectations.	Give up expecting things from life and from other people that they can't or won't give you. You can hope for health, love, and friendship and work hard to get them, but you do not have the power to make them happen.
7. Understand where to put your energy.	Create positive ways to meet your goals in ways other than the one that hurt you.
8. A life well lived is the best revenge.	Rather than focusing on wounded feelings and giving power to the person who caused you pain, look for the love, beauty, and kindness. Put energy into appreciating what you have rather than what you do not have.
9. Alter the way you look at your past.	Remind yourself of your heroic choice to forgive.

Adapted from Greater Good in Action at Berkeley. Nine steps to forgiveness. Available at: https://ggia.berkeley.edu/practice/nine_steps_to_forgiveness.

Work done at Berkeley has identified activities to increase our spirituality through practicing forgiveness of others and especially ourselves[8] (Table 28.2). Carl Thoresen and Frederic Luskin at the Stanford Forgiveness Project,[9] suggest separating feelings from an actual experience versus feelings evolving from someone making us wrong or doing something negative toward us. It is also possible that as we reflect on the episode, our anger escalates. An alternate approach could focus on reflecting on the effect of each perspective and letting go of the unhelpful aspects. We need to be gentle with ourselves and realize we do not have to interact with the person who wronged us. Forgiveness is for us, not the other person, so the other person does not control our lives. Just forgive.

SPIRITUALITY AND LEADERSHIP

What is the value of spirituality in health care leadership? A Catholic, Sister Joan Puls, describes spirituality as a force that focuses on "our human responses to the brokenness of our world, the threats to our planet home, the crisis points in our own lives, and the pleas and plight of human beings around us."[10] In health care we see the crisis points in the lives of our patients and their families, as well as our employees and our physician and allied health partners. As a servant or transformational or authentic leader, we cannot help but be affected by the enormity of these processes and wonder, "How do we cope?" In part, an answer to such questions comes with incorporating spiritual practices: meditation, prayer, yoga, reflection, empathy, and compassion. Part of our personal growth is reaching the calm that is the central focus of such practices.

LL ALERT

- Don't hang onto anger, upset, or hate.
- Don't demonstrate anger, upset, or hate.

SUMMARY

Increasing our knowledge and understanding of spirituality will increase our thoughtfulness as a leader. Whether we are religious or not, a better understanding of our thinking and our values and beliefs will serve to unite us in how we view the world and the human beings we encounter. We become more centered and focused and less prone to upset or emotional reactions to people and situations. Our very lives become more valuable.

LL LINEUP

- Consider what would increase our spirituality.
- Practice adopting spiritual practices.
- Clarifying our values and beliefs will help us see how we interact with the concept of spirituality.

REFLECTION Reflect on the last time an incident occurred in which you were hurt or demeaned or wronged. How did you respond? What were your words and actions? Now rethink how you might have viewed this event differently? Use the nine steps of forgiveness (see Table 28.2) to consider other perspectives and how you might think differently about the event.

29

Timing

If you haven't heard the saying, "It's all about timing," you have missed a major point in life! We may have a great idea, but if the timing isn't right, the idea falls on deaf ears. If we have a half-baked idea and the timing is right, we will either look foolish for being incomplete or like geniuses because the idea sparked creativity for others and the idea took off.

WHEN IS THE RIGHT TIME?

Merriam-Webster's second definition of timing is the focus of this concept: the ability to select the precise moment for doing something for optimum effect.[1] The idea that we can predict when the perfect time is may be difficult to believe. However, we regularly receive cues that tell us about timing. For example, when one of us had to figure out just the right time to go talk to her boss, this wasn't wasted energy. Reading the situation was critical to gaining resources or approval for important work. We commonly hear stories about people seeing "the tell" in poker—the cues that tell others someone has a winning hand or is bluffing. This is what timing is about.

People send cues all day long about when they are receptive to information, or are upset, or don't want to hear one new idea. For example, if someone who normally is neat arrives at work appearing disheveled, now is not the time to present a new idea. It will just sound like one more distraction in an already distracted day. When we normally stand at a doorway to give our bosses important information because they are ready to leave for another meeting and they invite us in, that, too, tells us something—this might be the time to link some idea to the important information at hand because our bosses have time. Even in social settings we discern who is happy, sad, angry, bored, disengaged, or the life of the party. When we make the effort, we read other people as well as we read our patients. And if we read any number of negative messages, we tend to avoid that person.

Jo Ellen Koerner, a former chief nursing officer in South Dakota, tells the story of running to the lion. The gist of that story is that when the lion seems distressed, other animals flee. Yet the lion is often signaling danger or that it needs help. Thus we should run to the lion. When Jo Ellen heard comparable signals of distress in health care, she would go to the source rather than go away from it. When a physician, for example, is upset, many of us seek shelter out of the area so as to avoid having any of the negativism directed at us. Jo Ellen would say, however, that we should run to that person and ask what is wrong and how we might help. In addition to the potential of diffusing the situation, the physician may see us as supportive and listen to what we have to offer to help resolve whatever the upset was about initially. This unexpected behavior, in essence, creates a timing event when we might be better heard.

Mary Beth Kingston, 2019 President of the American Organization for Nursing Leadership, says that she never experienced the message of "it's time for a change" in terms of her career.[2] Rather, she indicates, she was attracted to something specific. So sometimes, changes we attribute to time are really more about other factors.

DECIDING THE CONSEQUENCES OF TIMING

If a decision has few consequences, and especially none that are negative, and we haven't set something in place that is difficult to retrieve or modify, we can easily make a decision. Why waste many people's time if whatever the decision is really doesn't make a difference? Should we subscribe to the *Harvard Business Review* ourselves, or should we access it electronically through our organization's library? That decision is easily changed and probably affects no one in a negative manner. The timing can easily be done quickly because we didn't have to "read" other people or place a major budget request or consult someone regarding how to accomplish this. On the other hand, when a decision has major consequences, especially ones with negative aspects or ones that cannot easily be changed, our timing should be such that we allow for a lot of input. As an example, as a fairly young nurse, one of us worked with a chief nursing officer who insisted that we have the architects build a replica (to scale) of a patient room before launching a major construction project:

"She received a lot of pushback for 'wasting time and money' until nurses providing direct care 'tested' the room by simulating (before simulation was known) admitting a patient from the emergency department or recovery room. Guess what? The patient transfer couldn't happen because the room was not large enough to accommodate the bed, people, and the patient on a moving trolley! We also discovered that if a patient attempted to go to the bathroom alone, the door opened the wrong way, and if a walker were used, the patient and the walker couldn't fit through the doorway. What a disaster that would have been to have built a whole extension with rooms that didn't work." (In the intervening years, many organizations did not take the time and support the expense to test new areas before committing to the plans. In an evidence-based world, we wouldn't allow this quicker timing to occur because we would rely on the evidence of avoiding these negative consequences.)

Even though the study we are about to reference focused on chief executive officers (CEOs), we can learn a lot in translating the findings to our profession and positions. The CEO Genome Project was a 10-year study involving 17,000 assessments of people working in what is known as the *C Suite* (any of the people with the title "chief something or other") with 2000 CEOs.[3] These researchers found four behaviors that related to successful leaders, two of which relate to timing. Table 29.1 identifies those four behaviors.

The first finding relates directly to timing. Deciding with speed and conviction suggests that being decisive leads to being successful. "They make decisions earlier, faster, and with greater conviction. They do so consistently—even amid ambiguity, with incomplete information, and in unfamiliar domains."[3] The findings indicated that being decisive and successful were highly correlated, which suggest that we may wait too long in reaching a decision or that we don't do so with conviction. Many of the CEOs reported actively garnering opinions, and those often came from what we would call our Circle of Advisors, highly trusted colleagues who readily tell us the truth about their perceptions.

TABLE 29.1 **The Four Behaviors of Successful CEOs**
1. Deciding with speed and conviction.
2. Engaging for impact.
3. Adapting proactively.
4. Delivering reliably.

REFLECTION When was the last time you called on your circle? If you are going to have such a valuable resource, you don't want to abuse their time and, equally important, you don't want to only call on them very occasionally. If it has been more than 6 months, consider why you are not using them on a regular basis. Maybe you need new advisors because you now have the problems under control that made you seek out your current group initially. Or maybe you have been muddling through without taking advantage of this wise counsel. Can your group of advisors help you reach decisions more quickly?

The authors point out that CEOs may also ask if a particular decision should be made at a different level. This point seems to be especially useful for us because we often enter leadership roles from being seen as a highly competent direct care nurse. It is easy for us to rely on our comfort zone of clinical decisions when we have a highly competent group who can make those decisions but may not be able to make the decisions that are ours to make.

The third finding also relates directly to timing. Adapting proactively suggests that timing is critical. We need to move quickly when presented with issues, and if we are really smart, we need to figure out what issues are likely to occur and prevent them from occurring or being so ready to respond to a situation so that it doesn't have the opportunity to escalate. Although much of being a CEO could be almost predicted behavior, the things that haven't happened before are the ones that require quick thinking and then using the situation to make an issue better.

Think, for example, when the first case of Ebola occurred in the United States. We weren't operating from past experiences because this was the first case. We had to quickly decide what the next steps were and help write the protocols for how to deal with such a situation the next time.

When September 11, 2001, occurred, hospitals, especially in the area near the World Trade Center, were inundated with demands never before experienced. They, too, were writing the new protocols for history.

The pandemic of COVID-19 highlighted how quickly adaptations needed to be made because this novel virus had no specific point of comparison with other viruses. Thus everything was learned as we moved through the crisis.

Finally, if we want to think about an historical example, we can think about Florence Nightingale in the Crimean War.[4] Once she figured out that washing hands was important, she made sure that became part of the knowledge shared with her staff in the war and later with her students in her school of nursing. Her quick decision about what was needed, plus her political influence, allowed her to obtain such basic supplies as soap, which saved thousands of soldiers.

REFLECTION If you were asked about an example of your adapting proactively, what would you offer?

Again, a difference with successful CEOs was the amount of time they spent on long-term issues. Although many of us in our leadership roles might not be expected to plan long term, we have a couple of good reasons to do so. First, we need to have a long-range view of what we might like to do in our profession. As one of us is prone to say, "we might have several jobs and even lose some, but we have one profession or career, and because of nursing's breadth and depth, we can change jobs numerous times and still be functioning as nurses." Also of note is the idea that setbacks or failures, as we said before, are seen as growth opportunities; when the setbacks were viewed as failures, those individuals were less likely to be seen as successful CEOs. In this study, 90% of the CEOs who were successful also had a positive attitude about growth opportunities! We, too, can learn from that perspective.

One final note about this study: "100% of low-performing CEOs in our sample scored high on integrity, and 97% scored high on work ethic."[3] In other words, even low performers were "good guys"; they simply weren't successful. Similarly, we all want nurses in any position to have integrity and a solid work ethic. Those two characteristics may not help us select the best leaders. In part, the idea that every nurse is a leader (and must be) is based on the reality that often the only person we have to rely on in a particular situation is ourselves. We must be able to take charge (at least of ourselves, and preferably others) to quickly move through negative situations. Simultaneously, we must rely on our colleagues because strength is in numbers.

TIMING IMPLICATIONS FOR LEADERSHIP

Timing has been a topic of interest in various fields and for some time. Fortunately, for busy leaders, Daniel Pink, author of several books and former speechwriter for Vice President Al Gore, did our work for us when he wrote *When: The Scientific Secrets of Perfect Timing.*[5] He culled the literature related to timing and offered important conclusions for our consideration. Our cognitive abilities vary throughout the day. Those variations are dramatic enough to dictate that we should do certain tasks at certain times in the day. Further, the very nature of our performance varies with the type of tasks. As an example, for those of us who are chief nursing officers (CNOs) with reporting relationships with the board, Pink found the best time for the CEO to report to the board was early in the day. Would it be logical that this timing is best for CNOs too? Well, likely it is, and that is good because many boards don't meet all day and would likely not return for a meeting with someone at a different time of day for another portion of the organization.

"When" also depends on the type of people we are: early bird (lark), owl (late night), and the "middle" or as Pink dubbed them, third birds. Throughout the day we have peaks, troughs, and recovery, and part of our challenge is to figure out who we really are—and who others are. Rather than forming a stereotypical thought about someone who looks too tired to be at work, consider that person may be struggling to make it through a trough period of the day. We don't get to control when meetings occur, unless we are the ones calling the meeting. Otherwise, we need to learn to adapt sufficiently to perform at an acceptable level and know if that is our peak, trough, or recovery period. It isn't as if we can't function unless we are at our peak levels; it is, however, that we do our best if we are.

If we are trying to be creative, we probably shouldn't be doing that work first thing in the morning! That is when we are much more analytical. The synthesized research suggests that we would do better work on budgets, on balancing our checkbooks, or on detail-type tasks such as proofing a policy if we did it in the morning. If, however, we need to devise a new process for providing care or think about the future (of us or our organization), we are far better doing that in the afternoon.

REFLECTION What part of the day do you control? Are you maximizing your time? Are you a lark, an owl, or a third bird? Are tasks such as those described earlier matched to your peaks and troughs?

RECOVERY

So much of timing is considered in terms of peak performance. Less time and effort are devoted to considering the time of recovery. Clearly, sleep is one of the recovery strategies, and few of us get sufficient sleep. Yet other strategies can be used to recover. These restorative periods are guided by five principles, as shown in Table 29.2.

The idea of something beating nothing can mean something so simple as taking a quick break from some intense work rather than pushing through to the expectation of a big break. Maybe that activity is to just pause, close your eyes, think about breathing (and actually do some deep breathing), and clear your mind for just a minute. This information is the basis for some of the smartphone apps designed to remind you to breathe or move.

TABLE 29.2 The Restoration

Secrets	Examples
"Something beats nothing" (p. 60).	If you have a smart watch, stand every time it tells you to do so.
"Moving beats stationary" (p. 61).	Go for a walk (preferably outside).
"Social beats solo" (p. 61).	Do a quick video or audio consultation or phone a friend.
"Outside beats inside" (p. 62).	While you are outside (see the second point above), breathe deeply.
"Fully detached beats semidetached" (p. 62).	Set aside a "detach" period. No phones, computers, notepads, tablets, or nonfiction books are allowed (and maybe even no coworkers if they only talk about work). Read a general magazine, sit back and close your eyes, sew, knit, garden or anything else unrelated to the work you do.

Data from Pink DH. *When: The Scientific Secrets of Perfect Timing.* New York, NY: Riverhead Books; 2018.

Moving beats stationary suggests that maybe standing desks aren't the answer. We are just stationary in a vertical position. Pink suggests "microbursts" of activity.[5] These might be a quick set of stretches or a quick jog around the desk or taking a walk down the hall or back. Or stepping outside might allow us the advantage of fresh air in addition to movement.

Social beats solo means that the opportunity to interact with others at work about topics not related to work is a way to rejuvenate ourselves. It is almost like distraction therapy. Talking with others about topics such as family and community allows people to destress for a few minutes.

We love the idea of outside beats inside. One year two of us were presenters at Chautauqua, the Colorado Nurses Association's summer conference. The lights went out in the hotel, so we all went outside and gathered around a common area and finished the course—and yes, everyone loved it.

Fully detached beats semidetached may seem to contradict the first statement about something beating nothing. Yet if we remain only semidetached, that means we are still semiattached and consumed by the pressures of today's world. All of our electronic devices almost call to us (and some actually do) to pick them up and use them multiple times a day. We therefore are only in a semirecovery mode. Going "electronics free" for a designated period has great potential to allow us to be fully detached so long as we are able to not spend that time worrying about what messages we are missing.

LL ALERT

- Don't schedule your entire day with meetings.
- Don't let the potential for work drive your day.

SUMMARY

Timing is critical. From the perspective of finding the perfect moment, to the idea of choosing the time of day to do certain activities, to actively considering recovery, the concept of timing offers a lot of substance for controlling our energy and capitalizing on opportunities.

LL LINEUP

- Be as diligent about recovery as you are about engagement.
- Capitalize on research findings about determining the best time to do certain kinds of tasks.
- Remember: Timing may not be everything, but it is a highly influential factor in our success.

REFLECTION For just 1 week, keep a log of how you spend your time. Consider how many hours you sleep and how much time you devote to personal activities (grooming, eating, etc.). How much time do you spend getting to work and back? How much time is spent at work? What are you doing the rest of the time? Texting? Gaming? Taking care of your family? Taking a course? Visiting with friends? Meeting your goals? At the end of the week, review how you spent your time and if that review fits with how you value spending your life. If it doesn't fit, what will you plan to do?

30

Truthfulness

We have all had experiences where those with whom we work—leaders or colleagues—do not tell the truth. Sometimes the lack of honesty can be considered exaggeration, perhaps when people overstate their experience or accomplishments. At other times, the statements are profoundly untrue, designed to mislead or cover up mistakes. Regardless of the type of untruth, negative consequences affect the person telling the falsehood, as well as those with whom they work. Of particular concern, dishonesty can erode the trust that others have in us. Equally important, dishonesty triggers a stress response in the body, which activates our "fight or flight" response, reducing blood flow to the portion of the brain that handles high-level, logical thinking. When we are dishonest, we are less likely to think clearly and make good decisions.[1]

WHY DO PEOPLE MAKE UNTRUTHFUL STATEMENTS?

Estimates vary about how frequently people say something that is not true; most of these estimates are surprisingly large in number. Why is dishonesty part of our daily behavior? Table 30.1 outlines some possible reasons for these types of behaviors.

Trustworthiness is critical to a leader. We may have the best ideas in the world, the ability to choose a team, an excellent strategic plan, outstanding communication strategies, and sufficient resources to accomplish our goals, but if leaders are not considered to be truthful, their colleagues will not feel comfortable in following their lead. Consistent truthfulness leads to a trusting relationship. Since truthfulness (as well as trust) is one of the personal characteristics included in the Legacy *Leaders*-Ship Trajectory model, we need to understand ways in which the truthfulness of a leader (or lack thereof) can affect the processes and outcomes of a group and organization.

EXAMPLES OF DISHONESTY IN ORGANIZATIONS

One of us has had a couple of instances in her career, once in an educational environment and once in service, where the leader of the organization was found to have mismanaged funds and in both cases did not tell the truth about a

TABLE 30.1 **Potential Reasons for Dishonesty**
1. Avoiding the truth to prevent hurting themselves or another person
2. Perceiving the truth is shameful or embarrassing
3. Fearing the resulting "drama" in response to the truth
4. Believing that: a. The truth is too boring b. Telling the truth would give away too much information c. Dishonesty will result in some sort of financial or social gain
5. Perceiving the truth is not sufficiently grandiose
6. Avoiding punishment
7. Protecting position or status
8. Maintaining delusions of reality

From Universal Class. The role of truthfulness in collaboration. Available at: https://www.universalclass.com/articles/business/the-role-of-truthfulness-in-collaboration.htm.

situation. The leaders lost their jobs, although neither was criminally charged. Their actions resulted in the loss of a career and a great deal of pain for the leaders and their families.

The organizations they led did not get off "scot-free" either. Employees felt betrayed and confused, and the work of the organizations suffered because everyone's attention was on the scandal rather than on their mission. In these circumstances, when the mismanagement of funds was identified, the loss of the leader's job was inevitable, and the employees, as well as the leader, were affected. However, in both cases, the leaders compounded the problem by lying about their culpability. As a result, the trauma for the organization stretched on much longer than necessary. Some employees supported the leaders and others did not, resulting in internal conflict at all levels of the organization. You can imagine what could have been accomplished in the organization in the time after the discovery of the mismanagement had the leaders told the truth, taking responsibility for their actions.

REFLECTION Have you ever been in a work situation where a leader was not truthful? What was the result? What did you learn from this situation?

TRUTHFULNESS: ITS IMPACT ON RELATIONSHIPS

Truthfulness implies honesty, trustworthiness, and integrity. It denotes complete sincerity and accuracy in all details. It is not a trait that we are born with; instead, we must learn to tell the truth. Fortunately, telling the truth actually fosters truth-telling in others. Effective encouragement and role modeling by the leader can encourage such behavior in all relationships.[2]

Truthfulness is central in all relationships—the connection between two individuals in a personal relationship, between leaders and their colleagues, and the way employees feel about the organization where they work. Similarities can be found in the processes of being truthful in individual personal and professional relationships and the perceptions of employees (and other stakeholders) in the truthfulness of the organization as a whole. It is helpful to consider the impact of truthfulness in these two broad characteristics separately.

TRUTHFULNESS IN INDIVIDUAL RELATIONSHIPS

A personal or professional relationship requires a foundation of truthfulness. A number of behaviors can help us to develop a reputation of truthfulness, including the following:

1. Thinking before you speak.
2. Saying what you mean and meaning what you say. We should make our actions, including body language, match our words. For example, agreeing to be responsible for a particular piece of work, knowing full well that we have neither the time nor the skill to complete the assignment, and then being defensive or blaming others when the deadline for completion arrives and we have not done the work is untruthful. How much better it is to tell the truth—"I don't have the time to learn the skills necessary to do a good job." Similarly, holding people accountable when their words do not match their actions indicates our awareness of the importance of truthfulness.
3. Telling it like it is rather than sugarcoating the situation (in a kind and tactful way, of course). In presenting both sides of each issue, we can ensure objectivity. Of course, if we have a personal bias or a conflict of interest, we should make it known.
4. Telling people the rationale behind our decisions so that our intent is understood. If something is misinterpreted, we must quickly correct the record. We must also willingly accept responsibility by admitting a mistake or an error in judgment in a timely fashion.
5. Never compromising our integrity and reputation by associating with people whose standards of integrity we mistrust.
6. Being sincere about our reactions. Certainly, we do not want to be hurtful or cruel, but when a colleague asks us, for example, to review a flawed piece of work, we must find a tactful way to tell the truth. This is particularly true if we have supervisory responsibility for another's work.
7. Being open to feedback regarding our own work or position. We must always be willing to see things from others' points of view by asking "What are they trying to tell me?" Looking for the kernel of truth in the criticism allows us to see ourselves from a different perspective. We may not completely agree, but being defensive or reactive or punishing others for being truthful will only promote a lack of truthfulness on the part of those giving the feedback.[3]

Two examples from one of our pasts illustrates the effectiveness of these behaviors and how things might go wrong if we don't keep them in mind.

Scenario 1

"I was having a conversation with several employees about a change in policy that would specifically affect a part of the

organization led by a new employee. One of the employees said, 'We really like this new employee—we don't want her to be blamed for this necessary change in policy. Perhaps you should make sure that everyone believes this decision is yours alone—after all, you're the leader and no one likes the leader.' Needless to say, this was hard to hear—I had thought that I was generally liked, or at least respected.

"Fortunately, I took some deep breaths and didn't react in a negative way. Later, as I thought about the situation (OK, maybe I ruminated about this for some period of time), I realized that this comment was not about me personally. Instead, it was a message that in this particular context, the leader was obligated to take the heat for the decision. This was a wonderful learning opportunity for me to realize that a leader taking responsibility for decisions was a necessary part of the role, and the results (or fallout) were not an indictment of me personally."

Scenario 2

One of our colleagues—a new leader—was asked to participate in a 360-degree evaluation offered as part of a leadership development program. The opportunity to participate in this development opportunity was stimulated because of some concern by the hierarchy that the leadership style of the new leader was more autocratic than that practiced consistently in the organization. In fact, the evaluation documented these perceptions. Unfortunately, the new leader did not react well to this assessment, arguing that her style produced results, even though there was a relatively high turnover in her department. In addition, she berated those whom she supervised for giving her a negative evaluation. You can imagine how uncomfortable the work environment became.

> **REFLECTION** Can you relate to either of the examples provided? What experiences have you had where truth was told, resulting in behaviors (yours or others) that enhanced (or hindered) a reputation of trust? What did you learn?

TRUTHFULNESS BY AN ORGANIZATION

Individual relationships often make up the reputation of trustworthiness within an organization. The experiences that an employee has regarding truthfulness usually are driven by the relationships with their supervisors and other leaders. The more often employees recognize that the messages they receive within the organization hierarchy have the flavor of truth, the more likely they are to believe that truthfulness is integrated into the culture of the organization.

In addition, organizations have a public persona, which represents the organization's values and mission to all stakeholders and the public. Because of the relative complexity of organizations, it is often difficult to know what is happening on the inside. *Organizational transparency* often provides access to information that can shed light on the organization's willingness to be truthful with their stakeholders. Andrew Schnackenberg and Edward Tomlinson suggest that transparency by an organization is the perceived quality of intentionally shared information from a sender.[4] From this definition, we can see that the *intentional release* and the *quality*, including the *accuracy* and *clarity*, of the information are key to how well the transparency is accepted by the employees and other stakeholders. Schnackenberg and Tomlinson also acknowledge that transparency is not equal to truthfulness, but for organizations, it is an antecedent. Thus the extent to which an organization is transparent influences the trust employees and stakeholders have in the organization.[4]

Because of the impact that intentional transparency has on the perception of employees and stakeholders, many for-profit and nonprofit organizations have transparency policies. For example, Nuru International (http://www.nuruinternational.org), a nonprofit organization that helps build local organizations in areas of extreme poverty to create effective solutions that are sustainable and scalable, has such a policy.

William Arruda, a contributor to the Forbes blog, suggests that transparency encourages employees to become active in problem-solving within their role and scope. When employees feel "in the loop," they are able to see ways in which they can contribute to the organization.[5] So what markers identify that organizations are serious about being consistently transparent to represent their outcomes in a truthful manner? They:

1. Communicate and act upon the company's vision and mission statement.
2. Tell the truth and include employees in discussions of ways to solve problems. This approach will encourage employees to "rally around the goals," thus strengthening the entire team.
3. Communicate in a manner that encourages teamwork.
4. Do not delay dispensing information to avoid "workplace surprises."
5. Make important documents, including financial information such as salary data, available to employees.[5,6]

> **REFLECTION** Is the organization in which you work transparent? Does administration provide you with information that is valuable to you? Why or why not?

LIMITS TO TRANSPARENCY

Although most current authorities believe that transparency is important for organizations, remember transparency is not truthfulness. As a result, people may have concerns when organizations release information, particularly to those outside of the organization. Perhaps the greatest is that releasing data without context is risky.[7] In order for stakeholders to understand the "big picture," data and information must be put into context. For example, one of us was asked to provide ideas related to an organization's response to the 2020 novel coronavirus pandemic:

"Because I had no prior interaction with this organization, I had no context to understand their questions. The organization was trying to be timely in clarifying how it would address its role. All of my responses started or ended with 'if it is appropriate for the organization.' Maybe I was brilliant, or maybe I was irrelevant. I had no idea because I didn't have the context."

A perfect example of the need for context was the discussion of the Texas Nurses Association's Board of Directors in 2008–2009 in preparation for the 81st Texas Legislature:

"The center of the discussion was the Nurse Staffing Committee policy we hoped to offer, along with other Texas nursing organizations, for consideration by the Texas Legislature. The discussion that illustrates the concern of the context of data in transparency was the question, 'Should we propose that the staffing numbers of each nursing unit be posted for the perusal of patients, families, and the general public?'"

Multiple reasons were generated for not posting the goal staffing numbers for each unit. The two most common were (1) the general public won't understand what the staffing projections mean, and (2) if the appropriate numbers of nurses are not available at a particular time, the hospital might be liable, even if the number of nurses staffing the unit was appropriate for the needs of the patients on that unit. The opposing group was equally sure that the nurses, patients, and students had the right to know the staffing goal the unit was trying to achieve. In the end, the nurse staffing legislation was passed. It required that hospitals report to the state department of health the extent to which each follows the nurse staffing regulations. However, the legislation was silent on whether the proposed staffing pattern should be posted on each unit."[8]

This example illustrates the difficult questions that arise when specific information to be released as a part of the transparency effort has to be determined.

What are some of the markers of an organization that does not hold truthfulness as a value and does not incorporate that expectation into its culture? Here are some behavioral clues that employees may demonstrate:

- Little trust for the organizational hierarchy or among the workers themselves
- A high incidence of absenteeism—people who tell the truth are more likely to be healthier than those who are not, because they are happier and have less stress in their lives
- Less pride in the work by individuals and groups
- Poor productivity (more mistakes and time wasted)
- Little confidence in themselves and in the workplace[2,8]

LL ALERT

- Don't confuse transparency with truthfulness.
- Don't add to a problematic situation by lying about it!

SUMMARY

Truthfulness is a core value that influences all of our relationships: personal, professional, and organizational. Having a reputation for truthfulness requires time and effort to establish and can be lost very quickly. Truthful people understand themselves and know—and own—their strengths and weaknesses. They present themselves in a way that shows who they are. They are the same in public and private. They describe themselves and others as accurately as possible, and they keep any promises they make and meet their obligations.[9]

The role of a reputation for truthfulness in developing a Legacy *Leaders*-Ship Trajectory model is foundational—without truth, other attributes lose their impact. Let us always strive for truth.

LL LINEUP

- Being truthful promotes trustworthiness and engagement.
- Be as transparent as reasonable.

REFLECTION Reflect on your behavior and rate yourself according to the following questions:

- Do you understand and own your strengths and weaknesses?
- Are you the same in public and in private?
- Are you rigorously honest in your descriptions of yourself, others, and events in which you have participated?
- Do you keep your promises and meet your obligations?
- How are you able to speak truth when doing so has great consequences?

31

Trust

When we work in an organization—as most of us do—we find many things we can't control. We depend on those who are above us in the hierarchy, those who are our colleagues, and those whom we supervise to act in the best interest of the organizational mission. In short, we trust those with whom we work to do their part, just as we do ours.

Trust in organizational structures in today's environment (government, businesses, health care, education, and religion) has been falling over the last several decades.[1] This lack of trust on all sides affects the ways in which we all lead our lives and makes it crucial for today's leaders in all organizations to prioritize developing a culture of trustworthiness.

Martie Moore (2019), a Chief Nursing Officer at Medline Industries, Inc., suggests that trust is an outcome—the consequence of an action. In organizations where trust is central to the functioning of the organizational culture, a healthy culture is defined by what we say and do each day.[2] In an interview, Neesha Hathy, Executive Vice President of Charles Schwab, quoted former Herman Miller Chief Executive Officer (CEO) Max Dupree who said, "The first responsibility of a leader is to define reality. The last is to say thank you. In between the two, the leader must become a servant."[3] This, in our minds, is the essence of a culture of trustworthiness.

THE DEFINITION OF TRUST

The presence—or absence—of trust in any human relationship is critical to effective interaction. The Oxford English Dictionary defines trust as "a firm belief in the reliability, truth, or ability of someone or something."[4] Trust is an expectation that we can rely on another person's actions and words and that the person has good intentions to carry out their promises. Further, trust is most meaningful in situations where we are vulnerable in relation to another, such as in the boss–employee relationship. After all, the boss does control the evaluation of our performance and our pay!

Trust among colleagues requires time and intention to develop. Unfortunately, we all have had experiences where organizational leaders have not appeared trustworthy. Perhaps they do not seem to act in a consistent way; perhaps their words do not "ring true"; or perhaps they seem to act in ways that benefit themselves rather than the team or the organization. Similarly, we may have had experiences where we see these same behaviors in our colleagues—or even on occasion in ourselves.

> **REFLECTION** In your experience, what happens when you work in an environment where distrust is rampant? How do you feel? How are the outcomes of your work affected?

THE NEUROSCIENCE OF TRUST

In the early 2000s, Dr. Paul Zak, the founding director of the Center for Neuroeconomics Studies at Claremont Graduate University, hypothesized that a neurologic signal in humans must indicate when we should trust someone. He implemented a long-term research plan to see whether this idea was true. Based on the finding that a brain chemical oxytocin (yep—the same oxytocin so important in labor and delivery) had been shown to signal that another animal is safe to approach, Dr. Zak and his research team developed a protocol to draw blood before and after people chose an amount of money to send to a stranger via computer, knowing that the money would triple in amount when it was sent back. The research subjects could choose to keep the money or send it on the chance that they would receive three times the original amount of money if it was sent back. The risk, of course, was that the research subjects would lose the money if the phantom person was not trustworthy. Subjects were randomly given synthetic oxytocin via a nasal spray or a placebo and then were asked to make the decision to send or not send. The results demonstrated that oxytocin appeared to reduce the fear of trusting a stranger.[5]

Over the next 10 years, the researchers completed qualitative and quantitative experiments in the laboratory and in the field designed to identify the promoters and inhibitors of oxytocin. The results of this research trajectory found that when oxytocin hits the brain, the following occurs:

- Oxytocin increases a person's empathy.
- High stress is a potent oxytocin inhibitor.
- The relationship between oxytocin and trust is universal.[5]

Based upon these findings, Dr. Zak developed a survey instrument to measure behaviors that are stimulated as a result of oxytocin release. This survey was used to study several thousand companies.[5] The behaviors identified to be associated with trust are found in Table 31.1.

REFLECTION Review the behaviors in Table 31.1 that are stimulated by oxytocin and the resulting trust we feel. Which of these behaviors do you believe that leaders in your work environment demonstrate? How does the presence or absence of these behaviors affect the workplace? Which of these behaviors do you exhibit in your own leadership activities? Are there areas in which you would like to improve?

TRUST IN ORGANIZATIONS

Several studies have validated the importance of trust in the workplace. Trust is the building block upon which successful relationships—and ventures—are based. Research has demonstrated that the presence of trust in teams and organizations influences job satisfaction and the achievement of goals[6]; prevention of burnout[7]; and commitment to the

TABLE 31.1 Behaviors Stimulated by Oxytocin Release

Components	Related Evidence
Recognize excellence	The neuroscience shows that recognition has the largest effect on trust when it happens: • Immediately after a goal has been met • When it comes from peers • When it is tangible, unexpected, personal, and public
Induce "challenge" stress	Providing a difficult but achievable job results in release of oxytocin and adrenocorticotropin, which intensifies team members' focus and strengthens social connectives. This only works if the job is attainable and has a "hard" end.
Give employees discretion in how they do their work	After training, managers need to allow employees to manage their work in their own way, if possible. Being trusted to plan actions and figure things out is a big motivator, and autonomy promotes innovation.
Enable "job crafting"	When employees choose which programs they work on, they focus their energies on what they care about most.
Share information broadly	Employee uncertainty leads to chronic stress, which inhibits the release of oxytocin. Being open about plans through ongoing communication reduces uncertainty.
Build intentional relationships	When people intentionally build social ties at work, their performance improves. When managers demonstrate concern for team members' success and personal well-being, social ties are built.
Facilitate whole-person growth	Managers should function with the goal of "How can I help you get your next job?" This approach includes discussion about energy balance, family, and time for recreation and reflection.
Show vulnerability	Asking for help from colleagues is a sign of a secure leader. Encourage everyone to be involved in reaching goals.

work, team, or organization.[8] Given the evidence that trustworthiness in the leader (and the follower) is important, how can we make sure that our behavior demonstrates that we are to be trusted?

Steven Covey believes that trust actually represents the confidence of the group that the leader will lead them in the right direction. This confidence is the result of two dimensions of the leader's behavior: character and competence. Character includes the integrity of leaders, their motive, and their intent in interacting with people. Competence includes the leaders' capabilities, skills, past track record, and ongoing results. Both character and competence play a role in followers' decisions to trust the leader's direction; neither alone is sufficient.[9]

David Horsager, in the Forbes Leadership Forum, outlines eight characteristics that we must demonstrate to develop trusting relationships.[10] These "characteristics" can be used as a roadmap to evaluating trustworthiness in our own careers. They include:

1. *Clarity*—Being clear about the mission, purpose, priorities, expectations, and daily activities so that others will know what to expect.
2. *Compassion*—Sincerely caring about others; having their best interest in mind.
3. *Character*—Doing what is right rather than doing what is easy.
4. *Contribution*—Delivering real results, rather than just talking about them.
5. *Competency*—Continuing to be "teachable," learning new ways of doing things, and staying current on ideas and trends, even in the midst of "chaos."
6. *Connection*—Developing relationships by asking questions, listening, and being grateful for others' contributions.
7. *Commitment*—Being willing to be committed to the work and sacrifice for the greater good.
8. *Consistency*—Doing the small but important things that reflect your values on a regular basis.

We are trusted because of our way of being, not because of the external facade we portray. Most of us have had the experience of being "wowed" by the credentials of a new colleague, only to find that underneath this polished exterior is someone who does not demonstrate the characteristics for building trust. Trust is built and maintained by many small actions over time. As Warren Buffett has said, "It takes 20 years to build a reputation and five minutes to ruin it. If you think about that, you will do things differently."[11]

REFLECTION Compare Hosager's "Eight Cs of Trustworthiness" and Table 31.1. In what ways are these lists similar and in what ways are they different? Consider situations in which you have recognized the lack of trust. Which of these characteristics or behaviors would have improved the situation?

APPLICATION OF THE "THE CHARACTERISTICS OF TRUSTWORTHINESS"

Most of us have examples of occasions when implementation of one or more of the characteristics of trustworthiness resulted in an increase in trust within a team. One of our colleagues was the dean of a nursing program that was preparing for an accreditation visit when she discovered that someone in a key leadership position had not completed the necessary preparation for the accreditation visit. With only a few weeks to prepare, the rest of the leadership team jumped into action and completed the necessary preparation for that visit. These demonstrations of commitment in the face of significant challenges strengthened the bonds of the groups. Similarly, when the coronavirus pandemic hit the US in 2020, many non–direct care nurses jumped into action to provide more direct care within their organizations.

Those who were involved in the preparation could have said, "Fixing this problem is not possible in such a short time frame. We will just have to weather a poor outcome to our visit and make changes later." Instead, they worked many hours, under a great deal of stress, to prepare for the visit. They were honest with the team of visitors regarding the difficulties they faced, holding their breath that this honesty would not have a negative consequence. Interestingly, a highlight of the visitor's report was their analysis of the trust among the faculty and their awareness that the leadership team had gone to great lengths to repair the potential damage to the program. Their commitment paid off!

David Grossman suggests that what leaders *say* in relation to what they *do* has the most impact on the followers' perception of an organization.[12] When the leader's words are different from the way he or she acts, our feelings about the organization are negatively affected, which results in a decrease in engagement and commitment by the employees. For example, when the company leadership sends out an employee survey asking for suggestions regarding ways the company operations could be improved, followed shortly by a massive layoff or "downsizing," it is unlikely that the remaining employees will be inclined to honestly answer any future employee surveys, and their commitment to their work will be governed *only* by their own values.

One of us had an experience that highlights the need to be congruent in word and speech:

"I once worked for an organization that was experiencing significant reduction in revenue. This, coupled with a complete leadership change, caused everyone in the organization to feel uneasy. Although the leader (who was new to the organization) spoke of team building, innovation, empowerment, etc., a number of layoffs were made in the upper levels of the organization unrelated to competence, at least in the opinion of those who remained with the organization. (In short, the view was that all of the 'good' leaders were fired.) At the same time, senior leadership wanted to demonstrate to stakeholders, such as board members of the larger system, that the work environment was positive. So, on a regular basis, seemingly timed to be several months after the latest layoff, we were expected to complete an employee survey regarding the work environment.

"You can all imagine the results of these surveys—they were all very negative! The most amazing part of this story was that after several survey results continued to be negative (as the layoffs continued), the managers of each department were asked to tell their employees not to talk among themselves about rumors that we heard because it hurt the morale of the employees when many of the rumors were not true. Although this advice was probably good—rumors are typically not true—the admonishment felt like the victims were being blamed for the negative perception of the work environment. A better approach would have been for administrators to be sensitive enough to understand why the employees were uncomfortable and to speak honestly about the current and future plans for the company."

WHEN TRUST HAS BEEN LOST

All leaders are human, and we make mistakes that may cause those who work with us to question our trustworthiness. What should we do in this situation? Joel Peterson, the chairman of Jet Blue, notes that you have to apologize as quickly as possible and correct things when trust has been lost. Forgiveness of yourself and by others is also necessary to move forward. However, he also notes that some betrayals are unfixable. If, for example, value differences among the parties are too great, the priorities are too different, or the betrayals are too profound, fixing is unlikely. In these situations, moving on in another environment may be the best option for one or both parties.[13]

CHOOSING WHOM TO TRUST

Our confidence with trust over time is varied—some of us are more likely to trust than others. As we discussed earlier in the chapter, when oxytocin hits our brain, we are more likely to trust an individual. However, the choice to trust is also mediated by our previous experiences. Once we have the experience of being in a situation where lack of trust is prevalent, we often are reluctant to extend our trust in other situations, regardless of the persons involved. Joel Peterson provides us with three tests for deciding who to trust. First, do they have character? Do they demonstrate integrity? Can we count on them to do what they promise? Second, do they demonstrate competence over time? Third, do they have the authority to do what they say they will? Are others above them in the hierarchy consistently preventing them from taking action?[13] Of course, when we are initially building a trusting relationship, answering these questions may be difficult. However, they do provide us with a format for assessing the trustworthiness of someone over time.

THE IMPACT OF TRUST ON OUR OWN LEADERSHIP TRAJECTORY

Aspiring leaders must recognize that trustworthy behavior is key to developing leadership skills. Such behavior is not a "sometimes thing." Instead, we must be willing to apply the criteria Joel Peterson suggests for determining who to trust to our own behavior.[13] What is our reputation among those with whom we work? Do others see us as honest or as someone who "shoots straight" when difficulties arise? Are we seen as someone who can be depended on to do what we promised? Are we seen as competent, particularly related to effective decision-making? As an example of the importance of being viewed as competent, one of us was hired (at least in part) because one of the references the hiring manager spoke to said, "Oh you must hire her. When she speaks about a problem, everyone listens."

In addition, leaders must work to create positive relationships among their teams. Helping team members cooperate and resolve conflict are effective strategies to develop positive team relationships. Checking in with team members and giving honest feedback are equally effective. As leaders develop trustworthy behaviors, they are better able to support trustworthy behaviors in their team members. In short, development of individual and team trust is a reciprocal process.[14]

To avoid making mistakes that lead to a reduction in trust, consider the behaviors that *do not* engender trust. Steven Covey developed a chart of "The 13 Behaviors of High Trust Leaders" and included fake or fraudulent behaviors of each behavior.[9] Table 31.2 outlines this negative behavior, which serves as things not to do and highlights those behaviors we should avoid.

TABLE 31.2 Negative Behaviors Associated with Covey's 13 Behaviors of High Trust

Behavior	Fraudulent Behavior
Character	
1. Talk Straight	Spinning, positioning, posturing, manipulating
2. Demonstrating Respect	Faking respect or concern
3. Creating Transparency	Having hidden agendas, meanings, or objectives
4. Right Wrongs	Covering up or disguising instead of repairing
5. Show Loyalty	Being two-faced
Competence	
6. Deliver Results	Delivering activities that don't demonstrate the desired results
7. Get Better	Continuing learning, but never producing
8. Confront Reality	Focusing attention on side issues, while never dealing with the real one(s)
9. Clarify Expectations	Failing to pin down specifics that facilitate meaningful accountability
10. Practice Accountability	Pointing fingers and blaming others
11. Listen First	Listening only to form your reply
12. Keep Commitments	Overpromising and underdelivering
13. Extend Trust	Extending "false trust"—giving people the responsibility without the authority or resources

From Covey F. The 13 behaviors of high trust leaders mini session. Relationship Trust. 2020. Available at: https://archive.franklincovey.com/facilitator/minisessions/handouts/13_Behaviors_MiniSession_Handout.pdf.

LL ALERT

- Don't assume all people and organizations are trustworthy.
- Don't ignore the eight characteristics Horsager identified.

SUMMARY

Trust is critical in most important relationships in our work (and in our personal lives). To develop a Legacy *Leaders*-Ship Trajectory model, we must pay attention to the trustworthiness of all with whom we interact. In particular, we must monitor our own behavior to be sure that we are seen as trustworthy. To do otherwise is to short-circuit our leadership potential.

LL LINEUP

- Do what you say you will do.
- Recall daily that trust is key to developing and exhibiting leadership skills.

REFLECTION Think back to a situation where your trust was misplaced. How did this feel? What did you do? Knowing what you know now about trust, what would you do differently in a similar situation? Using the results of your reflection, develop a proactive plan for uncomfortable or difficult situations. This plan should include potential steps you will take to maintain trusting relationships with your colleagues, even when the environmental factors support a less open and vulnerable position.

32 Vulnerability

The formal definition of *vulnerability* suggests a defenselessness against nonphysical attacks. In other words, someone (or something) can be vulnerable to criticism or failure. Often leaders develop protections against criticism and failure, which can be likened to the armor worn by knights and fighters in previous eras. The workplace has been characterized as a hostile place, and those who rise to the top must protect themselves from the attack of others attempting to rise to the top and take their place. The workplace has been conceived as a very competitive milieu. This perspective can lead to disconnection and low levels of engagement with employees.

CONNECTION

From a social perspective, human beings are about connection. Connection with other human beings gives our lives purpose and meaning. For connection to occur, we must allow ourselves to be "really seen."[1] Our greatest fear is that we are not worthy of connection, which leads to protectiveness or a façade of leadership. In the workplace, this fear counteracts the ability to be connected to staff or employees. Yet workers long for this sense of connection with leadership and with coworkers. It is a motivator for coming to work.

The key to connection is the ability to be vulnerable. Brene Brown believes that vulnerability is simply defined as uncertainty, risk, and emotional exposure.[2] This means acknowledging that life and work are filled with uncertainty. None of us knows what tomorrow brings. We may get sick, the stock market may fail, our organization or workplace may suffer unanticipated reversals, or a pandemic may suddenly emerge. Life is full of uncertainty, and to pretend that these uncertainties do not exist is foolish. In the American system, we take risks every day; in business or the workplace, in driving our cars, in eating at restaurants (who hasn't had a case of food poisoning?), or in sending our children to school or out to play. The world is full of risks, as we have most recently experienced with the novel coronavirus pandemic. Emotional exposure is also vulnerability. Those of us who became nurses in the mid-20th century were taught never to cry in front of a patient or family. We were supposed to be professional, which translated to being "in control" at all times, to wearing our "armor" and ignoring feelings of fear, anxiety, disappointment, and "not knowing." We learned to numb vulnerability. The problem with numbing is that it cannot be selective. When we numb vulnerability, we also numb the positives in our lives, the joy, the gratitude, and the happiness. The numbing can result in being miserable while looking for purpose and meaning. For leaders today, "armor" and numbing simply don't work.

In Brenë Brown's keynote address to the American Organization of Nurse Executives (now the American Organization for Nursing Leadership) at the 2017 annual meeting, she talked about the armor that many nurse leaders wear so that we can act tough and project an image of indestructibility.[3] She believes true leadership does not exist without vulnerability, and she emphasized that it is terrifying, dangerous, and scary. She believes that due to the fear of being vulnerable, we choose comfort or the status quo over courage. She believes that these leaders are the ones who end up getting annihilated. In contrast, she described courage as consisting of four skill sets: being vulnerable, trusting, clarifying values, and "rising" (resiliency or the ability to get back up after being knocked down). As leaders, we will get kicked, criticized, made fun of, and be misunderstood. Every day nurse leaders will have to choose courage or comfort.[4]

THE LIMITS OF VULNERABILITY

Being vulnerable doesn't mean sharing every aspect of our personal lives, our divorces, or our crazy relative or friend. It doesn't mean "spilling your guts" in the workplace. It does mean expressing not knowing all the solutions; it means asking for help; it means refraining from blaming others for issues or failures. Instead, we need to ask about what was learned from a challenging situation. Being vulnerable means focusing on growing others and supporting them—being open and admitting our mistakes. This kind of vulnerability creates a work environment that is healthy, more like a family, a place where people can take risks and, if they fail, know they will not be crucified. Rather, the focus is on learning.

THE MYTHS OF VULNERABILITY

David Williams[5] has synthesized the four myths of vulnerability identified in Brown's research.

Myth #1: Vulnerability Is Weakness

In her research, Brown asked people to tell her about the times they felt vulnerable. They talked about starting their own business, the first date after a divorce, owning mistakes they made at work, or cheering for a child who wants to make the football team and it is highly unlikely to happen. In considering these stories, it became clear they had nothing to do with weakness. Actually, Brown identified that these vulnerable situations were measures of courage.

Williams believes that every entrepreneurial endeavor is courageous and risky. For example, in 2003, one of us described the beginning of the Colorado Center for Nursing Excellence out of the chief executive officer's (CEOs) kitchen:

"Although most people and organizations concerned about the nursing shortage wanted this new entity to solve the workforce issue, the nursing community was not happy that a social worker had been selected to lead the group, and financial support was limited. I was introduced to the CEO because I had just learned of the new Health Resources and Services Administration (HRSA) Title VIII funding for nursing professionals' continuing education and I wanted Colorado to be awarded some of the money. A mutual colleague arranged the meeting, and the CEO was very clear with me that she didn't know anything about my great idea but she had secretarial support (we had to write an 85-page, single-spaced document in just under 6 weeks). When we discovered we were funded, the future of the center was so precarious that the CEO said she didn't think we should accept the funding because she wasn't sure we would be in business in 6 weeks. I told her that we never turn down funding or we wouldn't ever be funded again. I convinced her to take the risk. We worked all contacts, beginning with board members, until we solicited enough funds to cover operations until we could get the grant up and running. We recruited additional grants from the Department of Labor, and by 2019 we were on our 10th HRSA grant and had received over \$5 million in program grants from local foundations. We were open, vulnerable, and direct about our needs and what we could accomplish. This experience is about a willingness to take risks, to be vulnerable, and to develop teams that exemplify what Brown teaches. This approach creates strong teams that achieve great outcomes."

> **REFLECTION** Consider how you have thought about vulnerability. How did the idea that vulnerability is not a weakness strike you?

Myth #2: You Can Opt Out of Vulnerability

As discussed earlier, vulnerability is the combination of uncertainty, risk, and emotional exposure. This is the basis of any startup organization. Vulnerability is a natural condition of the work that we do. Every time we write a grant, create a new process, or devise a product, we are vulnerable. To believe we are not vulnerable would be inauthentic and would leave us in a perpetual state of denial and stress. So we must be vulnerable, know we are vulnerable, and take the risk anyway.

Myth #3: Vulnerability Means Letting It All Hang Out

Purposeful vulnerability without boundaries, "spilling your guts," is attention-seeking behavior that creates the image of being desperate. One must ask, what would be the objective in sharing information that creates vulnerability? Is it a desperate cry for attention, or does it actually work to solve a problem?

Sharing private feelings and information that leaves you vulnerable should occur only with people who have earned the right to learn about sensitive knowledge. For example, businesses hold their "secrets" closely. The secret "recipes" or models are known only to a few high-level organizational representatives. On the other hand, those of us in health care often share more openly but generally not to the point of making the organization vulnerable. Leaders might even want to share if they are feeling vulnerable but not to the extent that others become anxious.

> **REFLECTION** Think about a negative message you saw on social media. What reaction did you have to reading that message? Have you ever provided a negative message about your employer or the profession? How did others respond?

Myth #4: I Can Go It Alone

Most of us understand none of us can "go it alone." When we ask team members or others to help with a project or if we ask a friend to help in role-playing a difficult conversation with a third person, vulnerabilities are being risked in a courageous and positive way.

Asking for help can be scary for many of us. But knowing that all of us are vulnerable and that owning our vulnerability is a form of true courage, the fear can be overcome. True sadness and grief would result if we reached the end of life and had to ask ourselves what we could have accomplished if we had truly shown up. Were we ready to give our all and, if necessary, sacrifice all? What would be the regret over failing to function in this way?

REFLECTION Consider if you have ever felt as if you had to do something completely by yourself. What went into your thinking about that choice? Did you feel vulnerable anyway? What prevented you from sharing that situation or issue with someone else?

WHEN VULNERABILITY ENTERS THE WORKPLACE

Some surprising benefits evolve from leaders being vulnerable and encouraging workers to be vulnerable in the workplace.[6] Table 32.1 summarizes these benefits.

In the workplace, both leaders and employees display vulnerability each time they bring a new idea to a meeting or challenge the traditional way of thinking—when the "we've always done it this way" approach is abandoned. As Brown would say, vulnerability is the birthplace of innovation, trust, and engagement. Employees feel safe to suggest risky ideas in such an environment, and they know they will not be ridiculed for a suggestion, even if it fails.

Further, creating a workplace practice of openly supporting one another as human beings allows all to share challenging personal situations, feel supported by peers, possibly do some problem-solving, and then return to engage in the work. Taking 10 minutes to listen to coworkers discuss a tough situation and ask what they need from you shows empathy and caring. This behavior allows people to process feelings and move on to the work of the day.

When human beings experience empathy from coworkers on tough days, they are more likely to connect to their teammates and to work well together. It makes the workplace and environment more fun, and team members bond and connect with each other. The team is strengthened.

TABLE 32.1 **Benefits of Vulnerability**
1. Fostering innovation
2. Improving motivation
3. Boosting teamwork
4. Promoting identification with leadership

Adapted from Seppala E. What bosses gain by being vulnerable. *Harv Bus Rev.* 2014. Available at: https://hbr.org/2014/12/what-bosses-gain-by-being-vulnerable.

When organizational leaders share their feelings and disappointments and their vulnerabilities or when bad news such as failed profitability or potential layoffs is in the offing, all tend to close ranks and support leaders. When passion and excitement for an organization's new direction or new funding are shared, others identify with people who set this new direction or gained the funds.

In trusting organizations, when people see no emotion or minimal information about what's occurring and the workload increases, they have difficulty understanding what leaders face. When leaders exhibit passion for the work of the organization, as well as the challenges, a true connection can be made in a group.

LL ALERT

- Don't ignore struggling colleagues who fail to understand vulnerability.
- Don't avoid feeling vulnerable—it is not negative.

SUMMARY

Leadership is not about titles, status, or power; it is about taking responsibility for identifying the potential in others and in ideas. It is about having the courage to develop the potential in both the people and the ideas. Leaders don't pretend to have the right answers—they ask the right questions. Leaders know that power becomes infinite when it is shared. A significant aspect of leading is to be vulnerable with others—to connect with them—to be real and authentic. A personal trait of effective leaders is the ability to be vulnerable in the workplace, to make mistakes and then own those mistakes, and to be open with others and encourage them to be open and vulnerable with you. Connections with others make all the difference in the perception of the workplace. The vulnerability that produces these connections is the key element.

LL LINEUP

- Consider when and with whom you can be vulnerable.
- Create the mindset that being vulnerable is an act of courage.

REFLECTION Think about a leader who did not demonstrate vulnerability. What did you learn from that experience? What types of interactions would you have with colleagues to demonstrate vulnerability?

Environment Overview

If you were really engaged in the first sections of the book, you probably kept saying to yourself, "Yes, but...." In other words, you were considering different environments where you have had experience and you knew that in a situation in environment A you did something different than you did in the same situation in environment B. The environment in which we exist and exert leadership influences how we use our personal strengths and can impede or accelerate our trajectory to gain and hone skills of leadership. For example, who comprises our alliances influences how we behave. Gangs, for example, are often not described individually one by one. The group is described, and that description is often based on the worst behavior and applied to all. Similarly, Magnet nurses are described as a group—one that is often uplifting and reinforcing of nursing's best professional descriptions, and all affiliated with a Magnet organization benefit from the perception we have about what it means to be a Magnet organization. The same can be said about nurses who have been designated as Daisy nurses.

Your mother may have said what our mothers said: You are judged by the company you keep. That means you can be the best-behaved person and not be seen as such if you are with people who are being disruptive or negative. You also can be judged as living your values if you exhibit belongingness rather than simply stating you believe in diversity. Both of those examples can derive from the environment in which you live—and the environment in which you work. Choose wisely would be good advice!

As you enter this last section, you may think finding communication and relationships in a section about environment is strange. Our rationale for placing these elements in the environment is that we are greatly influenced by our setting in how we execute the personal skills of communicating and building relationships. If the organization tolerates gossip, we find it easier to gossip. If the environment mouths civility but exhibits incivility, we are more likely to be swept up by the culture and join in being uncivil.

The environment also contributes greatly to our engagement in work. If we see our role at work as filling a job, we aren't going to become actively engaged in the mission of the organization. However, if we see our role as one filling our passion, we likely can give multiple examples of how what we (and others) do at work fulfills the mission of the organization. The organization either promotes innovation and quality or it does not. Our task is to evaluate what we see and sense so that we can be effective in our roles and modify our behavior, or know we won't be a fit, or determine to change the environment.

The last chapter in this section is devoted to something most of us experience and yet seldom discuss. We all exit a position—we may have found a new role in the same organization or we found a new opportunity in another organization. Or, we may have retired from a position. How we leave is as important as how we arrive. What we put in place to support something really important (a legacy) helps the remaining leaders envision what they can and need to do to continue a legacy and to build on it. Legacies don't just happen. They are the result of commitment of many people to a vision about how some particular thing can be. The work of Florence Nightingale and Lillian Wald, to name two of our past leaders, provided us with numerous legacies about nursing and about being a professional. The work of four nurses in the American Academy of Nursing gave us the legacy of Magnet-designated hospitals. The work of Clair Jordan, former Executive Director of the Texas Nurses Association, gave us the basis for what is now Pathways to Excellence–designated organizations. Linda Aiken provided numerous studies that supported the idea of a well-educated workforce and having a sufficient number of nurses to affect morbidity and mortality. Although most of us don't leave a legacy of those magnitudes, we do affect others in the environment in which we work—and we are affected by the environment to be who we are professionally.

This section focuses on only the key elements of what we know as *environment*. As with other elements of the model, each of us may have something else we would want to add. We are free to do that to enrich our own perception of the value of understanding what the environment brings to our perspective of leadership.

33

Alliances

In Adam Grant's *WorkLife* podcast, "Become Friends With Your Rivals," he provides exemplars of working with people we don't normally view as part of our alliances.[1] If we reframe how to form alliances and with whom we might ally, we expand our influence and the potential to be influenced. Although inclusion is discussed elsewhere, alliances are really about the idea of inclusion, and the more inclusive we can be, the greater our potential for forming meaningful alliances.

WHAT IS AN ALLIANCE?

A bond or connection is at the core of an alliance. The word also means an association to further common interests of the individuals or groups. Alliances could also be seen as an alignment—it is the connection of others to us and our ideas.[2] An alliance is designed around the common interest in an issue, around a view of action to be taken, or to buffer or thwart a different view or approach. The common interest, although challenging, is often easier to accomplish than either of the other two. We may agree that global warming, as an example, is an issue and that it is multifaceted. Yet we have seen limited movement worldwide because among those who agree this is an issue, they disagree about how to resolve the issue. But if we align this group against those who want to do nothing, they align in a stronger manner. Alignments save time and energy, serve as a place to exchange ideas, and unite people for a common purpose.[2] Further, we can enhance those alliances (or alignments) by clarity, dialogue, and inspiration. Our purpose might be to secure Magnet® designation, reduce falls, secure effective legislation related to school health, or advance the science of nursing. These examples illustrate how complex alliances are.

Looking at alliances could be viewed as a dance with partners moving slowly, then quickly, then near, and then apart. For example, an alliance often moves slowly in getting established. Partners are busy evaluating the benefits and liabilities of partnering with someone else. Once they establish trust and a mutual perspective of their work together, partners move quickly. They come together to accomplish a task and achieve an outcome and then move apart to return to their primary reason for existence. Further, alliances that seem strong and consistent may in fact have multiple disagreements—but not in public. Although diversity of opinion can be enriching, that diversity can slow progress as those differences are explored to reach some mutual view or position. An important point for us to consider is this: the most effective alliances are those that have worked out differences outside of the public purview. They seem highly aligned even if that is not the case. The two of us who live in Texas are very familiar with the need to settle differences about advanced practice nursing issues behind closed doors, because when those doors open, nursing is facing medicine with its powerful, very well-funded lobbying efforts. When we aren't aligned, we are doomed.

REFLECTION Consider how the concept of alliances applies in nursing. Nurses are together when attacked externally. What are we like on a regular basis?

Collaboration, which is required for an alliance, is a strategy used to become more effective in aligning with others. A key tactic in gaining collaboration is to be focused on the other person or group. Obviously if the other person or group is using that same approach, no conversation can occur. However, the more likely outcome is that each person or group takes turns sharing insights and views. As a result, two people or groups, who might not have been able to communicate effectively before, now understand each other's viewpoint, which could lead to an alliance on part or all elements of a discussion. This commonality might reflect shared values or a particular interest.

REFLECTION Consider a group at work. Is it an alliance? In other words, is this group coming together around a common issue? Is the level of involvement merely agreeing to work together or has actual work occurred? If work hasn't occurred, how could you move this alliance toward action?

If those in favor of our ideas and viewpoints are the allies, then those against must be the "antis." When two or more groups can agree on a topic or an approach, they are more powerful than either group could be independently. The goal, of course, is to get multiple groups to agree on ideas and viewpoints so that spokespersons can say they are speaking for thousands.

An alliance of two strong groups is truly powerful. And if a group isn't seen as very powerful, its power can increase by being in alliance with a powerful partner. Additionally, listening to what the antis say and watching what they do allow for better understanding of how they view an issue. The goal in working with antis is to be as proactive in listening as possible. This allows us to be prepared to strengthen the alliance's perspective and tailor a message that can be heard.

Alliances can be formed from those who are more mature in their positions or organizations and with those relatively young in those positions or organizations with the intent of that interaction forming a way to build an alliance. The key, however, is that some value or mission or desired outcome has to be held in common with another group in order for an alliance to form.

TYPES OF ALLIANCES

In Robert Hackman's work related to teams, his division of types of teams can form a framework for thinking about the types of alliances.[3] The first of his four groups is *information sharing*. This is a minimal effort on the part of groups that agree to be in alignment. It requires active listening to be certain the ideas one group expresses represent the thinking of the other groups. If we aren't in alignment on our thinking about an issue or about actions to take, we can't sustain an alignment for long.

The second grouping is *consultative*. This, too, is a form of an alliance, although the approach is more of an expert group and a group that has less intensity. Not all unequal partners in an alliance are using the expert group in a consultative role. Sometimes these groups come together to learn before some critical situation arises that tests the position of an alliance.

The third group is *coordinating*. As an example, one group in an alliance may be the expert group, and yet it is small in size due to the definitive focus of its work interests. In nursing, those smaller groups could be a highly specialized clinical or functional area or a group devoted to a specific role, such as educator or researcher. That kind of group benefits when it aligns with a broad-based organization, such as the state nurses' association, which might have more members than any focused specialty group.

The last grouping is *decision-making*. This also can apply to an alliance. Some alliances merely exchange information so all members of the alliance are informed, and some are decision-making. These decision-making alliances are powerful, even if an inequity exists in terms of size and influence. The challenging part of building an alliance is deciding at what points everyone agrees and when certain groups will assume certain roles even though other groups will not participate actively. In some cases, an alliance might exist behind the scenes to achieve some outcome that is desirable for the group or the community.

Imagine how an alliance could crumble almost instantly if members thought they were participating because decisions were going to be made, only to learn the alliance was really about keeping various groups informed! Being clear about the nature of alliances is critical to their success.

Another way of looking at alliances is to consider the work of Mike Leavitt and Rich McKeown.[4] They identify eight key elements for collaborative efforts to succeed, as shown in Table 33.1. A group assembled to assess an issue, for example, would likely not address every one of the elements, yet many of those elements have great implications in nursing. Having a common information base is another example of an element that is critical in nursing's efforts, because we may see an issue differently depending on our position in an organization or our clinical focus. Their expectation is to have a critical cadre of leaders (stature, substance, and committed are their words). To engage the "right" people in the issue, careful consideration about which individuals or groups are allies should be undertaken.

THE INDIVIDUAL LEVEL OF ALLIANCES

Perhaps your mother never said to you: you are judged by the company you keep. As we said earlier, ours did! Thus we learned early in life the importance of with whom we wanted to affiliate. Our first affiliation, of course, is with the profession of nursing, the most trusted profession in the Gallup surveys.[5] Automatically, we are seen as valued members of a community. The idea of affiliation can include the organization where we are employed. If we work

TABLE 33.1 **The Eight Elements of Alliances and Coalitions**

Elements	Description
1. A common pain	A shared problem that incentivizes action
2. A convener of stature	An individual or group with sufficient influence to cause others to want to engage in work
3. Representatives of substance	Influential stakeholder groups
4. Committed leaders	Influential individuals who are determined to see the action to fruition
5. A clearly defined purpose	The agreed to and desired outcome of the work done together
6. A formal charter	The agreement for how to work together
7. The northbound train	Belief in the effectiveness of the group
8. A common information base	Transparent knowledge of the issue and the process

Leavitt M, McKeown R. Finding allies, building alliances: 8 elements that bring—and keep—people together. San Francisco: Jossey-Bass; 2013.

for a Magnet® organization, we have an elevated status in nursing. If we work with an organization that has repeatedly been cited for violations of some standards, our reputation is lowered.

Affiliation also includes which professional organizations we affiliate with—if any. We make that last comment because our profession's participation in external professional societies is low in comparison with many other groups, such as physicians and lawyers. When we join a professional society, we extend ourselves beyond our work and support the work of the profession, not just our individual work. Those groups form alliances with other groups for a variety of purposes, often related to legislative influence. For example, the American Nurses Association often works closely with AARP (formerly called the American Association of Retired Persons) because together both groups are concerned with protecting and advancing the health of older persons. If our specialty in nursing is gerontology, we have just extended our influence through this organizational affiliation.

In any organization, people tend to work with a small group of people. That might be a unit-based group or a role-based group, for example, neurology (clinical) or clinical nurse specialists (role). If the group is good, that aura transfers to us and we are obligated to help maintain and advance that perspective. If we are further identified in some way, such as being recognized as a DAISY Foundation recipient, we again enter into a smaller and more prestigious group. The 2020 pandemic response by frontline nurses cast an aura over all of us.

All of these relationships help form the opinions of others about our influence and ability to bring about change. For example, each of us (the authors) advanced in our professional work not just because of our own work but because we knew the key leaders in various areas to be able to contact them at any time. We had instant consultation available to us from the experts in the profession. That is a goal we should all have in order to have the best thinking available to us.

Unless an individual is highly influential, being able to speak for an alliance of people is more effective than speaking merely as one's self. If you aren't in a true relationship with others, this is a task to assume for your own development.

CREATING ALLIANCES

Creating alliances with others is not rocket science! It involves being willing to listen to others, to consider what you have in common with them, what your mutual goals might be, the rationale for establishing a relationship, and the commitment of time to be effective. In some ways, that is what we do when we form friendships or work teams. We figure out not who is like us (although some of us do that some of the time) but who has values that relate to ours for the intent of achieving some betterment of the service known as nursing. (Note that we also form other affiliations such as educational, religious, gender, lifestyle, and so forth.)

Creating alliances involves deliberative thinking not in terms of how to use someone else, but rather how working together toward a common goal can be eased or made more effective.

"You might remember that in the chapter on advocating, we shared the story of the Colorado Center attempting to resolve the issue of APRN new graduates leaving the state because they couldn't find physicians to supervise them in

acquiring prescriptive authority. I realized early in this effort that the center could not do this alone. The key to successfully revising the legislation was creating an alliance of not only nursing organizations, which included the state nurses' association, the Colorado Organization of Nurse Leaders, nurse midwives, nurse anesthetists and additional specialty organizations (e.g., perioperative nurses), and school nurses, but also community organizations, such as AARP, the state hospital association, the community mental health group, the federally funded health clinics, and the rural health association. All these organizations united in support of 'access to care.'

"These community groups all needed APRNs and immediately saw the advantage of supporting our efforts. With the political acumen of a key center staff person, Ingrid Johnson, who served as a volunteer intern to the state senator sponsoring the legislation, these groups lobbied state legislators in support of decreasing the hours required for obtaining prescriptive authority and allowing APRNs with prescriptive authority to also supervise the new graduates. Members of the alliance met regularly at the Colorado Center to strategize and clarify and organize the efforts of all the group members to ensure everyone was united and their hard work was both focused and effective. It was a major learning moment regarding the power and effectiveness of groups uniting to form an alliance."

Alliances such as these allow us to extend our influence beyond ourselves because we are seen as a member of a group. When we have the opportunity to make a difference at a more impactful level, who of us doesn't want to do that?

LL ALERT

- Don't join just any alliance.
- Don't dilute your effectiveness by joining too many alliances.
- Don't rely on alliances to do the work because this allows us to shirk our individual accountability.

SUMMARY

Forming alliances is a tool that allows leaders to be more effective. That ability to relate to others and other groups allows us to expand what we do to advance the health of the nation in different ways than we could do individually.

LL LINEUP

- Identify groups that relate to your specialty and role.
- Contribute something to one or more of those groups so that you are seen as broader than whatever your title and role are.

REFLECTION Identify all of the groups (including those external to your profession and role) that you could say were groups in which you are allied. Consider if a theme emerges and if it is in alignment with what your values and goals are. If a theme does not emerge and you want to use the important approach to expanding your influence, what do you need to do to expand your alliances? How do you or will you maintain the alliances so they are effective?

34

Communication

Being able to communicate effectively is perhaps the most important of all leadership skills and one we devote the least time to. Successful leaders are continuously attempting to improve and grow this skill set. Basic communication concepts can be found in many undergraduate leadership texts. Leadership communication, however, requires taking those skills and applying them in different contexts and developing them at a higher level.

Communication is a process by which information is exchanged between individuals through a common system of symbols, signs, or behaviors.[1] The only thing human beings do more often is breathe. Unfortunately, some people seem to think that communication is as natural as breathing and thus don't improve this skill.

The American Organization of Nurse Executives (AONE) (now known as the American Organization for Nursing Leadership [AONL]) Nurse Executive Competencies stress the importance of excellent communication skills in its first competency. This competency identifies the importance of effective communication as it relates to managing and resolving conflict, facilitating group discussions, demonstrating skill in interpersonal communication, making oral presentations to many different audiences, and producing cogent and persuasive written communication.[2]

When considering the complexity of communication, we think about what constitutes communication—not just words but also facial expressions and body language. Although the thought that communication is 58% body language and facial expression, 35% tonality, and 7% words has been exposed as old and inaccurate, we understand how important tonality and body language are to effective communication.[3] For example, sometimes tonality actually changes the meaning of the words so that they are opposite of the dictionary definition. Emphasizing a word in a different manner can change the meaning. For example, saying "really!" is very different in meaning from saying "really?"

Facial expressions and body language are integral to communication. If we didn't believe that before, think about the day-long, back-to-back electronic meetings we endured in 2020 as many jobs moved to the home and Internet. When we seldom see body language and sometimes even have difficulty seeing faces, full communication can be a challenge. For example, if we say we are calm but wave our arms around as we talk or have an anxious look on our face, we communicate a different message. Communication is complex, and yet it's the primary tool for connection with other human beings in creating relationships.

MENTAL FILTERS

One aspect of what makes communication complex is we all create interpretations of the world based on our own realities, which evolve from our life experiences, socialization, genetic heritage, attitudes and opinions, emotions, and life choices. These aspects can form communication filters through which people interpret the world and other human beings. Clearly, distorted communication is common. These distortions (filters) affect how people send and receive communication. As a trivial example, consider how a carbonated beverage is referred to in different parts of the country: pop, soda, soft drink, and coke (a generic term).

The classic work of Thomas Crane identified several primary communication filters, such as mental state, assumptions, attitude, hidden agendas, belief systems, judgments of self and others, emotional states, and the current state of the relationship. Any or all of these can have a major influence on communication. Each can be a filter and can work with other filters to further obfuscate communication.[4]

A frame of mind (*mental state*) exists during an interaction and includes positive and negative attitudes. When we feel overwhelmed and stressed, we experience difficulty in shifting to a clear mental state. However, being upset, stressed, or overwhelmed usually exacerbates a difficult situation. Excellent leaders use a tactic to be able to focus. They ask for 5 minutes and turn away from the stressful situation, take a moment to clear emotions, then return and remember that everyone watches the leader.

REFLECTION Recall a recent example where you felt upset. How did you behave? How did others respond?

One of the most significant issues in communications is failed expectations, which are often based on unclarified *assumptions*. To become conscious of assumptions and expectations requires constant self-examination and reflection. It also requires frequent contact with the other person to identify any expectations and/or assumptions based on opinions about the other person. The best approach is to begin an interaction with a "clean slate," or no preconceived considerations. Focus on what the real message is.

Many stories exist about *attitude*, such as looking at a glass of water filled halfway and emphasizing the difference between those who describe the glass as half full versus those who describe the glass as half empty. The difference is indicative of how individuals see the world. Do you want to spend time with someone who has a different story every day about how tough or bad life is or someone who is positive and sees the world as full of possibilities? The Harvard Business School found that success in life is 7% aptitude, knowledge, or skills and 93% attitude and talent. Your attitude as a leader is "catching."[5] Do you want your people to be positive or negative? Human beings are not always aware of what motivates behavior. In fact, we may have *hidden agendas and intentions*. Therefore habits, conditioning, and underlying needs and desires may dictate behaviors. Habits and unconscious needs and desires can dictate a person's reaction to a situation rather than creating an appropriate response or an effective assessment of the communication interaction. One strategy would be for leaders to spend a few minutes clarifying intentions for the day before beginning interactions.

Hidden agendas can be either positive or negative. Many people have an agenda when seeking interactive time with another person. As an example, one of us constantly asked questions of someone in a leadership position because she was secretly nominating that person for an award (a positive agenda). Unfortunately, however, most hidden agendas are not positive. Receiving the message may be insufficient—we might have to seek the intention by asking about the purpose of a statement or question.

We have found setting goals and expectations for the most important conversations tends to produce better results. As an example, conversation should have an agreed-upon purpose, confirmation of the time allotted, agreed-upon agendas, and a goal or outcome at the end of the conversation. When we add the component of mutual agreement at the beginning of those important conversations, we are better able to control the direction and therefore the outcome of the conversation.

Belief systems comprise personal values acquired throughout life. These belief systems expand or limit thinking, actions, and responses. Many people operate from a positive, upbeat perspective of "live life"—anything is possible, so learn, laugh, and love. On the other hand, some people believe that much of life will be negative; they feel they must protect and defend against all the terrible events in the world. Those who approach life positively are open to change, easy to communicate with, and receptive to others. Those who are waiting for the next disaster are difficult to work with or enroll in new ideas. People like to be around positive people, and such people function well in leadership positions. Every interaction can be affected by our belief systems.

Who is toughest on you? When learners are asked this question, consistently, the response is a form of "me." *Judgement of ourselves and others* is a difficult issue. Judgment is the process of forming an opinion or reaching a conclusion based on the available material. Thoughts produce related feelings, such as anxiety, anger, and depression. We often confuse our own perceptions of situations and events with reality. Judgments of events and behaviors can be said to trigger anxiety, anger, or depression. When applied to people, these emotions usually result in relationship breakdown. Likewise, self-judgment results from thoughts we have about ourselves and the meanings attached to those thoughts. Many of us have a little voice that sends messages, such as "you really blew that interaction" or "what made you say such a dumb thing?" Judgment of ourselves does not support growth and learning; rather, it focuses on self-criticism and negativism.

Emotional states significantly affect the thinking process. Consequently, emotions of upset, anger, and hurt affect our ability to think clearly and logically. Negative feelings such as insecurities, threats, stress, fear, need to be right or perfect, and unhealed interpersonal "wounds" affect a person's ability to communicate and think clearly. Conversely, positive emotions such as delight, joy, hopeful expectations, and humor affect communication and thinking in a positive way that allows us to overlook issues that require attention. If we are sufficiently self-aware and trust is sufficiently high, think what might happen if we disclosed our emotional state. Might the other person not try to help us get the message right?

Any nurse who has been in a clinical area and listened to the conversations knows how important *the current state of the relationships* is within the work setting. These unit relationships affect the team and the performance of the individual and thus the organization. Negative feelings and interactions, unfinished business, unresolved conflicts, and emotional residue are poisonous to communication, relationships, and team functioning.[4] If leaders have relationships with others that are in a state of disrepair, every interaction can be significantly affected by the negative issues.

COMPENSATION FOR THE FILTERS

To compensate for these communication filters, we need to practice becoming centered and self-aware and to work at being less reactive or less judgmental. Communication breakdown can be avoided by listening carefully to others and striving for awareness of these filters. The goal is to neutralize them as much as possible. This is a process or journey in communication growth and improvement, requiring time and energy.

> **REFLECTION** What do you use to compensate?

Effective leaders seek a quiet place, take several deep breaths and refocus their energy, center themselves, and choose the objective, thoughtful response. They are able to "let go" of the negative and choose a different approach. It's about "choosing," and it requires practice.

EFFECTIVE COMMUNICATION SKILLS

Common leadership communication skills that extend beyond the basic ones focus on oral presentations, writing, emailing, texting, social media, and deliberative listening. Oral and written communication requires the ability to be concise without being terse, to convey caring without losing the essence of the message, and to convey confidence without seeming aloof. That is not easy to accomplish! Listening requires the overlay of politics, discrimination, and the expectations of others to be heard. One of the aspects of communication that such interaction establishes is rapport, which is described as mutual understanding or trust and agreement between people or a close connection.[6]

Another aspect of effective communication is the ability to summarize the ideas and feelings of others. It requires complete attention and 100% focus on the interaction to be able to accurately summarize what was shared. This can also help to clarify, as the person will agree with the summary or clarify what might have been omitted or misunderstood. One of us has often sat in meetings and then conveyed a message that others thought was great:

"They are surprised when I respond that the message consists of their ideas, and I have merely condensed and synthesized the essence of their comments into a summary statement. The reason I can do this is because I am a laser-like listener in these situations."

GUIDELINES FOR CREATING A POSITIVE COMMUNICATION ENVIRONMENT

Creating an environment that is conducive to a positive interaction facilitates effectiveness. Even if the person with whom we are interacting has an official, high-level leadership position, we can still take the lead. Several aspects can be thoughtfully prepared in the 10 minutes or so before the interaction. Table 34.1 lists the aspects for creating a positive communication setting.

COMMUNICATION BARRIERS

Barriers to communication are often unconscious.[7] For example, *judgment* is a barrier where another person is found to be wanting in some area. As an example, many of us intuitively know when someone is judging us as less than an undisclosed standard. This approach destroys any chance of a meaningful interaction between two people.

TABLE 34.1 Aspects for Creating a Positive Communication Environment

Specific aspects	Descriptions
Create a positive mindset	Take responsibility for creating positive communication.
Be vulnerable	Don't be afraid to reveal yourself to others unless you have specific reasons to be distrustful.
Begin with questions	Ask questions about a local event or family/mutual friends, unless you know the person to be very business focused.
Be positive	Acknowledge and encourage the other person.
Set goals and expectations	Use important conversations to lead to improved outcomes.
Choose the message	Consciously fit the message with the receiver's style.
Share the responsibility	Remember that each person shares equal responsibility for communication.
Use language conveying trust and openness	Imply equality, even if a status or title difference exists.

Not *paying attention* when the other person is talking or sharing is classic. Many times, leaders are busy (as are others!) and believe time can be saved by multitasking. This approach can be exemplified by checking a phone or computer emails as someone arrives, checking their watch, or allowing interruptions by phone calls or other people. All of these activities are disrespectful of the person attempting to convey a message he deems important.

Overuse of *technical language* and acronyms to impress or confuse the other person is also a disrespectful barrier to effective communication. This can happen with new employees who have yet to master all the terminology, abbreviations, or idioms specific to the job. One of us worked with a new employee who developed a "dictionary" of frequently used terminology and abbreviations that was shared with other new employees so all could benefit. This was a creative positive approach to learning a new job.

Fixing the problem or giving unwanted advice may be a more prominent issue for nurses, because nurses are taught to solve problems and "fix" whatever confronts them. We do this with patients and families and team members. It's easy to see how this approach would bleed over into other conversations. Figuring out the approach to take is a perfect example of the art of leadership.

Avoiding an issue or concern brought to a leader is problematic. When communication is about an issue that is clearly important to the other person, ignoring the issue and moving on to another topic is disrespectful to the person's concerns.

Although avoiding the behaviors just described can increase effective communication, any one of them can create significant communication breakdown. Because we all tend to fall into communication patterns—some of them negative—let's look at communication breakdowns and how to move forward when leaders are involved in a breakdown.

REFLECTION Look at the barriers again. What do you do? How will you plan to change that behavior?

COMMUNICATION BREAKDOWN

In complex situations such as those encountered in health care organizations and related facilities, multiple stressors feed communication breakdown. Communications are more apt to break down when crises are apparent, such as state inspectors appearing unannounced due to some complaint or sentinel event. Everyone involved is stressed in these intense situations, and the tendency is to have a more muddled mental state. We can make assumptions, judge and blame others, and have negative emotions. In such situations, most of us know what physical responses occur when these situations arise. Some yell, some turn red in the face, and some withdraw from the situation. The Awareness Model depicted in Fig. 34.1 demonstrates the difference between conscious responses and unconscious reactions to stressful interactions.

The upper circle demonstrates that when we are in an *automatic "reaction,"* we spontaneously go to Blame, Judgment, and Demand. It may be reassuring to understand that nearly everyone experiences a meltdown at some point in their lives. Regardless of how difficult situations are, each human being decides, even at an unconscious level, how he or she will respond. No one "makes" a person feel anything. Each person chooses various responses. It is possible to work toward a communication interaction that produces a positive, constructive outcome.

When a person reacts to a situation at the *feeling* level, he or she focuses on blaming others for whatever has happened. By taking responsibility for at least part of the breakdown, the communication shifts from one of blame to one of ownership for a specific piece.

Likewise, when a person is caught up in reaction at the *thinking* level, he or she easily can make a judgment. When

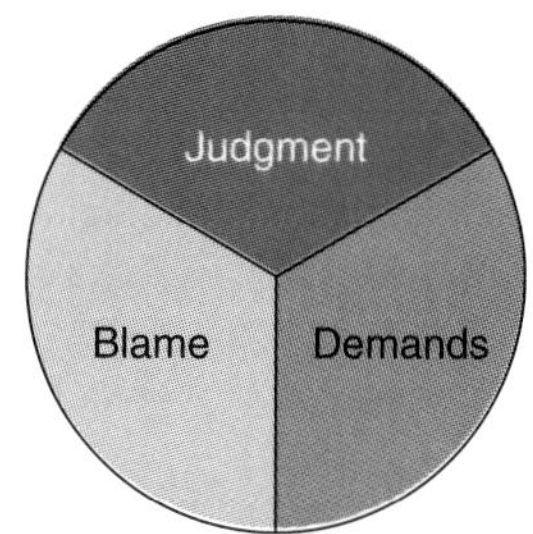

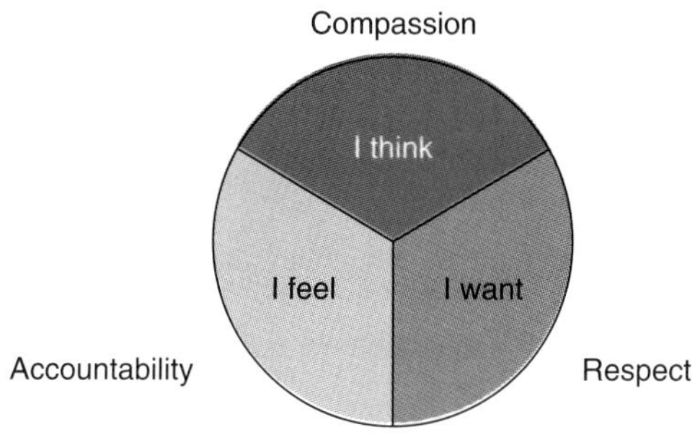

Fig. 34.1 **Awareness model.** From Yoder-Wise. Leading and managing in nursing. 7th ed. Amsterdam: Elsevier; 2019.

it is possible to breathe deeply and become calm, a respectful way to make a request to the team member becomes possible.

Most broken relationships, whether with coworkers, physicians, or family members, are focused on blaming another person, judging them as wrong, and demanding that something mean and hurtful happen to them (the "perpetrators"). Accountability, compassion, and respect in interpersonal interactions are much more likely to create situations in which each person's needs are met and the work is done. We can role model such behavior with others because they watch how we manage difficult situations. That is a key part of how others learn.

REFLECTION When the coronavirus affected almost every country in the world, lots of communication breakdown occurred. What did you experience?

ACTIVE LISTENING

Listening, as we have said before, is the other half of the communication process. We speak and then we listen to the other person. Our experience is that active listening is much more than just looking at the other person and nodding! By reflecting what the other person said, we issue a restatement of the communication, including both words and feelings such as tone of voice and facial expression. This reflecting ensures we are understanding what others are saying and the underlying intention. This translates to good listening skills complementing good questioning skills. When we are unsure of what the other person is asking or saying, we must question until we are clear.

Human beings continually strive to feel "heard" and understood at a deep interpersonal level. This striving is about being connected to other human beings.[8] In other words, many people are so busy talking and attempting to convey their story or point of view, they may not take the time to listen to the other person. A colleague once shared that her 6-year-old crawled up on a chair adjacent to the kitchen countertop and took her face between his hands, looked into her eyes, and said, "Calling Mom, this is Kevin calling Mom." She was embarrassed that she had not been listening to him but instead was focused on making dinner and reflecting on a key problem at work.

One of the greatest gifts leaders can give to others is one-on-one time in which they focus 100% on the other person. The focus on listening purposefully to understand demonstrates to the speaker that (1) the message has been heard, (2) the intensity of the speaker's emotions is understood *and* accepted, and (3) he or she should continue to share even more deeply. Actively listening requires specific actions, as shown in Table 34.2.

Listening is critical for leaders. From nearly 3500 participants in a coaching development program, Zenger and Folkman selected the top active listeners as determined in a 360-degree assessment.[9] They selected the top 5% and compared them to others in the data set and identified

TABLE 34.2 Aspects of Active Listening

Techniques	Descriptions
Establish rapport/build trust	Listen carefully and distinguish between the message content and the underlying emotional and nonverbal cues.
Demonstrate concern	Exhibit facial expressions and statements such as "That must have been very difficult."
Paraphrase to show understanding	Restate what you think you heard by saying, for example, "Let me see if I understood you correctly…"
Use nonverbal cues	Use eye contact, lean forward, nod, and smile to demonstrate understanding.
Use brief verbal affirmations	Use verbal cues that convey the person was being attended to: "I see," "I understand," "I know."
Ask open-ended questions	Ask something that cannot be answered with yes or no or a one-word response: "What are you thinking now?"
Seek clarification through specific questions	Use specifics to convey active listening: "What made you think X?" "Can you tell me more about Y?"
Wait to express an opinion	Support the other person to talk until they are complete, then express yourself.

Adapted from Doyle A. Learn about active listening skills with examples. 2018. Available at: https://www.thebalancecareers.com/active-listening-skills-with-examples-2059684.

those behaviors that made the most difference. The findings indicated significantly more active listening than the other group, not talking over others, conveying listening through facial expressions and verbal sounds, and being able to repeat what the other had said. They then grouped these findings into four categories.

First, good listening is much more than not talking over the other person. The leader asks questions that lead to *discovery and insight* into the other person's thoughts and emotions. Asking really good questions indicates active listening and understanding far more than a nodding head or an interested facial expression. Active listening was seen as a dialog rather than a speaker–listener interaction.

The second finding was listening that *builds self-esteem*. The leader made the conversation a positive experience by making the other person feel supported and conveying confidence in the other person. The leader creates a safe environment in which issues and differences are discussed openly.

The third skill is listening as a *cooperative conversation*. The interaction flowed smoothly, and neither the leader nor the other person became defensive about any comments made. Comparatively, poor or less sophisticated listeners were viewed as competitive. They seemed to listen to find errors in thinking or to problem-solve, and they constructed arguments or responses while the other person was talking. Good leaders can challenge assumptions and disagree, but the person still finds the interaction helpful as opposed to an attempt to "win" an argument.

The fourth skill is *making constructive suggestions*. This involves providing some feedback in an acceptable manner that opens possible paths for the receiver. Making these suggestions needs to be done in a skillful way rather than being perceived as "jumping in." It may also be possible that the person is more likely to want suggestions from someone who is viewed as a good listener rather than seen as a leader who has been critical and gives advice. The critical listener may not be seen as trustworthy, and thus the advice is not seen as useful.

"YOU, YOU, YOU"

Mark Murphy created a negative word analyzer that analyzes email, written speeches, and communication for the number of negative words. The program has highlighted more than 2000 words that can be framed as negative.[6] These words can create conflict and defensiveness. The one that appears most commonly of the 2000 is "you." It can indicate a lack of empathy on the part of the leader. And it requires being very purposeful in eliminating "you" from your vocabulary. While working on this, consider writing down key sentences before speaking with a person to be certain you avoid the use of "you" in difficult situations.

REFLECTION Have a colleague count the number of times the word "you" is used in your conversation or record yourself delivering a message to another person. How often was the word "you" used?

LL ALERT

- Don't use words such as "should", which implies control and could initiate feelings of guilt.
- Don't use the word "but", which negates everything said before it.
- Don't say "always" or "never" because hardly anything is always or never and thus you appear to be exaggerating.
- Don't say "can't," which is usually less truthful than what you mean, which is won't.

SUMMARY

Communication is one of the most powerful tools leaders have. It is used every day in multiple ways, such as verbally in talking with nurses and others; written communication, including both reports and emails; and listening actively to everyone involved in an interaction. We have made many suggestions as to the most effective way to communicate, and effectiveness leads to mutual respect between leaders and everyone who encounters them. Our focus has to be on how effectively we apply the tools.

LL LINEUP

- Think carefully about how you listen and how effective you believe you are.
- Watch others' facial expressions and body language for cues as to how you are able to connect with them.

REFLECTION Reflect on the tonality used in an interaction with a colleague. What was conveyed with the tonality? Consider what the underlying intention of the message was. How was the intention conveyed in the tonality of the message? Did you convey the message during a disagreement? What was "unsaid" in the interchange? What was the underlying message? Were your words and body language congruent in delivering the message?

35

Contribution

Professionalism is one of the two critical elements that inform the Legacy *Leaders*-Ship Trajectory model. Part of professionalism is the contributions we make to our profession and the community. Professionalism is central to our nursing practice; we begin to hear that word and apply it in various contexts beginning with our first nursing course. It is threaded through all our practice standards and the ethical principles that govern being a nurse. An important component of professionalism is altruism/advocacy. Altruism/advocacy refers to unselfish regard for and devotion to the welfare of others rather than our own well-being. Professional behavior requires that our self-interest does not interfere with decisions regarding our practice.

As we move through our Legacy *Leaders*-Ship journey, we must continually recognize that self-interest should *not* be the driving factor in building a legacy, nor in developing leader skills. Of course, those of us interested in leadership typically have a healthy self-concept and hope for various accolades in our careers that say to the world "I am successful." However, that need for recognition cannot be the main driver for our striving for achievement. Our primary focus must be on "What can I contribute—to patients, my community, and to the science and practice of nursing?" In addition, we must derive joy from the work we do—otherwise, what is the point?

Most of us can think of people within our sphere of influence who appear to be primarily interested in improving their position in the organization or profession. One of us once worked with a chief nursing officer (CNO) of a large community hospital, who, after an emergency where the power went down at the hospital, was discussing (bragging) about how she had handled the situation. One of her staff asked her exactly what steps she took to solve the problem. She quickly responded, "Oh, I don't give away my secrets. I don't want others to be able to do what I know how to do." Granted, this is an extreme case, but it was clear to everyone in the room that this CNO was not primarily interested in the welfare of the patients, her staff, or the organization where she worked. She simply wanted to be the "top dog." This type of behavior does not build a Legacy *Leaders*-Ship trajectory. Similarly, another of us worked with someone who later, and in a different state, used state funds illegally. As a colleague said, "Exactly how much money do you have to make to be satisfied?" This person was focused on things that weren't to the organization's benefit.

By contrast, one of the ways to build a career that does lead to a legacy is to consider what nurses individually and collectively have done over time to make teams, organizations, communities, and health care in general better. This can inspire us to consider how we might do the same. One of us once worked with a provost at a university who often said, "We stand on the shoulders of those who came before us." Another of us had experience at the American Nurses Credentialing Center that was shaped by the executive Director, Dr. Jeanne Floyd, who always focused on what was best for nursing. She would ask: "What would Gretta (Dr. Margretta Styles, a past president and visionary) do"? As a result we all had a view of what was possible. It is hard to focus only on ourselves when we recognize the contributions that our colleagues have made over time. Let's explore this idea in more depth.

REFLECTION How often have you worked with nurses who seemed to be motivated by self-interest and the need for recognition? How were the interactions with this person and the resulting work of the team or organization affected by this behavior? Conversely, have you worked with nurses who were most concerned with their contribution to the bigger goal? Were the interactions different?

FRAMEWORK FOR NURSES' CONTRIBUTION

Differentiating the unique contributions that nurses make to the care of individual patients (and their significant others) is difficult because the "tasks" required of each health care discipline in the interprofessional team are often similar or perhaps even the same. (After all, we all take some sort of health history.) Teddie Potter, in *Reflections in*

Nursing Leadership, provides us with a wonderful framework to answer the question, "What unique contribution does a nurse make to health care?" She describes a conversation with a physician who was writing about interprofessional collaboration and wanted to know more about what nurses did. He said, "Physicians diagnose or treat. In two words, what do nurses do?"[1] Dr. Potter couldn't answer in two words (nor can we, and we expect you might not be able to do so either). So she answered with a question:

"Imagine you have a medically fragile patient in the hospital. You have correctly diagnosed the condition and ordered the appropriate medications. If nurses weren't present, what would happen to your patient? The physician thought for a while and then said, 'He'd die.' I looked him in the eye and responded, 'And that is what nurses do.'"[1]

> **REFLECTION** Could you say in two words what you do? If not, could you create a scenario, such as Dr. Potter did, to let others know what you do? What is that scenario?

From this experience, Dr. Potter developed a framework called the BASE of Nursing Practice, which illustrates nursing's contribution to healing.[1] The paradigm has four domains. Nurses must be proficient in all domains, applying them in whatever aspect of practice in which they are involved, both in acute care settings and in the community. The domains are defined in Table 35.1.

You may wonder if Dr. Potter came up with a short answer to the physician's question, "What do nurses do?" In fact, she did. In her article in *Reflections on Nursing Scholarship*, Dr. Potter said, "I could have responded with certainty and confidence that Nursing is *being* and *knowing*."[1]

As people who love stories and come from story-telling families, we found this answer very meaningful. As Dr. Potter's framework demonstrates, evidence generated from research gives us a direction to choose the appropriate interventions we provide through active caring. Of course, we cannot depend upon one personal experience alone to determine the best strategies for care. However, being present to really hear the stories allows us to use what we hear to provide patient-centered care in the context of the patient's experience *and* the evidence.

AN EXAMPLE OF BEING PRESENT

One of us remembers a time during her graduate school experience when she was working with an older adult couple at their home as they dealt with the husband's treatment for bowel cancer:

"On one home visit, the patient indicated that he was going to have exploratory surgery, because the physician suspected that there was potential blockage in the bowel. Both the patient and his wife felt hopeful about this surgery, because they understood that the surgery would significantly prolong his life. They were both nervous about the procedure and asked if I would be willing to be in the operating room during the surgery. Of course, I said yes, and the surgeon agreed.

"As I was standing on a stool at the patient's head during the operation, the surgeon said to others in the room, 'It appears there is no blockage. That is disappointing, but in any case, I am sure that the patient and his family are aware that this procedure would not save his life.' He then looked to me for confirmation. I had to say that the patient and his wife were hoping that this surgery would, in fact, prolong his life. Because I had been in their home, spending time with the couple, I was able to hear the full story of their hopes for the surgery and share this couple's perspective. I hope that my statement helped the physician to interact with the family and the patient after the surgery was over."

> **REFLECTION** Do you have an example of a circumstance where you were able to be present? What was the result for you and the recipient(s)? What would you do differently in another situation?

TABLE 35.1 Components of Potter's BASE Framework

Domains	Characteristics
Being present (a way of being)	Therapeutic use of self—*really* being present and listening
Active caring (a way of being)	Caring that requires action
Stories from narratives (a way of knowing)	The stories come from those we care for and often provide clues to what is needed, thus providing direction to choose interventions from the evidence
Evidence from science (a way of knowing)	Evidence-based practice

From Potter TM. In two words, what do nurses contribute to healing? Reflections on nursing leadership. Sigma. 2016. Available at: https://www.reflectionsonnursingleadership.org/features/more-features/Vol42_4_in-two-words-what-do-nurses-contribute-to-healing.

DOCUMENTATION OF NURSES' IMPACT ON HEALTH CARE

Defining what a nurse does is difficult because of the myriad potential roles and functions that are available. Following are some of the major responsibilities of nurses, regardless of the care setting:

- Performing assessments, whether the client is an individual, group, community, or population
- Interpreting assessment data and making judgments to determine the appropriate nursing interventions or programs to promote health and protect patients from risk of harm
- Providing health promotion, counseling/coaching, and education
- Administering medications, wound care, and numerous other personalized interventions
- Advocating for appropriate treatment protocols, policies supporting safety, timely symptom management, and consultations with specialty services and other stakeholders
- Coordinating care across the health care system
- Conducting or participating in research in support of improved practice, education, and patient outcomes
- Serving as a manager and/or leader in a variety of teams or organizations
- Teaching others to improve the health care processes[2]

> **REFLECTION** Can you think of other broad functions nurses might have? Which of these could be implemented in a variety of care settings or practice environments?

NURSES' IMPACT ON HEALTH CARE OUTCOMES

Over the last 20 years, research has documented the impact of nursing practice on outcomes. In 2002, Aiken and colleagues reported in the *Journal of the American Medical Association* (*JAMA*) that in hospitals with insufficient patient-to-nurse ratios, surgical patients experienced higher risk-adjusted 30-day mortality. Failure-to-rescue rates were also higher, and nurses were more likely to experience burnout and be dissatisfied with their jobs.[3] This led to a plethora of studies that explored the impact of nursing care in hospitals. In 2015, the American Nurses Association (ANA) published a literature review outlining the impact of nursing staffing—the role of nurses—on patient care in acute care hospitals. Following are some of the results of these studies regarding both inadequate and adequate nursing staffing.

Inadequate staffing in nursing resulted in:

- Increased mortality
- Missed care
- Waste of health care dollars (costs from termination, unfilled positions, advertising/recruiting, hiring staff, training and orientation)
- Nurse burnout
- Nurse job dissatisfaction

Improved staffing in nursing and work environment resulted in prevention of:

- Avoidable and costly readmissions
- Hospital-acquired infections
- Medication errors

Improved rescue of patients from deterioration and death also was an outcome of improved staffing and work conditions.[4]

The impact of nursing in outpatient and community settings on health outcomes is also being evaluated, although to date, the research on the relationship between nursing and patient outcomes in community settings is not as robust as that related to nursing practice in inpatient settings. However, a review of program descriptions and evaluations in the literature gives hope that research regarding nurses' impact in these settings will continue to grow.

CARE COORDINATION

The role of care coordination is an area where the nurses' role and related outcomes is showing promise. An early example of the effectiveness of care coordination is the evaluation of the transition care model, which complemented primary care by ensuring continuity of high-quality care across settings by multiple providers. In this approach, the team is led by an advanced practice registered nurse (APRN). Various clinical trials of this model demonstrated that patient care experiences and health outcomes were improved, while hospitalization from all causes and total health care costs were reduced.[5]

A more recent example of such innovative programs designed to improve care coordination is at Massachusetts General Hospital. In this program, when a patient is admitted to the hospital, he or she is assigned to an attending registered nurse (ARN). The ARN is assigned to the patient while in the hospital and after discharge and is responsible for promoting continuity of care as the patient moves through the health care system. This is not the only program involving nurses in new roles that are designed to improve patient experiences and lower costs. These new roles may involve health promotion activities; strategies to reduce hospital readmissions, thus lowering costs; and providing more affordable, more convenient, and patient-centered care in the community.[5]

On a larger level, you might want to return to the chapter on advocating (Chapter 10) and review the information about how nurses are the only group trusted to fix the health care insurance issue in the United States. Historically, nurses have been called the glue in an organization. We hold it together as others move in and out. How differently might countries have responded to the coronavirus in 2020 if nurses had been able to apply this glue to the whole system as opposed to individual hospitals. Our contributions must be beyond the organizational level, which by itself is an area in which we can have great impact.

REFLECTION What area in your professional practice (or personal life) do you advocate for policies that positively influence the health of the citizenry? What have you learned in this work? What issues are important to you that you would like to be involved with in the future?

NURSING CONTRIBUTIONS AT THE ORGANIZATIONAL LEVEL

Nursing organizations across the country, fueled by the work of individual nurses and groups of nurses, contribute significantly to the health of US citizens through legislative, regulatory, and policy initiatives. Many local, state, national, and international nursing organizations are involved in this work, addressing a wide variety of topics ranging from health care reform to the care of women and children. However, four national organizations, the American Academy of Nursing, the American Association of Colleges of Nursing, the American Nurses Association, and the National League for Nursing spring to mind as examples of advocacy. Table 35.2 provides an overview of the topics addressed.

TABLE 35.2 Advocacy Efforts by Selected US Nursing Organizations

American Academy of Nursing (AAN) http://www.aannet.org	American Association of Colleges of Nursing (AACN) https://www.aacnnursing.org/Policy-Advocacy	American Nurses Association (ANA) https://www.nursingworld.org/practice-policy/advocacy	National League for Nursing (NLN) http://www.nln.org/advocacy-public-policy
AAN serves the public and the nursing profession by advancing health policy and practice through the generation, synthesis, and dissemination of nursing knowledge. Outputs of this work include policy proposals, testimony, manuscripts, policy briefs, recommendations, and advocacy papers, as well as position statements and research agendas. Process includes the use of expert panels on areas, such as: Advanced care planning Care coordination Genomics Global health Health care reform Health equity Violence	AACN's advocacy work centers on the highest education for nurses. Areas of concern include: Federal policies Nursing Workforce issues and the opioid crisis This work is carried out by Capitol Hill visits and testimony by staff, deans, faculty, and students.	ANA's advocacy work centers on legislative and regulatory activities, advocating directly with decision makers and representing nurses on Capitol Hill. The focus on priorities for practice and policy include the areas of: Nursing excellence Nurses' Work Environment Health policy, including patient safety State and federal issues, including agencies and regulatory bodies	NLN focuses on nursing education policy in the following areas: Access Education Diversity The Workforce The NLN organization includes an advocacy center and collection of statistics related to nursing education at all levels. This work is carried out by NLN advocacy work, including position papers, blogs, and testimony before legislatures and regulation bodies. Topics of interest include: Health care reform Scope of practice High-stakes testing Diversity Academic progress Faculty shortage

LL ALERT

- Don't let impending burnout redirect your energy, your time, and your career.
- Don't limit the impact you can have to only "the job."
- Don't forget to attend to self-care so you can make your greatest contributions.

SUMMARY

A colleague of ours tells the story about her tenure as the nurse manager of a busy inpatient pediatric service of a large metropolitan health center. She had been in this position for a number of years and she was tired! She describes making rounds one day and realizing halfway through her rounds, that while she talked to patients and their families, she was not paying full attention. She was mentally reviewing her "to-do" list.

This was a watershed moment for her. She realized that she had to do something to re-engage with her nursing practice—and the patients. She quit her job, went back to school, and changed the trajectory of her career.

When you feel burned out and disengaged—remember your leadership legacy depends upon your interest in your work. Take steps to recommit so that you can contribute to the practice of nursing.

LL LINEUP

- The contributions that all of us make to nursing practice, patient outcomes, and the profession have a profound influence on the health care delivery system and on our own leadership legacy. Let's all continue to put our desire to contribute to this important work first. It will benefit us both individually and collectively.
- We have stood on the shoulders of those who came before us. Through our leadership legacy, we can provide wide shoulders for those who follow.

REFLECTION What is your contribution to nursing practice? What do you hope for in the future?

36

Culture

Edgar Schein's emphasis on culture is focused on what groups learn. He seeks to explain how leadership and culture are two sides of the same coin.[1] The Scheins (father and son) define culture as the accumulated shared learning of a group as it solves problems of external adaptation and internal integration. This learning has worked well enough to be considered valid and taught to new members as the correct way to perceive, think, feel, and behave in relation to those problems. This accumulated learning is a pattern of beliefs, values, and behavioral norms that come to be taken for granted as basic assumptions. Another way to think about these aspects is "the way things are done around here."

HOW IS ORGANIZATIONAL CULTURE CREATED AND COMMUNICATED?

In recent research, nurse leaders were surveyed and asked to indicate how they spend their time. The number-one response (35%) was developing relationships and fostering the culture.[2] Attending to culture is clearly an important aspect of leadership. Specific aspects of culture that affect its style include behaviors that can be observed when people interact, such as greetings and interaction patterns, customs, and traditions such as what happens when there are promotions or project completions.[1] What are the publicly identified espoused values, the group norms, and the implicit or explicit rules by which employees relate or interact with one another? What special competencies are displayed, such as the skills needed to function in the behavioral health areas or the labor and delivery area? Are symbols or root metaphors or even a distinct language needed for new people to be able to function? Consider acronyms or mental models that guide how events are governed or described.

Leaders are vital in creating and changing cultures. Leaders shape cultures by what they say and do, as well as what they reward and discourage. If a leader wants a culture that supports employees to learn and grow, behaviors must reinforce that focus. If a leader thrives on competition and believes that competition creates the best results, the culture could evolve into cutthroat or fairly destructive behavior between those in the competition. If a leader chooses to confront each instance of uncivil behavior in a supportive way that doesn't demean the transgressor but encourages him or her to find another strategy to address concerns, the culture soon will change to one that does not tolerate uncivil behavior. Peers may even address behavior with each other when taught how to do so in a civil way. Oftentimes, at the behest of the leader, behaviors are seen as part of a value system regarding how we treat one another, as well as patients and families.

REFLECTION What does your organizational culture say?

CULTURAL STYLES

An example was given of culture by asking if it was a bear culture or a penguin culture. According to Schein and Schein, the delineation is how the group or team responds to an incompetent or weak member of the group. Bears attempt to nurture the weak to improve performance, whereas the penguins respond to the weak by pecking them to death. In nursing, most of the profession respond as Bear Culture, whereas some situations or areas tend toward a Penguin Culture, or getting rid of the weak member. This is somewhat simplistic but an interesting allegory to demonstrate how different cultures can be. Boris Groysberg and colleagues, through their research, have identified eight critical elements of organizational life/culture.[3] These cultural styles are caring, purpose, learning, enjoyment, results, authority, safety, and order, and each of these styles has strengths and weaknesses. In Table 36.1, the styles are identified and the advantages and disadvantages of each style are described. In the review of the literature, two primary dimensions of culture were identified: people interactions, which were focused on highly independent vs. highly interdependent attributes, and response to change,

TABLE 36.1 Positives and Negatives of Culture Styles

Cultural Style	Positives	Negatives
1. **Caring:** warm, sincere, relational	Focuses on relationships and mutual trust; milieu is warm and collaborative; members help and support one another and are loyal	Focuses on consensus; may reduce possible options; could also stifle competitiveness and slows decision-making
2. **Purpose:** driven, idealistic, tolerant	Focuses on idealism and altruism; milieu is tolerant and members try to do good; focuses also on sustainability and global communities and shared ideals	Focuses on long-term purpose and ideals, negating practical and immediate concerns
3. **Learning:** open, inventive, exploring	Focuses on exploration, expansiveness, and creativity; milieu is inventive and curious and options are explored; knowledge and adventure emphasized	Overemphasizes exploration, leading to lack of focus and inability to exploit existing advantages
4. **Enjoyment:** instinctive and fun loving	Has a lighthearted, fun, and exciting milieu and members create happiness and stimulation with a sense of humor	Focuses on autonomy and engagement, leading to lack of discipline and resulting in issues of compliance and governance
5. **Results:** achievement, goal focused, driven	Focuses on achievement and winning; outcome oriented and merit based; members strive for top performance and drive for success	Overemphasizes results, leading to communication and collaboration breakdowns; increased stress and anxiety
6. **Authority:** bold, decisive, dominant	Focuses on strength, decisiveness, and boldness; milieu is competitive and members strive for personal advantage; strong control and dominance	Overemphasizes authority and bold decision-making, leading to politics, conflict, and a psychologically unsafe milieu
7. **Safety:** realistic, careful, prepared	Focuses on planning, caution, and preparedness; milieu is predictable, risk conscious, and careful; members desire protection, and change is slow	Focuses on standardization leading to bureaucracy, inflexibility, and dehumanization of the milieu
8. **Order:** respectful, cooperative, rule abiding	Focuses on respect, structure, and shared norms; desire to fit in and play by rules and customs	Overemphasizes rules and traditions, reducing individualism, stifling creativity and limiting agility

Adapted from Groysberg B, Lee J, Price J, Cheng Y. The leader's guide to corporate culture: how to manage the eight critical elements of organizational life. *Harv Bus Rev.* 2018:49.

which identified cultures emphasizing stability, consistency, predictability, and status quo vs. those emphasizing flexibility, adaptability, and receptiveness to change. From this work, the eight styles were conceptualized. The study of these styles has evolved over the last two decades and helps us understand the variations in culture.

HOW AND WHY DOES ORGANIZATIONAL CULTURE CHANGE?

Cultures are not stagnant. Members of the unit, area, or organization learn over time what behavior is acceptable and what is not. They learn how to act within the culture to be successful. However, to set a course to purposefully change a culture is not easy. Intense energy and perseverance are required because most employees have learned to survive, or even excel, by adapting to the "old culture," and they do not wish to change behaviors. They are comfortable in the current pattern. We may even have encountered a situation where resistant employees have said, "I've been here the last 15 years. This won't last, I will simply wait the new leader out. He or she will be gone in the next couple of years." This is a sign of resistance to the change the new leader is attempting to engender. Leaders must invest the time and energy to persuade the employees of the advantages of the new culture.[4]

Groysburg's team describes four interventions leaders can use in shifting a culture[3]:

1. *Articulate the aspiration.* A nurse leader can begin this change process by an analysis of the current culture, using a process and framework that is open to the entire organization. An assessment of the outcomes of the current culture and their alignment or not with the stated values and goals is essential. This must be shared with others.
2. *Select and grow leaders* who are aligned with the new stated values for the culture. Leaders encourage other leaders and colleagues at all levels to discuss and describe how patient care will align with these values. In addition, leaders can create a safe environment where nurses can experiment with how to meet the new cultural values and the goals. Nurses can be educated about the new strategies to meet the goals and values and engaged in how the change will be implemented.
3. *Use organizational conversations about culture* to underscore the importance of the change, including rounds, town hall meetings, listening tours, structured group discussions, newsletters, and other methods of communication.
4. *Reinforce the desired change through organizational design.* When the organization's structures, systems, and processes are aligned and support the aspired to culture, the process proceeds much more easily. One example of the alignment is performance management. The tools used in this process, whether it is quarterly or annual evaluation or peer review, are redesigned in a way that supports the implementation of the new cultural values. Orientation and employee training can also be a vehicle for reinforcing the new culture values.

REFLECTION Assume you work in a less-than-desirable culture and you aren't in a key leader role. What can you do as an informal leader to shift a culture, even if no one else is doing anything?

WHAT ARE SUBCULTURES?

Subcultures also exist. In health care, an organization has an overarching culture; yet subcultures exist in various areas or units of the organization. We could denote the differences in various units of a hospital as soon as we exit the elevator to a specific area—even when blindfolded. That indicates the strength of subcultures, which can be quite different. These subcultures have a shared norm or belief system in, for example, how care ought to be delivered to patients and families. These subcultures can be delineated as enhancing, orthogonal, or counterculture.[4] An enhancing subculture is one that aligns with the organizational cultural values and demonstrates even a bit more enthusiasm for these same values. The orthogonal subculture adheres to the organizational overview of the values, yet holds its own distinct values that do not conflict with the overall culture. In contrast, the subcultures that are considered a counterculture hold values that are in conflict with the organizational values. Cultures with deeply embedded values are fairly well aligned across the organization, which are frequently viewed as higher performing. However, organizations that tolerate and embrace orthogonal and enhancing subcultures may demonstrate more agility and adaptability to the rapidly changing health care landscape. For example, when one of us was attempting to change the culture of patient-focused obstetrical care, innovation was a core value. Not only was obstetrical care changed, but also many other innovations followed, such as a women's resource center, healing touch for patients across the facility, and national education conferences focused on innovation. One of the key values was innovation. All of the leaders were focused on "How can we improve the care we give?"

INNOVATIVE CULTURES

Characteristics of innovative cultures include willingness to experiment, tolerance for failure, psychological safety, highly collaborative, and nonhierarchical structure.[5] Such cultures are hard to create and sustain, and in Silicon Valley, these cultures came to be known as "skunk works." Often these cultures are cited for their free-flowing, fun environments, yet three important, not-so-fun aspects of these cultures must coexist with fun and relaxation. The first is a *tolerance for failure,* which mandates an intolerance for incompetence. High standards are set for the team, and the best talent is recruited. Mediocre technical skills, sloppy thinking, or bad work habits are not part of the standards, and team members who exhibit any of these are moved out of the team. Risky ideas that fail, even with highly competent team members, are true failures, and the focus is then on the learning from the project. This highlights the difference between productive and unproductive failures. Productive failures lead to learning, and the celebration is for the learning. How does a leader create a healthy balance between productive failures and incompetence resulting in possible termination? These situations are quite stressful. It is not easy to determine how much of failure is a bad idea or an idea that encountered a problem no one could have anticipated. Especially in health care, all providers make human mistakes, and the issue is are they repetitive or did learning occur?

The second key aspect is a *willingness to experiment* while being highly disciplined. The team members experiment to learn. Disciplined teams select experiments in order to learn. They create rigorous, detailed plans to learn as much as possible while containing costs. Although the women's center idea, described earlier, had many successes in patient and family education, parent bereavement support groups, a breast center, lactation program and human milk bank, staff education, and national meetings, they also had major learning experiences, such as a failed osteoporosis screening program.

The third aspect identified was to focus on *collaboration, but with individual accountability*. Collaborative cultures naturally seek help from colleagues, which comes from a sense of collaborative responsibility. But do not confuse collaboration with consensus, which requires significant amounts of time. Consensus can be poisonous to navigating the complex chaotic situations associated with today's innovative processes. A culture of accountability (individual and group) is based on the expectation that each member is accountable for making his or her decisions and the associated consequences of the decisions. These three aspects are crucial to innovative cultures. Leaders encourage others to be innovative.

REFLECTION How many of the three effects exist in your organization? How can you affect each, especially any that are missing?

WHAT CREATES A TOXIC CULTURE?

The first element of creating a toxic culture is for leaders to totally ignore culture and allow the culture to evolve, resulting in fragmentation across the organization and a patchwork of subcultures ununited under a whole organizational vision.[6] This translates as acting as though they know nothing about culture and that it doesn't matter. At the same time, we must be conscious of the level of influence leaders have. And frontline leaders always look to the senior leaders for signs of what is acceptable and what isn't. At the same time whatever the leadership team does is emulated. And when bad habits are tolerated, the organization suffers.

Ron Carucci identifies three strategies used by leaders that consistently create a toxic culture.[7] What may be the most common, is how *scattered* some leadership teams can be. They set agendas haphazardly and frequently only shortly before the scheduled meeting. They veer off topic and focus on minutia rather than important decisions or problem-solving that needs to be addressed. This can lead to wasted resources, wasted effort, and widespread confusion. In contrast, effective teams have clearly defined charters, focusing on the most strategic priorities and utilizing well-articulated decision-making strategies. And they ensure these same strategies are used throughout the organization.

The second approach that ensures a toxic environment is creating *unhealthy rivalries*. This arrangement positions senior leaders to be individualists, competing for resources, influence, and even their boss's job. This approach can lead to information hoarding and vicious character assassination. This kind of competition decimates trust within the team because the behaviors and agendas of the teammates are counterproductive, which creates self-protection and risk-taking avoidance. This disrupts team alignment, and the rest of the workers are hesitant to follow because they know the team is not in agreement.

The third issue is *unproductive conflict*. When the leadership team role models behavior, either consciously or unconsciously, in which conflict is mishandled, the remainder of the organization is aware. Speaking negatively about other team members and gossiping about them when they are not present stimulate the rumor mill, which spreads throughout the organization. Such behavior is not acceptable for employees and therefore is unacceptable within the leadership team. Employees do what they see the leaders do, and consequently leaders must always be aware of their behavior. Leaders have immense influence, either positive or negative, on the culture. A toxic culture is abandoned by people with strong positive values and a growth mindset. Many of these desired employees do not want the hassle of chaotic organizations and misaligned leadership. They desire meaningful work in growing, innovative, productive organizations.

TOXIC CULTURES IN HEALTH CARE

In health care, toxic cultures can often be categorized as hostile environments where teams do not know how to work effectively together and coworkers mistreat one another. In these organizations, the subcultures may vary widely depending on the frontline leadership. It wouldn't be unusual to have a "nursing culture" and a very different culture in pharmacy, environmental services, or physical therapy. Within nursing, the culture on medical-surgical units can be quite different from the neonatal intensive care unit or outpatient services. Joe Tye and Bob Dent[8] talk about importance of the "invisible architecture" of an organization consisting of core values as the foundation, the culture as the superstructure, and individual workplace attitude as the "finishing touches" of the interior of the structure. What the people bring to the organizational culture is more important than the attractive physical plant or the visible architecture of the physical structure. Successful organizations understand that the core values, the organizational culture, and the people's emotional attitude create the work environment that focuses on the care of patients and their families. Leaders would not build a physical plant without detailed blueprints and gifted builders. But once the new building is occupied, many organizations pay little or no attention to the invisible architecture, the shared values of the organization, the human structure by which those values are embedded into the organization, and the process by which they are implemented. And individuals are recruited and grown in the context of those shared values.

Toxic cultures that are allowed to evolve haphazardly may have no shared agreements about how coworkers behave toward one another. They result in emotional negativity and uncivil behavior. As Tye and Dent so eloquently described, when leaders convey expectations for cheerful customer service and yet don't confront emotional negativity in the form of curt, disrespectful behavior toward either patients or family members, the negativity becomes the accepted standards. When leaders say the value is respect for coworkers but gossiping and eye rolling are not addressed, respect of other human beings is only a good intention. The result of no follow-through regarding the stated values of the organization is the message to "never get caught" as opposed to "always do the right thing."

Have you been ignored or treated impersonally by a bureaucrat? You may have seen gossiping, eye rolling, or bullying, or you may have been completely ignored rather than receiving reasonable customer service. When you witness these behaviors, you know a toxic culture exists. Most of us have seen such behavior in nursing units. In such situations, where the values of the organization and the individual practitioners are unclear and toxic behavior is ignored, no clarity exists around the values. The values exist only on the wall or on the back of the individual's identification badge—they are not embedded in the culture of the organization. Examples of deeply enculturated values include organizations such as Southwest Airlines, where flight attendants provide the safety briefings (often in a comedic routine) that encourage people to listen (and even have the passengers applauding). The focus is on engaging the passengers to be aware of safety and not just reading the script because it is part of the job. Likewise, in health care facilities where professional staff are committed to promoting the highest level of health, regardless of the diagnosis, the nurse interacts with the patient and family in a positive, supportive, personal way, rather than discussing "the knee replacement in room 413." A commitment to a positive model of care and nurses who believe in the model create a positive constructive culture based on value for the patient and family.

GRITTY CULTURES

High achievers aren't usually the smartest people, but they have extraordinary stamina and are continually striving to improve. They are passionate about what they do and gladly sacrifice for their goals. More than anything, they are focused on what they need to learn to reach success. They might have chosen an easier option but remain committed to these goals. This incredible combination of characteristics is identified by the researcher, Angela Duckworth, as grit.[9] She conducted extensive research at West Point and found that grit was a better predictor of success than achievement scores or athletic ability. She and Dr. Thomas Lee have expanded the thinking about grit from an individual perspective to teams founded on grit. They evolve and develop based on cultures that value grit.[10] Because health care is so complex, it isn't possible to function as a lone provider, either as a physician or as a nurse. We must work in teams, and the strongest teams are those that are bound together due to the individual grit of the members. Building a culture based on grit begins with recruiting and developing individuals who have grit. These are professionals who have a strong sense of purpose and commitment to their "calling." Their work is a passion, and they will persevere regardless of the obstacles. This behavior takes the form of resiliency in the face of adversity with a focus on continuous learning and improvement.

When searching for these individuals, a careful review of their work history, looking for extended years of commitment and loyalty to institutions or projects with evidence of advancement and achievement, is necessary. Search for evidence that these professionals have been resilient with failures in the past, have been agile in dealing with obstacles, and have sought continuous self-improvement through either formal or informal learning. Look for evidence that the person has a purpose bigger than themselves (it's not about me) and that aligns with the mission of the settings. These gritty teams have similar traits to the individuals, in that they work hard, learn, improve their skills and their performance, create something positive out of failure, and are learning and growing. Gritty health care teams view the group effort as a way in which improved care can be brought to patients and families. Thomas Lee believes that every gritty health care organization has a mission that puts patients and their families first—before research or education. These organizations establish social norms that support the mission. They have a restlessness with the status quo and, instead, focus on the drive to continually improve patient care. Crisis events are viewed as an opportunity to learn and grow, as well as strengthen the culture. Gritty people gravitate to gritty teams, which leads to a gritty culture.

LL ALERT

- Don't associate with people who aren't civil.
- Don't support arrogance or people and organizations that are competitive and pit one another against each other.

SUMMARY

Designing and building a successful, caring culture is one of the most important legacies a leadership team can leave. The job of leaders is to promote and develop strong, supportive learning organizations that have stated values supported by most of the employees. Employees who do not support the stated values and goals can be taught to support the organizational culture or can be supported to find an organization in which there is a better fit with their goals and objectives.

LL LINEUP

- Commit to designing and building a successful, caring culture.
- Plan the culture to be a legacy.

REFLECTION Ask yourself if your work culture supports uncivil behavior (gossiping and eye rolling) and consider what you would like to do regarding any changes in the culture. Consider if you meet the description of gritty and whether you are currently on a "gritty" team. Does the organizational culture support you? How?

37

Engagement

No leader is able to accomplish a successful team or organizational outcome without *engagement* from both the leaders and their colleagues. Engagement is a voluntary activity that we choose, usually if our work environment encourages our involvement. The question for leaders eager to encourage engagement is: What are the internal and external factors that encourage engagement among those with whom we work?

We have all been a part of teams or organizations where we were excited about the work in progress, those who were leading the effort, other colleagues, and the potential outcomes. As a result, we were willing to work as hard as necessary to achieve the goal. In contrast, we have been involved in situations where we felt unwilling to commit our time or energy to the process. Unfortunately, the Gallup poll data over the last 20 years have demonstrated that a large percentage of American workers are not engaged in their work.[1] With so many people furloughed in 2020 as a result of the COVID-19 pandemic, a strong possibility exists that engagement in the coming years might remain low—or become lower. In these circumstances, is this reluctance to engage the result of our own motives, the behaviors of the leader(s) and/or other colleagues, the unattractiveness of the potential outcome, or some combination of all of these? Discovering the factors that influence engagement (or lack thereof) is an important factor in achieving our own Legacy *Leaders*-Ship Trajectory model, as well as supporting our colleagues in their journey.

WHAT IS ENGAGEMENT?

The concept of engagement first was introduced in the leadership literature by William Kahn, who defined personal engagement in the work environment as "people employed and expressing themselves physically, cognitively, or emotionally during role engagement."[2] Over time, other descriptors that illustrate the concept of engagement have emerged. For example, engagement may be characterized by an enthusiasm for the work, as well as positive attitudes of the workers toward their work and their workplace.

CHANGE AND ENGAGEMENT

Inevitable change in the work environment often has a profound impact upon the engagement of leaders and members of the team or organization. As we are experiencing escalating change, we often feel as if we are facing an oncoming train. Dealing with this rush of expectations as a result of change may be too much to bear. In these difficult circumstances, leaders must encourage themselves and others to expend the energy necessary to confront the change and work toward an outcome that meets the agreed-upon mission of the team or organization. In this context, engagement is the combination of the group's perception of the changing environment and the level of energy that is generated by the change.[3]

Wilson Learning Worldwide (https://www.wilsonlearning.com/wlw/articles/l/engagement-leaders) suggests that the leader can NOT engage others—the employee must do this for themselves. The leader can only provide an environment that entices followers to engage in the work of the organization. Followers (and leaders) have three choices regarding engagement in their work, including the following:

1. If individuals have a positive perception of the potential change in the environment, they take ownership in the work, putting a high level of energy into their activities. They are engaged.
2. If individuals are resistant to the potential change in the environment, they might comply grudgingly and demonstrate a "wait-and see" attitude. These individuals can be considered inactive; they have yet to actually engage, although the potential for them to become engaged is present.
3. Individuals who are against the potential change often become actively disengaged. This type of individual is often the most disruptive as change is occurring.[3]

In a large Gallup poll of US employees taken from January to June 2018, the percentage of "engaged" workers in the United States was 34%, the highest percentage since Gallup began reporting the national figure in 2000. In contrast, the percentage who were "actively disengaged" was 16.5%. Despite the fact that this was the most positive report on engagement in 18 years, slightly less than 50% of employees were in the "inactive" stage.[1] Given that organizational performance (and productivity) is highly related to increased employee engagement, significant opportunity remains to improve the engagement of US employees through effective leadership and coaching, particularly in the post–COVID-19 world.

> **REFLECTION** How would you describe your organization in terms of engagement? What "evidence" leads you to that statement

AN EXAMPLE OF DISENGAGEMENT

One of us had the opportunity to have a leadership role in the development of a county-run psychiatric hospital for the seriously and persistently mentally ill:

"Sponsored by the county mental health authority (MHA), this facility cared for patients who were court committed for treatment for up to a 30- to 90-day period. We placed significant emphasis on collaborating with the outpatient component of the MHA to transition these clients into a supportive living and working environment. This was an opportunity to provide coordinated care to clients who suffered a great deal. Internally, shared governance, relatively new at the time, was the model of care delivery, resulting in significant differences in the roles of physicians, nurses, social workers, and other providers. Many of those who were hired as the hospital opened were deeply committed to this approach of care, and their engagement was hugely responsible for the success of the program. However, some physicians, nurses, and social workers felt uncomfortable with the new roles and the requirement for close collaboration among disciplines, resulting in disengaged behaviors. For the most part, these disengaged staff ultimately left the organization, although not without being inactive and throwing some roadblocks into our drive toward success."

> **REFLECTION** Have you ever been totally engaged in a professional endeavor? What factors supported this engagement? What were the outcomes for you and the project? Have you ever experienced times where you were not particularly engaged? What were the factors that influenced that behavior? What were the outcomes?

ENGAGEMENT AND THE LEADER

Developing engagement in others requires leaders to first consider their own level of engagement in the project, team, or organization. As these leaders become more engaged, they can role model this behavior for others. Although leaders cannot *make* others become engaged, this role-modeling behavior and related coaching by the leader, will certainly provide encouragement for others to become engaged.[1] Gallup would suggest that coaching by the leader can significantly impact the middle (and largest) group to shift their behavior and become actively engaged.

A number of studies have identified a variety of organizational drivers that address employees' rational, emotional, or motivational needs, thus encouraging employee engagement. The findings of these studies reiterate that employee satisfaction is not simply driven by concrete benefits (salary, benefits, and other resources). These factors provide the basis for initial satisfaction, but the emotional and motivational benefits support the full engagement of the employee. The findings of these studies are found in Table 37.1.

On a practical level, leaders can make four promises to their followers that will encourage empowerment.[4]

Promise 1

I will show you how much you and your work matter by…

- Talking about how important our work is.
- Recognizing how your work contributes to the goals of the organization in ways that are meaningful to you.
- Emphasizing ways your interests can be enhanced by your work.

Promise 2

I will support your growth in your job by…

- Articulating the organization's goals, plans, and accomplishments clearly.
- Asking for and receiving your feedback.
- Listening to your opinions.
- Allowing you to choose the way you do your job.
- Providing you with challenging tasks.

Promise 3

I will encourage innovation by…

- Encouraging risks and supporting your decisions.
- Being accepting of failures.
- Asking what can be learned from mistakes.

Promise 4

My leadership will encourage your engagement by…

- Treating you with dignity and respect.
- Celebrating accomplishments.
- Following up on promises and commitments.

TABLE 37.1 Research-Based Factors Enabling Employee Engagement

Type of Needs	Findings	Reference
Rational	Effective leadership	Roth[3]
	Adequate pay and benefits	Roth[3]
	Overall job satisfaction	Roth[3]
	Necessary resources	Markos and Sridivi[5]
	Adequate training and development	Markos and Sridivi[5]
	Incentives	Markos and Sridivi[5]
Emotional	Feeling involved and valued	Roth[3]
	Connections with others	Roth[3]
	Optimistic environment	Tims et al.[6]
	Opportunity to commit fully to their work; investment of self in work activities	Seaton[7]; Gruman and Saks[8]
	Self-efficacy (the belief that one can attain specific performance behaviors) fostered and rewarded	Tims et al.[6]
Motivational	Opportunities for employee empowerment and growth	Roth[3]
	Other-oriented leadership styles (e.g., transformational, servant, authentic)	Tims et al.[6]
	Clarity of role expectations	Carasco-Saul et al[9]
	Leadership behavior that stimulates identification with supervisor	Carasco-Saul et al[9]
	Psychological ownership in the team or organization	Carasco-Saul et al[9]
	Strong feedback	Markos and Sridivi[5]
	Effective two-way conversations	Markos and Sridivi[5]

REFLECTION Consider each of these promises in light of your current position. No matter where you are in your individual leadership development, you can use these promises.

DISENGAGEMENT

Why are people disengaged in their work, and what can we do about this attitude? When we see employees who are not motivated, involved, or committed emotionally, we are likely seeing a group of disengaged employees. These employees may demonstrate a lack of enthusiasm and curiosity. They may also offer only complaints, instead of ideas for improvement. They blame others and seem to avoid taking responsibility for their own mistakes. Others often characterize the "disengaged" as "passive-aggressive." The more disengaged employees in a group or organization, the less likely the environment as a whole will be seen as an engaged environment. Table 37.2 presents a checklist that can be used as an assessment of an environment in which a significant portion of employees might be disengaged to determine engagement within that environment.

CustomInsight (https://www.custominsight.com/employee-engagement-survey/research-employee-disengagement.asp.) identifies five drivers of engagement and disengagement that are related to the behavior of the manager. The five disengagement drivers associated with the behavior of the manager include:

- Inadequate definition of goals and expectations by the manager.
- Emphasis on cooperation and teamwork by the manager.
- Lack of autonomy because of the manager.
- Not feeling valued by the manager.
- Lack of respect for management.

Addressing factors that cause disengagement may not immediately lead to engaged employees, but it may lead these employees into the middle group and encourage them to perform their job duties. Clearly the role of the manager, who may or may not be a leader, is critical!

TABLE 37.2 Environmental Assessment of Engagement

Characteristics for Assessment	Yes	No	Unsure
1. Are the values and vision stated in the team or organization mission and other documentation obvious in the day-to-day work? Do the leaders just "talk the talk" or do they "walk the talk"?			
2. Does accountability mean that someone at the bottom of the hierarchy receives the blame when something goes wrong?			
3. Is competition among colleagues rampant in the environment?			
4. Is the focus on efficiency rather than effectiveness?			
5. Does the senior management team demonstrate competition rather than collaboration?			
6. Do employees avoid providing suggestions to improve the work for fear of retribution of potential "criticism"?			
7. Is emotional intelligence (the social grace to monitor one's own or others' feelings and emotions and use the information to guide one's thinking and action) rarely a consideration in the work environment?			
8. Do the leaders by word or action discourage interruptions by employees who need to have significant conversations related to work issues?[10]			

Adapted from CustomInsight (https://www.custominsight.com/employee-engagement-survey/research-employee-disengagement.asp).

EFFECTS OF ENGAGEMENT SURVEYS

Because of the importance of employee engagement, many organizations survey their employees to identify their level of engagement. In the quest to achieve higher engagement scores, some leaders have exerted pressure on others to respond positively. This may result in higher "engagement scores" that can be shared with the organization's board or other stakeholders, but in fact, it diminishes the actual engagement of the employees.

LL ALERT

- Don't respond to pressures to "increase engagement scores."
- Don't break promises to others.

SUMMARY

A variety of strategies are available for leaders to support their own engagement, as well as the engagement of those around them. This content can be used as a self-evaluation to determine how engaged you and your colleagues are in your own work environment and the potential next steps, should additional action be necessary.

LL LINEUP

- Remember that leaders influence how others feel about where they work.
- Know that no matter what your job description says, you have the potential to influence engagement—for yourself and others.

REFLECTION Do you believe that you are currently engaged in your work? Why or why not? Do you believe that your colleagues are engaged? Why or why not? Use the Environmental Assessment of Engagement checklist provided earlier to identify possible situations that are present in your work environment. What changes would you like to see in your work environment to increase the level of your own engagement or that of your colleagues? How might you contribute to this change?

38

Governance

Have you ever been enthralled by the rhetoric of a leader, stimulated by his or her plans for the future of an organization, only to realize as time moves on that very little change has occurred within the organization? Although the leader was dynamic and able to articulate an enticing future, that person was not able to follow through in implementing the vision that was so appealing to you—and probably many others. Why is this so?

Multiple factors may contribute to the failure of the organization to reach aspirational goals. The personal characteristics of a leader may get in the way of achievement, and resistance from others both internally and externally to the organization may also impede progress. However, frequently, an ineffective *governance structure or process* plays an important role in the lack of success or forward movement of the organization. Two major considerations relate to governance. One is when we serve on boards identifying the skills we need to be effective as board members. The other is for those of us who are in formal, high-level leadership positions to identify information we need to know and what to expect of the board governing our organizations.

THE ROLE OF GOVERNANCE

What is the role of governance? Regardless of whether the organization is for-profit or nonprofit, governance provides a structure of relationships and processes that direct and control the enterprise to achieve the goals established.[1] Abigail Noble, head of Latin America and Africa, Schwab Foundation for Social Entrepreneurship, suggests "any leader and all teams, organizations and even nations, succeed in the long run because of accountability mechanisms that make sure that the leadership is on the right course. Governance, which includes boards, monitoring systems, and mechanisms like codes of conduct, ensures success."[2]

REFLECTION Are you familiar with the functions of the board of directors for your organization? Do you know the answers to the following: How many members are appointed to the board in question? How long is a director's appointment to the board? What stakeholders do these members represent? How are the decisions made by the board communicated to the employees and other stakeholders? Do you believe that the actions of this board affect your role and function? If you do not know the answers to these questions, how would you find them? What should you do to learn more about the structure and function of the board?

COMPONENTS OF A GOVERNANCE PLAN

The purpose of the governance plan of any organization is to ensure control of the organization, independent of the top executives. This ensures that the executives will behave ethically, considering the best interest of the organization ahead of their own. The governance plan also outlines processes to ensure objectives are met and organizational processes are not neglected, skirted, or altered for the benefit of individuals.[3]

Board of Directors

The board of directors of an organization is the most important component of a governance plan. The board is a group of highly accomplished individuals who have expertise in various areas necessary to operate the organization. The broad and overarching responsibilities of the board of directors usually are to:

- Ensure the vision and legacy of the organization
- Demonstrate credibility of the organization to external stakeholders
- Provide strategic support and expertise to reach the relevant mission and goals

- Compensate for a lack of in-house competencies or expertise through board members
- Provide access to networks that can assist with activities such as fundraising, advocacy, and recruitment of talent[4]

In specific terms, the board of directors must:

- Preserve and, when necessary, revise the mission of the organization
- Select the chief executive officer
- Ensure that the organization is well managed
- Represent the external world to the organization and the organization to the external world
- Protect the organization from external threats
- Exercise financial stewardship
- Make sure the board has the right skills and practices to do its job
- Ensure that the organization is in compliance with all laws and regulations[1]

Individual board members are responsible for:

- Being present at board meetings and other required activities
- Preparing for the work of the board
- Asking hard questions
- Voicing their own opinions
- Acting with integrity
- Being a good steward of the organization's assets[1]

Board members are chosen through an organized system (e.g., elections or appointments), typically on a rotating basis. Because board members are the only group in the organization who can exercise oversight and control of the executives, they should demonstrate highly ethical behavior. The most effective board members are those who are immune to personal influence from company executives and are committed to the organization and the mission.

The lack of public and stakeholder trust in the integrity of corporations' financial statements and business conduct has escalated as a result of for-profit organizations' misconduct in the early 2000s. In addition, charitable organizations have faced challenges to the legitimacy of their tax-exempt status. To combat this mistrust, the Sarbanes-Oxley Act, passed in 2002, set new standards for governance accountability, independence, effectiveness, and transparency. Although some of the provisions of this act apply only to publicly owned companies, nonprofits (including health care organizations) are adopting at least some of the provisions outlined in the act. These call for:

- Establishing provisions that protect whistleblowers and policies on document retention and destruction (required for nonprofits)
- Establishing an independent audit committee, with at least one trustee being a financial expert and keeping auditors independent
- Adopting a written code of ethics formally
- Adopting and implementing policies and procedures related to conflicts of interest
- Defining criteria for independent directors (trustees cannot serve directly or indirectly as a partner)
- Holding meetings without management present to evaluate performance and independence of management
- Adopting specific procedures to evaluate performance and independence of management
- Adopting specific procedures for recruiting and nominating qualified board members, making these publicly available[5]

Nurses On Boards

The impact of the work of a board is central to the effectiveness of the governance of the organization, and the need for diversity on the board has been identified as vitally important in achieving this effectiveness. Elena Bajic, founder and chief executive officer (CEO) of Ivy Exec, asserts that the best boards have a wide variety of skills and experiences that encourage the organization to move forward. Her company, IvyExec.com, helps recruit and build diverse boards for clients. She says that "it is like putting together pieces of a puzzle; they are all different but in the end, fit together perfectly."[3] Bajic believes that boards that are too culturally homogenous may miss important cues about market trends or internal problems. Thus a diverse board should be made up of at least some women (a statement made due to the number of boards that historically—and yet today—have an all-male membership), people of color, and a wide variety of ethnic backgrounds.[3]

Particularly, in health care and social services, this diversity should include nurses. Unfortunately, for years nurses were rarely recruited for board positions. In fact, even today, some organizations do not expect the nursing leadership to *even attend* the board meeting. Leaders of the Center to Champion Nursing, brought together by the results of the 2010 Future of Nursing report by the Institute of Medicine (IOM) (now the National Academy of Medicine), recognized the historical underrepresentation of nurses on boards of directors and organized a movement to encourage the appointment of nurses to boards across the country. In November 2014, 12 national organizations (AARP, Robert Wood Johnson Foundation, and 10 other national organizations) announced the formation of a nationwide effort to get 10,000 nurses, with their frontline perspective, onto boards of directors by 2020. This initiative

TABLE 38.1 Skills Nurses Bring to Boards of Directors

Advocacy/Policy	Audit	Communication
Compensation	Finance	Fundraising/ Development
Investment	Management	Product Development
Product Development	Quality Assurance	Strategic Planning

became known as the Nurses on Boards Coalition (https://campaignforaction.org/join-effort-get-10000-nurses-onto-boards-2020/). The Nurses on Boards website provides resources for nurses who wish to be on boards, as well as organizations who want to recruit nurses to their boards.

You may wonder what expertise nurses bring to a board of directors. Certainly, nurses have excellent communication and decision-making skills that are assets in any board situation. However, the Nurses on Boards Coalition has identified some specific skills that nurses bring to boards. Table 38.1 provides an overview of these skills.

An Example of a Nurse on a Board

As of the beginning of 2019, more than 6000 nurses held appointments in organizational boards across the county. When one of us was appointed to the board of a specialty hospital with a national reach, she was excited and eager to see the inner workings of this unique hospital. Her appointment followed another nurse's term on the board. Both of these nurses were suggested to the nominating committee by the chief nursing officer, who felt strongly that a nurse would provide special expertise that was needed on this board.

"The first meeting I attended was somewhat overwhelming. Other members of the board represented men and women with a variety of expertise: law, finance, philanthropy, medicine, and governmental affairs. I knew that I was competent in nursing care of the population being served, management, staffing, quality management, and advocacy of patients and nurses. I had been on professional and community nonprofit boards and understood a board's general functioning, but would this be enough? Fast-forward several years, and I can say that my expertise has been valuable in a number of circumstances, because my perspective was that of a nurse. For example, when changes in patient care or safety were considered, I was able to provide the perspective of nurses—and other nonphysician staff—which was valuable in an organization connected to a residency program. In fact, my questions regarding the impact of any policy on staff raised the awareness for the rest of the board regarding the important role staff played in patient outcomes."

> **REFLECTION** Do you know a nurse who is a member of a board? Consider questions you would ask him or her about the experience in that role. Would you want to be on a board? Why or why not? If you know a nurse who serves as a member of a board, make an appointment to interview this person. Then ask yourself if that is a role you would seek.

Accountability Framework for Executives

In addition to the board of directors, an organization must operate under a framework that outlines the functioning of the organization to ensure that decisions made by the executive team are made on behalf of the organization. This framework should include a streamlined organizational chart that outlines the accountability for all decisions made in the organization. Specific rules regarding executive decision-making should be established as policies. One of these policies should direct the board to initiate formal reviews of executive decisions that result in a significant impact to the organization. The implementation of such a review process supports ethical decision-making. Finally, proper governance requires that all financial decisions and actions be audited routinely by a completely independent organization.

Implementation of good governance practice includes structures and policies that ensure that the board and management will continue to attend to business throughout the year. For example, it is important to maintain corporate minutes of all board meetings to document activities. Orientation of new board members at the beginning of each year can help new members become aware of good governance practices from the start.

On an annual basis, the board should go through a self-assessment process to compare its practices to benchmarks of similar organizations, thus prioritizing the activities of the board. A conflict-of-interest policy should be discussed before a conflict arises so that board and staff can identify the types of situations when a conflict of interest might occur and consider how they might be handled.[2] Annually, the board should also approve the executive director's/CEO's compensation and benefits and document how the board determines if the compensation is appropriate and not excessive. Finally, Table 38.2 outlines the written policies required as part of good governance.[6]

TABLE 38.2 Required Written Policies
Whistleblower protection policy
Document retention/destruction policy
Gift acceptance policy to govern receipt of "noncash" gifts
Review of Internal Revenue Service (IRS) filings annually

SHARED GOVERNANCE

No discussion about organizational governance is complete without some consideration of the concept of shared governance. *Shared governance* is defined as a structure and process in an organization that puts the responsibility, authority, and accountability for decisions into the hands of the individuals who will operationalize them. Shared governance most often affects nurses who work in clinical practice where shared governance is operationalized, as well as in higher education.[6]

Over the last 30 years, shared governance has been emphasized at times, and at other times, the approach has been less popular. The literature suggests it seems to be integrated in the leadership model for transformational or servant leadership in health care.[7]

Although shared governance supports the professional practice of nurses by increasing their opportunity for decision-making, as well as their accountability, it may be confusing in practical situations. Being able to make decisions regarding their practice may well enhance the professionalism of the nurse—and hopefully patient outcomes. However, what if the decisions made by the individual or group of nurses conflict with the goals of the organization? How do the decisions get made?

The truth is that all legal authority in an organization originates in its governing body. Regardless of the organization's for-profit or nonprofit status, mission, or location, the legal right and obligation to exercise authority over an institution are vested in and flow from its board. The board then formally delegates authority over the day-to-day operations to the president/CEO, who, in turn, may delegate authority over certain parts of management or practice to specific groups within the organizations.[7] When intentional sharing of responsibility and accountability exists, it is easy to see how roles and responsibilities can be confusing.

Gen Guanci, a consultant at Creative Health Care Management, recognizes the role confusion that can occur when implementing some form of shared governance, particularly around the question, "Who is in charge?" She identifies some criteria for what is and is not shared governance.[6] Table 38.3 outlines these differences.

Perhaps the most important point to be made in this table is that the shared decision-making is related to *professional practice*. Although management/administration may ask for staff input regarding other decisions (e.g., budgeting or strategic directions), they are not obligated to follow this input, because these decisions are ultimately the responsibility of the board of directors.

An Experience with Shared Governance

In the late 1980s, one of us was responsible for developing a nonprofit psychiatric hospital for the seriously and persistently mentally ill:

"The model of shared governance was on the upswing, and because of the structure of the ownership of the facility and the peculiarities of state law governing the practice of physician employees, it seemed like a perfect opportunity to integrate shared governance into the processes of the hospital. Imagine my surprise when the concepts of shared governance were not as enthusiastically received as I had hoped. This was made very clear to me when a small group of nurses made an appointment to see me to say that they were concerned because 'the social workers were running the hospital.' I would

TABLE 38.3 Criteria of Shared Governance

What Shared Governance IS	What Shared Governance Is NOT
• A model to allow people working at the point of care (or interaction with others, such as faculty in higher education) to make necessary decisions • A strategy to develop leaders and identify future positional leaders • A tenet of professional practice for any professional group • An expression of organizational culture	• The replacement or elimination of positional leadership • A strategy to support downsizing of positions • Self-governance • Abdication of leadership responsibilities by the management team

not have been surprised if they had complained that the physicians were leading the care delivered at the hospital, but I was shocked by this development. I asked the group how we might change the processes so that the nurses would be able to control their own practice. Unfortunately, they had no suggestions. This experience taught me that much education is required for professional staff to understand (1) what their practice role is in any setting, (2) what it means to be accountable for one's own practice, and (3) how their practice responsibilities interact with others working in the same space."

REFLECTION Do the governance structures where you work allow you to make decisions about your own practice? Are you clear about what competences are part of professional practice? If not, what can you do to expand your knowledge in this area?

LL ALERT

- Don't assume that everyone in the organization understands organizational governance as an important part of leadership.
- Don't abdicate your role in supporting shared governance.
- Don't take a new position until you evaluate the effectiveness of the organization's governance structure.

SUMMARY

As leaders, we must be sensitive to the governance processes in any organization where we work. Developing an effective leadership trajectory requires an awareness of the impact of many factors in our environment, including governance, and the ability to respond to the specifics of the governance plan is a key component of successful leadership.

LL LINEUP

- If nursing does not report directly to the board, advocate for this.
- If you serve on a board, actively participate in board proceedings and ensure that the board is performing its legal duties.

REFLECTION Given your thoughts stimulated by previous reflections in this chapter, what steps will you take to integrate knowledge about organizational governance into your Legacy *Leaders*-Ship Trajectory model?

39

Inclusion

Inclusivity is often used with the concept of diversity, which is sometimes used in a narrow sense related to race, ethnicity, and gender. We believe that is a narrow view because the diversity of the profession, our patient populations, and the world is much broader. Race and gender are both well documented in the literature as being needed for diversity. But what about age, ways of thinking, religion, politics, disabilities, nationalism, lifestyle, and more? When we (the authors) think about diversity, we are thinking of additional ways to consider rather than ways to restrict. The broadest perspective of diversity is belonging, a condition where people feel not only acceptance but "wantedness."

FROM DIVERSITY AND INCLUSION TO BELONGINGNESS

In a sense, diversity is often about math. At least that is how we have commonly seen it presented in the general literature. The points most commonly raised relate to the percentage of people identified by some characteristics and then what percentage of a group or geographic area or profession represents those characteristics. The goal is typically that X% (of the profession/group, etc.) reflects that same percentage of the total population. That reflection seldom occurs. What may happen is tokenism: we add one of every characteristic we could see as diverse and "check the box" that says we addressed diversity.

Another way to look at diversity is what Laura Liswood calls Noah's Ark, which refers to having two people from each underrepresented group.[1] She describes the majority culture (white males of the United States) as an elephant and the others as the mice. To survive, the mice know everything possible about the elephant and know how to stay out of its way or to adapt. The elephant knows little, if anything, about the mice. As a result, asking the elephant to learn about mice is a major undertaking. The reverse isn't often asked because the mice have learned and practiced how to coexist with the elephant. If we all assumed the mice roles, we would learn more about people who were different from us.

Inclusivity is more about actions. Inclusivity has to be based on diversity in order to go further in the process of creating just societies, whether that happens on a nursing unit or in a health care organization or in a community. Inclusivity involves the act of going beyond representation and making people feel accepted in the group. The incorporation of these differences into consideration for who our friends are, who should be on our clinical team, who needs to rise in leadership positions, and who gets recognized for contributions to the organization creates bigger possibilities for what each of us can be as nurses—and as humans.

> **REFLECTION** Have you ever joined a new work or social group and felt as if you were standing on the outside looking in? Think what that felt like (or might feel like), and you will know it is not a good feeling. How do you get to be "in"?

In many situations, both social and work-based, people form "in groups." They typically comprise the "cool" people. And if an "in group" exists, we can likely find an "out group," which comprises those people who don't quite fit in the INs. People in the OUTs either try to get into the INs or they brush off the idea of anyone wanting to be in the INs. This type of exclusivity is sometimes based on appearance, knowledge, social status, or on a variety of other distinctions. This view almost always is not supportive of the best efforts the organization, or the individuals in the organization, can put forth. As Kat Holmes says in her book, *Mismatch: How Inclusion Shapes Design*, being inclusive often has additional benefits.[2] One of her examples is how curb cuts (those spaces where a ramp is made from the street to the sidewalk), although designed to accommodate wheelchairs, also help children riding bicycles, people with difficulty walking, and those of us who wheel carts or luggage to navigate the space. In other words, considerations for including people can often produce benefits beyond those who were the ones being included.

Normally we don't tell other peoples' stories; however, the closing words in this one are priceless. Lisa Wardell is the only African-American female chief executive officer (CEO) in a category of businesses known in the Standard and Poor listings as a mid-cap 400 index.[3] Bob Johnson, an investment advisor; Lisa Wardell; and various bankers were meeting. Bob introduced Lisa with an acknowledgment of the bankers not having one diverse person on their team. He then turned the meeting over to her. After she made her presentation, she asked why he had sort of dumped the meeting on her. "Because I want you to understand that until you believe that you belong in the room, you don't belong in the room." Wow! What a lesson for us all, especially those of us who might score on the high side of the Imposter Scale! (Briefly that means you are undervaluing who you are.) We have to gain sufficient self-belief to be clear we belong in the IN groups, and until we do, we won't be anywhere other than on the periphery!

In people's attempts to move diversity along to inclusion, they sometimes do the same "math approach." As Rumay Alexander, former president of the National League for Nursing, said in her first presidential address, people don't want to just be invited to the dance (diversity: you are "allowed" in), they want to dance (inclusion: you actually participate). We think that analogy can be pushed one step further. People get to design the dance event, create the music, and decide what happens next. That is belongingness. In the movie, *The Blind Side*, the story of Michael Orr, Michael is asked by the family he has been living with if he would like to officially become a part of the family. His response was that he already thought he was part of the family. What a great example of belongingness! When we feel we belong, we are surprised by a question about becoming a member of the group.

REFLECTION Consider a national or state meeting you attend where you aren't with your work colleagues or a friend whom you usually meet. How do you feel? Are you a person who was "allowed" in because you registered? Did people reach out to you to include you in some event or discussion? When you left the meeting, were you thrilled with the learning? Or were you thrilled with the experience because you felt, as we would describe from our personal lives, "at home"?

We would be remiss in speaking about inclusion and the movement to belonging if we didn't share with you findings from Google's Project Aristotle[4] and the work of Patrick Lencioni.[5] Project Aristotle's goal was to determine how best to form teams at Google. Among the five factors they found (psychological safety, dependability, clarity of structure and plans, personal meaning, and positive impact), psychological safety certainly relates to feeling included. We cannot feel safe if we feel someone nearby is "out to get us." That really has to do with trust, which is, according to Lencioni, the number one dysfunction of a team.[5] That psychological safety/trust in others is a huge factor in people feeling connected in an organization. We can talk about trust, and yet it is only believable when we reach out to others to exhibit trust in their abilities and confidences. Some of us have very good friends with whom we would not share a secret because we may trust them in some specific tasks, but we don't trust their confidentiality. That same kind of feeling is what veterans since World War II speak about when they described their experiences in combat. They were okay as long as they knew their "team" had "their backs."

EXAMINING BIASES

A bias is a slanted or preferential, often preconceived, view. It can have a positive connotation—for example, a bias toward success or intelligence. Commonly, however, it is thought of in a negative perspective, one often associated with prejudice. We all have biases, and as Jennifer Eberhardt, author of *Biased*, points out, many are unconscious.[6]

A bias can be explicit or implicit. Explicit biases are fairly easy to spot. They are exhibited in what we say ("Well what would you expect from a woman?") or what we do (walk on the other side of the street to avoid a group of people from an ethnically different group). Biases are explicit when we demonstrate our views in what we say or how we behave. Implicit biases, on the other hand, are harder to detect. Rachele Kanigel, author of *The Diversity Style Guide*, says that we tend to categorize the world.[7] In our fast-paced society, we often need to make quick assessments of a situation, and even when we don't, we size up a situation fairly rapidly.

Implicit bias occurs when we attribute to a characteristic a value about that characteristic. Perhaps the most commonly known example is found in the "dumb blond" jokes. People other than blonds do dumb things and not all blonds do things that might be called dumb. Yet the second we see a blond woman who isn't assertive, articulate, and confident, our brains go to the concept of the dumb blond. Beyond the jokes, people have views about the characteristics of almost every group, and when those stereotypes kick in without acknowledgment (at least to self), we categorize people, which may or may not be an accurate conclusion. Race is a common basis for biases, because it (along with gender) is among the most common ways we divide people into groups. In many cases, we can readily see skin color and body build (a characteristic often used regarding gender). What's in the heart takes time to determine.

Another currently "popular" bias to have is one against specific generations. Even though several studies suggest specific behaviors we can anticipate from any group, doing so forms a stereotype of an age group. And yes, for the past several decades we have stereotyped generations: baby boomers, Gen X, Gen Y, Millennials, and so forth. These generalized descriptions should convince us we shouldn't operate on the descriptors as fact for any individual. The same is true for national origin, gender, race, age, and almost any other way we classify people.

> **REFLECTION** Consider how you celebrate New Year's Eve, a fairly universal event worldwide, although the actual date may vary. What do you do? What foods and beverages do you consume? Who are the people you are with? Now find a few people who are not friends but are "like you" (gender, age, ethnicity, etc.) and ask them what they do for New Year's Eve. (The point of this is even celebrations are stereotyped and yet actual people behave very differently.)

When we form stereotypes, we can fall into the trap of excusing some behavior ("Well, you know how millennials have no real career goals.") or we are confused when we don't see the stereotypical behaviors. We stand the chance of alienating a whole group of people when we lack an inclusion philosophy.

These aren't the only areas of discrimination or biases we can see at work. As an example, physicians often have a separate dining room in hospitals, and different food is served there than elsewhere. One of us was reading a copy of *The Week* (March 8, 2019) and without deliberately seeking out articles that could fall into a category of discrimination, found the following:

1. "The Last Word: A Woman's Place in the Courtroom." This discussed battling sexism in the courtroom, where someone's trial outcome could hinge on the female attorney's behavior as a female.
2. "Best Columns: Europe: Give Your Kid a Name That Travels Well." This focused on the trend in Denmark to name children with a more worldwide name (e.g., William) rather than traditional Danish names.
3. "It Wasn't All Bad." A kindergartner girl with short hair was viewed by her classmates as looking like a boy. So the teacher chopped off her own hair, which gave confidence to the young girl and provided the opportunity to discuss differences.

Gender, names, and hairstyle—three simple things that can cause controversy even in kindergarten. How can so many forms of "what is right" appear in just one issue of one magazine? These writings also occur in other publications, such as *The Wall Street Journal* (Saturday/Sunday March 30–31, 2019), where three articles on the *same* page addressed issues of how people are seen in America. The first, by Peggy Noonan, discussed how our political divide in the country is more intense. The next article focused on a hunt for diversity "bias" at Villanova University, and the third addressed the issue of Jussie Smollett, a black, gay actor who was arrested for creating a hoax in Chicago about being attacked because he was black and gay. We could consider the fact that media make money to stay in business by reporting news people want to read, which is usually something that would not be called happy stories. However, the frequency of such articles could also suggest the potential that we are addressing biases more openly, or that more are being reported more publicly than was true in the past, or that we wish to create divisiveness on an ongoing basis.

> **REFLECTION** At this point, you might want to stop reading and do a self-assessment to learn about your own biases. If so, we encourage you to go to https://implicit.harvard.edu/implicit/takeatest.html. Harvard University has several assessments such as race, skin tone, weight, sexuality, age, disability, and religion. This insight, just as other self-assessment data, helps each of us understand where we are in the spectrum of perspectives. From that information, we can determine how far we need or want to progress in being more open to people who differ from who we are. If you chose to do this, what did you learn about yourself?

Although breaking these biases is a critical activity, the idea of inclusion pushes our thinking even further. For example, instead of stopping ourselves mentally from thinking whatever stereotypical messages we have given ourselves, we need to move beyond just stopping such thoughts and toward reaching out to others from any of the groups we could say are "not like me."

Inclusion is designed to break up the INs and the OUTs so that everyone is part of THE group. This cohesiveness of everyone being in THE group creates a sense of belonging, which exceeds the basic act of inclusion. Samuel Lalanne of Citigroup says this belongingness is an evolution of a journey, and the best way to have this depth of belonging is through storytelling.[8] This level of belongingness creates a sense of value. Think what happens when we tell a story about an experience that allows others to hear how we experienced something as opposed to merely hearing or seeing facts. That storytelling helps achieve two things:

1. Others get to understand who we are as individuals and not all (choose any way of dividing people) see something the same way.
2. We all get to learn different perspectives of the same event, which helps us understand we are products of our prior lives and thus interpret new experiences in light of our past experiences.

When we talk about those different perspectives, especially in story form, we gain a new appreciation for the complexities of life. Each of us (the authors) would be described as growing up poor. Yet we cannot match the stories of some of the young men and women in nursing today who grew up homeless. By listening to people's stories, we can begin to see how we can connect in a different way than simply focusing on a task before us.

CHANGING THE EQUATION

We already acknowledged that in health care, we need to reflect the people to whom we are accountable—patients. Typically, we are delighted when we fill an empty position or get someone to agree to take on a special project, and then we realize we forgot to consider what impact those choices have on our overall goal of creating an environment of belongingness. Even if we are not in a formal leadership position, we can start somewhere. Commonly, that starting point is ourselves. No matter what position we hold in our profession, we can contribute to changing the way in which we include others. Some of that change can be simple—whom we sit with at lunch, whom we hug when we see others suffering, whom we speak up for when a nasty situation develops—these are simple examples of how we can become more inclusive. But what about the complex?

We can't focus only on inclusion in the workplace, although we can include the concept of inclusiveness as a critical aspect of being an effective team. The authors of *The Best Team Wins*, Adrian Gostick and Chester Elton, say "diversity of knowledge and experience that good teams bring to assignments allows them to be more responsive to customers" (their term for what we would call patients).[9] In other words, the ability to not have just representation but to have a truly inclusive team of members who feel they belong has payoffs beyond how people feel about their workplace; they actually make a difference in their work. In our (the authors') view, this inclusion in teamwork also has the value of modeling for society what our potential as humans can be. If nursing is the most trusted profession, which it repeatedly has been, think how we can lead society through our demonstration of embracing all.

As Juliet Bourke and Andrea Espedido point out, being inclusive isn't just a good idea, it produces good results. For example, teams report they are high performing and collaborating.[10] Bourke and Espedido surveyed over 400 employees to determine what leaders needed to do to convey inclusion. Those six behaviors are listed in Table 39.1. An important finding of their study relates to how leaders perceived themselves in relation to these behaviors: they were typically uncertain about the impact of specific behaviors related to inclusion. Additionally, to be an inclusive leader, these behaviors had to be seen by everyone agreeing to the concept "this is what the leader does" and that the leader performs these behaviors consistently. The authors conclude their work with advice about developing as an inclusive leader. First, deliberately ask others about your style. Second, be visible and speak your mind about inclusion. Third, be inclusive of people who are not like you, and fourth, evaluate if you are making a difference. Becoming or maintaining an inclusive perspective is critical to the

TABLE 39.1 Six Behaviors of Inclusive Leaders

Visible commitment	Act authentic in commitments to diversity and inclusion
Humility	Admit mistakes, seek others' contributions
Awareness of bias	Admit personal blindness and system flaws
Curiosity about others	Listen without judgment, seek empathy in understanding others
Cultural intelligence	Be attentive to others' cultures and adapt as needed
Effective collaboration	Empower others and support diversity of thinking

Bourke J, Espedido A. Why inclusive leaders are good for organizations, and how to become one. 2019. Available at: https://hbr.org/2019/03/why-inclusive-leaders-are-good-for-organizations-and-how-to-become-one?utm_medium=email&utm_source=newsletter_weekly&utm_campaign=insider_activesubs&utm_content=signinnudge&referral=03551. Accessed April 5, 2019.

workforce of today and tomorrow, and as with many other skills, we can learn to be inclusive.

REFLECTION Have you excluded someone who was "different" (meaning not like you) at work? Consider what caused you to do so. Was it a lack of quick wit, hairstyle, tattoos, clinical knowledge, or color of skin or hair? What one step could you take tomorrow to include that person in your circle of colleagues?

LL ALERT

- Don't offend others as we seek to bring balance.
- Don't practice tokenism or quota counting.
- Don't tolerate values or behaviors that are disruptive in a desire to be inclusive.

SUMMARY

Moving beyond diversity to inclusion to create an environment of belongingness is critical to helping people feel engaged where they work. Inclusion is critical now and for the future. When we aren't inclusive, we limit what we can be, and we certainly won't create a sense of belonging. By increasing our circle of colleagues, we expand our view of the world and the impact our purpose can have.

LL LINEUP

- Acknowledge that bias (both explicit and implicit) exists.
- Determine what it would take to have an organization, unit, or team that could be called a belongingness example.
- Create a story that helps people see who you really are.

REFLECTION Think about the various people you work with on a regular basis. Are they homogenous or heterogenous? If you say heterogenous, is that at the tokenism level? Is it at the Noah's Ark level? Or is it at the belongingness level? How did you decide that? Consider a story you could tell about whatever level you indicated and what you might do next to solidify true belongingness.

40

Innovation

In a world where VUCA exists on a daily basis, doing our best just as we always have done is insufficient. If you remember from the chapter on lifelong learning, if you aren't learning, you are no longer just standing still, you are falling behind. VUCA (volatility, uncertainty, complexity, and ambiguity) is our new constant companion. Those four factors lead to disruption in what we do, how we think, and how we act. If we aren't thinking in innovative ways, we will have to rely on someone to shape our careers and work. If we are thinking, and subsequently acting, in innovative ways, we remain relevant.

Creativity is the concept; innovation is the implementation. Idea to Value asked 15 experts their definitions of innovation. Only two phrases garnered more than 50% agreement. Those words, each being used by 60% of the experts, were *having an idea* and *executing the idea.*[1] We used to think being creative was good, and with any other good business practice, putting an idea into action is the only way to test it and its value. We wouldn't just want to think about a new way to assist someone with activities of daily living. We would need to determine if our idea brought real value to someone who needed such assistance. And, let's be clear: some health care organizations do not support innovation. As Jeannette Crenshaw and Pat point out, the environment must be safe before anyone is willing to take a risk,[2] as Fig. 27.2 illustrates. An organization needs only a few risk takers, because they operate toward the unsafe end of the safety spectrum. They are the ones inventing something that has yet to be tested. In comparison to all the work that occurs in an organization, relatively little of the overall effort is devoted to risk-taking activities such as innovation. Relatedly, Scott Anthony says personnel are crucial, and if no one is in charge of growth, the organization is not going to be focused on growth.[3] If punishment occurs when one fails, the organization does not support innovation. Too many ideas have to be tested to produce winning ones, and if punishment occurs along the way, why would someone keep trying to be innovative?

REFLECTION How safe is it to take a risk in your workplace? How does your workplace culture support innovation? Could you offer a rather "off-the-wall" idea and have it received as a possibility? Are people who do things differently or point out a different way of thinking about something valued and supported? Or are they ridiculed and punished? Identify a risk you would be willing to take the next time you are at work. Is it really very different from the current norm?

THE HARD WORK OF HAVING FUN

If you scan the literature about innovation, you will see that many publications focus on the "fun and games" of innovation. Far fewer focus on how hard this work actually is. We have to think in new and creative ways, and that certainly sounds like fun. However, if we don't push with intensity the opportunity to challenge ideas, to be willing to quickly drop the first idea and pick up the second just as quickly, we miss the full benefit of being innovative.[4] The authors of *Collective Genius* make clear that the role of a leader is to create a culture where both willingness and ability are maximized. Willingness supports the culture by integrating purpose, values, and the rules of engagement (how we work together). Ability includes creative abrasion (generating ideas through the group process), creative resolution (integrating ideas to make decisions), and creative agility (testing, experimenting, reflection, and adjustment).

Balancing individual creativity with the need to create a group consensus is one of the greatest challenges of asking a team to work on something that relates to innovation. The authors identified six paradoxes related to innovation (Table 40.1). This push–pull tension can be exhausting. Think for a minute how challenging it is to feel as if you are being torn in two or swaying back and forth. Yet without either of the elements, a great idea could go nowhere. We would add one other tension to the list and that is the

TABLE 40.1 Paradoxes of Innovation

1. Affirming the individual—	—and the group
2. Supporting—	—and confronting
3. Fostering experimentation and learning—	—and performance
4. Promoting improvisation—	—and structure
5. Showing patience—	—and urgency
6. Encouraging bottom-up initiative—	—and intervening top-down

From Hill LA, Brandeau G, Truelove E, Lineback K. Collective genius. *Harv Bus Rev.* 2014:94–102.

tension created between the need to be a high-reliability organization and the need for flexibility. We make no progress without risk, and yet risk isn't a positive influence on reliability. All of us play some role in innovation, even if we aren't the ones with the idea.

HOW TO BECOME INNOVATIVE

As early as 2011, one of us wrote about the ability to think differently and futuristically. The Wise Forecast Model was designed to be simple and easy to remember so that any of us could apply it in any role we might enact.[5] The three-step process appears in Table 40.2.

Learning widely is a challenge in itself! We are overwhelmed with relevant literature related to our clinical and functional specialties. And now we learn, we must learn beyond those boundaries. We (the authors) have tended to provide references for this book from sources external to nursing and health care. That was a deliberate strategy to help readers value the fact that many others in the world have the same kinds of leadership experiences we do. Some are equally as demanding, where lives depend on what they do. If we are trying to develop (or strengthen) a skill, we need to look beyond our usual sources if we wish to be innovative in our approach to situations. Thus we need to turn to other sources of learning and not just the professional literature. Sometimes, what helps us understand what we need to do derives from a news item or TED Talks. As organizations become more inventive, they use multiple ways to disseminate their information, and if we are open to those various ways, we may gain insight into something we might not have understood in a traditional professional literature publication. How do we gain insight? The November 2014 issue of *Harvard Business Review* provides some insight—in fact seven insights.[6] Table 40.3 illustrates how those seven insights can be implemented practically. All of those ways allow us to learn widely.

TABLE 40.2 The Three Steps of the Wise Forecast Model

1. Learn widely: Read literature from outside the health care field and outside the United States.
2. Think wildly: Ask "what if" questions to combine disparate ideas and form something new.
3. Act wisely: Take the best of thinking wildly and decide whether it is likely to be possible. If it is too disruptive, it might not be possible to choose that option unless other disruptions are occurring.

From Yoder-Wise PS. Creating wise forecasts for nursing: the Wise Forecast Model©. *J Contin Educ Nurs.* 2001;42:387.

Often the things we take on in the name of innovation are the problems we see that haven't been addressed. Deborah Ancona and Hal Gregersen, both affiliated with the MIT Leadership Center, would call the people who champion these solutions "problem-led leaders." In other words, they take on problems that others also consider issues and in doing so they create a group of followers who are also passionate about finding a solution.[7]

According to the Innovation Resource Consulting Group (IRCG), we can follow a seven-step process to enhance our skills related to innovation.[8] First, embrace opportunity-mode thinking. The focus is being alert to possibilities. Second, be adept at critical thinking. The focus here is to end assumptions that we sometimes carry forward with any idea. Third, develop empathy for the end user. Although an idea might sound good to the creator, if it doesn't seem that to the person who has to actually do or use the innovation, the idea isn't likely to succeed. Fourth, think ahead of the curve. Put another way, be a consumer of information so you can draw on multiple perspectives. Fifth, fortify your idea factory. This requires thinking about what you know, talking with others, and brainswarming. Step six involves collaboration, and a good way IRCG suggests to do this is by joining a specific-purpose team. The intent is to have a successful experience in a rather low-risk environment. The last step is to build the

TABLE 40.3 Application of Seven Insights for Innovation

Insight	Application
Anomalies	Looking for the deviant can alert us to opportunities. Think about the potential of data that cue us to action. Falls, catheters, who works when—all have the potential to help us see something differently.
Confluence	When two or more things come together initially or in a different way, new opportunities present themselves. Consider the inventions nurses have made or products they have improved because the right patients were available who needed a different solution than was previously available.
Frustrations	These need no explanation, and if we want to start somewhere, look at the work-arounds. They tell us something doesn't work routinely because we have perfected some of the work-arounds. And, frankly, many of us are proud of how we figured out to make something work!
Orthodoxies	Traditions hold a certain reverence and yet when broken can lead to better ways of providing care. What could be broken where you work?
Extremities	Strategies are always developed to deal with the majority. What about the conditions we seldom deal with that irritate our patients or our colleagues and have not been addressed or addressed by only a few people?
Voyages	"Traveling" into another space (think a different clinical area, a different unit, a health care organization in another city) to see what they do can stimulate new solutions for back-home issues.
Analogies	As much as some of us don't want to think of the work we do as a business, in fact it is. So what is some business in town doing that might be adapted to your place of work?

Insights from Sawhney M, Khosla S. Managing yourself: where to look for insight. *Harv Bus Rev.* 2014:126–9.

buy-in. This step involves using influence to help others see a problem as you see it; to understand why a proposed action is the best solution; and to be willing to vest their energy, money, and reputation in working on this innovation.

REFLECTION What have you read or watched recently that piqued your interest and made you wonder how your patients or colleagues would benefit from such an approach or tool? If you can't recall anything, go pick up some magazine totally unrelated to nursing or health care and scan the articles to see what stimulates your creativity. Then consider what you could do with that creative idea.

Thinking wildly entails being able to say "yes and" rather than "no that won't work." As an example, brainstorming often allows people to throw out thoughts that someone else can squash before we have an opportunity to think about the potential of the idea. This step doesn't have to be done with someone else: just be as wild in your thinking as you can—and without judgment. Safi Bahcall suggests that the wild thinking that occurs in organizations is called *loonshots*.[9] A loonshot is recognized as such because it is a "fallen-out-of-favor" project that has been abandoned, and the champion of that work is seen as unhinged (his word) or looney (ours). In his *Harvard Business Review* article, he identifies seven ways to increase innovation, as Table 40.4 shows.[10] Those ideas apply to organizations—our challenge is to see how we can use them as an individual seeking better ways to lead. The items in italics are one translation of the relevance to individuals.

REFLECTION Consider some work-around you do on a regular basis. We all have them, and we use some so frequently we might not even recall that they are the work-around. What is the root cause of why you use that work-around? Thinking as wildly as you can, what strategies could you consider to fix the root cause of the issue? As Dan Weberg, nurse innovator, says, the workaround may be the solution. So why isn't it the policy?

Acting wisely entails the judgment phase of the process. We can now figure out what is totally impractical for a variety of reasons—it costs too much; it can only be done in laboratory conditions, not with live patients; only a handful of people in the world know how to do this; it's too complicated and few people would follow the process to complete the task; and so forth. This is not to say that sometimes we shouldn't move ahead even if only a handful of people currently know how to do something. The odds of being successful are much more limited, however.

TABLE 40.4 **Seven Ways to Increase Innovation in Organizations**

1. Celebrate results, not rank. Rewards go to results, not to rank.	*Focus on creating results rather than seeking promotion. Far more leaders exist in an organization than those indicated by title.*
2. Use soft equity. Rewards should be geared to what excites the person, including nonfinancial rewards.	*Let others know what you think are rewards, and if you don't know what those are, stop and think about what they might be.*
3. Take politics out of the equation. Lobbying a boss won't help; only results will.	*Don't waste your time impressing the boss. Focus on how well you can do with the work you have to do.*
4. Invest in training. If the people who learn new skills have the opportunity to use them, they work more diligently to enhance those new skills.	*If you are offered the opportunity to gain new skills, grab it! If not, find such opportunities on your own. Our development is our accountability, not that of some organization.*
5. Perfect employee placement. Put the right person in the right job!	*If you love your job, let others know. If you hate it, find something that works better for you. (This is not about shift or amount of work. It's about passion for a clinical area, a project, a role, and so forth.)*
6. Fine-tune the spans. Broader spans of control create fewer layers that become an incentive about rank rather than results.	*Even if your boss has a huge span of control, do something to let that person know who you are, and make it a point to convey what you are doing and want.*
7. Appoint a chief incentives (innovations) officer. This provides a central point for coordination.	*If this opportunity arises, consider whether you can do that job!*

From Bahcall S. The innovation equation: the most important variables are structural, not cultural. *Harv Bus Rev.* 2019:74–81.

REFLECTION Look back at your reflection regarding the work-around. Of all the wild thinking you did, what one or two strategies are the most likely to produce success in deterring the work-around and actually fixing the precipitating issue?

When a team of researchers in South Korea looked at factors influencing nurses' innovative behaviors, they found over a third of the variance in creative self-efficacy derived from self-leadership and individual knowledge sharing, and those two factors had a direct and positive effect on an innovative culture.[11] Self-leadership (for example, constructive thinking) related to those nurses who set goals for themselves and sought to improve their work. Individual knowledge sharing seemed to promote more creative thinking and exchanges of information. This study could suggest that we don't each have to spend time learning the same things. Rather, we can share the learning burden to stimulate wild conversations about what is possible. That is what innovation is about—the possible, not the what is—and an easy way to get to that way of thinking is to ask: What if? What if we took an idea from a fashion designer and made a better patient gown? (Yes, we know that a fashion designer has already done that, but patient gowns is a consistent topic—at least for patients!) What if we provided transportation home for a patient rather than waiting for a family member to arrive? What if we....

Almost all of the literature about innovation discusses culture; however, Gary Pisano says the kind of culture that supports innovation must be counterbalanced by intolerance for incompetence, discipline and candor, accountability, and a strong leader.[12] None of those ideas sounds like fun, and he doesn't intend them to be. The gutsiness of moving people along, in or out of the organization, for example, may not have been a goal before. Now we have to assume new commitment to high standards—and enforce them. What this means for each of us is that we have to assume the role of innovation-scientists with the same rigor we would expect of someone in a lab inventing a new medication or stopping an out-of-control organism. We must assume the diligence that is required to document what we are doing, to identify corrections we make midway, and to sharing with the larger organization the meaning of our findings. Others want to know WIFM: what's in it for me!

One scary thought, however, is this: Nurse leaders in general are not innovators! When two researchers surveyed 137 nurse leaders through the American Organization of Nurse Executives (now the American Organization for

Nursing Leadership), the majority of responses indicated nurse executives were in the category of early majority.[13] Using Everett Rogers's theory of diffusion as a framework, the researchers used a tool to determine how nurse managers/executives rated themselves in the five categories of innovation. Only two individuals were viewed as innovators. That number plus the 15 who were categorized as early majority (the two groups closest to the "cutting edge") totaled 17 out of 137 respondents. Although that number might be high in a general survey, we must consider the need to have nursing's leadership being more innovative. On the other hand, maybe they don't have to be innovative so long as they can create and support a culture of innovations where others are the innovators.

LL ALERT

- Don't lose everyone as your collaborators by getting too far ahead in your own thinking.
- Don't put down anyone who finds this work scary—they are potential collaborators.

SUMMARY

Not everyone will do something innovative, but everyone should be able to think creatively at least from time to time and to carry a concept to completion. Innovation can be a deliberative process, not just a moment of inspiration. The profession has to be innovative to stay relevant, and our individual task is to figure out how we contribute to that process.

LL LINEUP

- Assess your organization: How does it support innovation?
- Use the Wise Forecast Model to innovate or at least start the process.
- Test one idea and evaluate its process and outcomes.

REFLECTION Think about what you perceive your strengths to be in terms of innovation. Will you find the "out of the way" articles from another field that contribute ideas to some issue at work? Will you be the naysayer so those with the vision have the opportunity to strengthen their statements and vision? Will you be willing to step up when called upon to test a new idea or product? What is your role in innovating?

41 Politics

Just say the words *organizational politics* and people immediately roll their eyes, grimace, or otherwise show their disdain. No one wants to admit that they participate in political mechanisms in their work world. However, the reality is that we ALL participate in work-related politics as a means of accomplishing the goals of our institution. We are first introduced to "politics of the group" in preschool or kindergarten, when we learned that if we were helpful to the teacher, she would like us. Some of us also learned that if we told a joke during class, the teacher might not like us, but if the joke was funny, the kids in our class would. In short, we are programmed from our earliest days to respond to the political environment of the groups with which we interact.

All jobs are influenced by the politics of the organization. Some simply are more obvious or dramatic than others. Even if we work alone as a consultant or other independent contractor, we must be aware of the environment of organizations we advise. Michael Jarrett, in the *Harvard Business Review,* notes that most leaders in organizations tend to view political moves in a negative light and try to pretend that politics do not influence their decisions. Yet it may be that actions that consider the political implications may in fact be in the best interest of the organization and its members.[1]

Mary Wroblewski suggests it is futile to avoid political action in an organization; she describes political action as "not just a tool for the self-serving," but as "a natural, useful tool as part of strategy execution."[2] Assessing the political landscape and understanding the source of political capital in the organization is the first step in moving toward positive outcomes. Because we can't avoid politics, we have to capitalize on this important organizational characteristic.

THE DEFINITION OF ORGANIZATIONAL POLITICS

The various definitions of organizational politics reflect this conflicting view. For example, the Business Dictionary states that politics represents a pursuit of individual agendas and self-interest in an organization without regard to their effect on the organization's effort to achieve its goals. However, Michael Jarrett suggests that organizational politics refers to a variety of activities associated with the use of influence tactics, including power, to improve personal or organizational interest.[1] This difference suggests organizational politics can be used for either good or ill.

REFLECTION What do you believe about using power? Have you had experiences where others have used the political system of a team or organization to improve the organization's outcomes? What happened in these circumstances? Have you also had experiences where those with whom you worked used their power to promote themselves rather than improve the functioning of the organization? What was the result of this situation, and how did you feel?

SOCIAL POWER AND POLITICAL CAPITAL

Most of us are familiar with the categories of social power established by Bertram Raven and John French 60 years ago. These researchers found:

- **Legitimate or positional power** related to the position a person holds in an organization's hierarchy, particularly if the position is deserved. In relative terms, few of these positions exist in a health care organization, and the hierarchy of the organization dictates who (what position) has the final word.
- **Expert power** related to the knowledge or expertise of the person in a particular area. Many people in an organization have this type of power. Those people who are enamored of themselves may use a shorthand code to close down a conversation (e.g., I am the most seasoned surgeon). Experts who value being an expert and who don't need the limelight not only share their expertise but also invite others to share theirs.

- **Referent power** related to the interpersonal relationships that a person cultivates with other people in the organization. We likely all know someone who is a name dropper. Their motivation is usually based on conveying they know the "right" people.
- **Coercive power** related to a person's ability to influence others via threats, punishments, or sanctions. Probably the most common example that leaps to our minds is a manager who uses threats to staff a unit. This is a "do X or else" situation. It carries little influence when the "enforcer" isn't present.
- **Reward power** related to the ability of a person to influence the allocation of incentives, including salary, appraisals, and promotions, in an organization. We typically think of our nurse leaders who have this ability. But actually we all have this power. Here is an example: If two of us serve on a committee and I hate proofing our minutes and you love details, I have the opportunity to reward you for proofing the minutes with a specialty coffee, a rose, or something else that is something I know you like. (And it always has to be about what YOU like, not what I think you should have.)[3] Both the gift and knowing you like details are rewards; the latter conveys that I know and understand your talents.

Some of these categories represent formal power (legitimate, expert, reward) within the organization; others (referent, coercive power) are more informal in nature. Political power comes from the ability to understand what other people fear or desire and use this understanding to influence their behavior.[4] However, these categories do not address the motives of the person exerting the power. Certainly, we frequently see news reports of corporate power resulting in fraud and corruption where the motive was to gain power, resources, or win at any cost. However, evidence of leaders who use power in a moral way, in order to bring about good, also abound. The individual's or group's moral compass informs their motives, which can result in the positive use of power. In Table 41.1, Michaelann Quimby (2019) outlines three types of moral political power, defining for us which type represents a motive to achieve organizational goals.[4]

To be an effective leader, we must be vigilant that political actions we take on behalf of a team or organization represent the best interest of the group *and* are representative of our best selves. Two strategies can be helpful to keep us on the path of righteousness. First, we must keep our own values and mission and those of the organization that we represent in the forefront of our decision-making. Ask the question, "Does this action(s) reflect our values?" or "Will the action(s) help us achieve our mission?" If the answer to either of these questions is "no," a review of the action(s) is in order. Of course, if our own values and mission are in conflict with those of the organization, we must also analyze whether we can support the action. If we cannot, we might not be the "best fit" for the organization.

Second, we must examine our personal motives before we move forward with a chosen action. We need to ask ourselves if the action to be implemented enhances our position while negatively affecting other people or groups. If the answer to this is "yes," we are not acting from a moral perspective. Michelann Quimby suggests three questions, identified in Table 41.2, that we might ask ourselves to assess our motives in our actions at work.[4]

On a related note, this feeling of having to support a position that does not fit with our values may lead to moral distress. When we work in a hierarchy, we may be required to carry out orders from a supervisor that are against our own convictions. Over time, the resulting distress may accumulate and weigh on us. The residue of this discomfort can manifest itself in physical symptoms, including hypertension, fatigue and exhaustion, emotional symptoms, anger, frustration, sadness, and isolation. Ultimately, poor communication, absenteeism, lack of trust, and in the case of those in health care, poor quality or unsafe patient care and detachment from patients or the job can occur.[5]

TABLE 41.1 Types of Political Power From a Moral Perspective

Types of Political Power	Definitions
Amoral Political Power	Unconsciously understanding and manipulating others with no awareness of your own motivating fears and desires.
Immoral Political Power	Consciously understanding and influencing others without examining and understanding your own motives.
Moral Political Power	Consciously examining, understanding, and evaluating your own motivations, fears, and desires before using your understanding of others to influence them.

Quimby M. Organizational power politics: using your power for good. The Systems Thinker. 2019. Available at: https://thesystemsthinker.com/organizational-politics-using-your-power-for-good/.

TABLE 41.2 Assessment of Motives in the Workplace	
At work, what do I want to achieve?	(Examples: respect, money, control—add others)
At work, what am I afraid of?	(Examples: losing my job, competition, not being liked—add others)
What values guide my work?	(Examples: ambition, creativity, collegiality)

Quimby M. Organizational power politics: using your power for good. The Systems Thinker. 2019. Available at: https://thesystemsthinker.com/organizational-politics-using-your-power-for-good/.

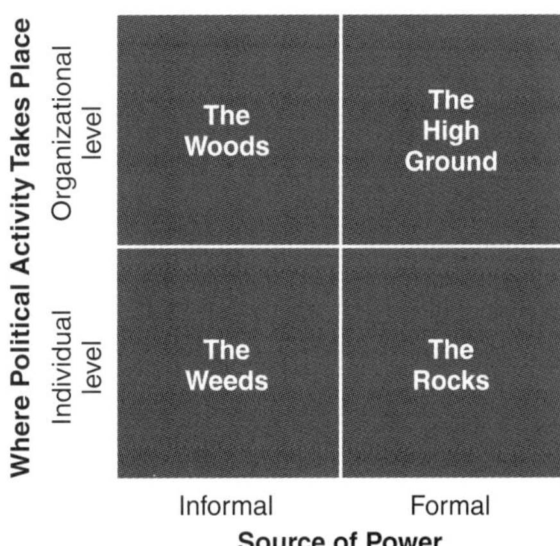

Fig. 41.1 The landscape of an organizational political environment. From Jarrett M. The four types of organization politics. *Harv Bus Rev.* April 24, 2017. Available at: https://hbr.org/2017/04/the-4-types-of-organizational-politics.

AN EXAMPLE OF "LIVING" THE VALUES AND MISSION OF AN ORGANIZATION

A colleague of ours was appointed the director of an associate-degree nursing program that had a history of plummeting enrollment and faculty attrition. He was hired to address both of these problems. He had not previously worked at this college but did have a great deal of experience in associate-degree nursing education. Upon assuming the director position, he took time to meet with each faculty and staff member, learning their perspectives on enrollment, faculty attrition, and their day-to-day challenges. He asked them their perceptions of the strengths of the department, as well as their own. The new director also talked to students, alumni, and other stakeholders to discover their perceptions of the program.

From this assessment, the director drafted a plan of action and reviewed it with faculty and staff, as well as the provost to whom he reported. He used this feedback to revise the plan before sending the plan to the provost (again) and to the president for their approval to move ahead with the plan. Throughout the process, he was transparent in his actions and publicly credited team members' important contributions. The result was a swift drop in faculty attrition and a gradual increase in the enrollment, and the reputation of the program improved.

REFLECTION What is your analysis of this situation? Can you hypothesize what the motives, values, and mission of our colleague might be?

SOURCES OF POLITICAL POWER OR CAPITAL

In the *Harvard Business Review*, Michael Jarrett suggests that the first step to feeling comfortable with organizational politics is to understand the sources of political power or capital. He conceptualizes the organizational political environment as a landscape or nature spot. This nature spot includes an area of the **woods**, full of thick trees; **high ground; weeds;** and a **rocky** section. He believes that these four metaphorical domains describe various potential political environments within any organization. His metaphor offers us a framework for assessing our own political environment and developing moral political actions for a positive outcome.[1] Fig. 41.1 and Table 41.3 illustrate these metaphorical domains.

These metaphors not only offer a creative approach to describe the political environment in our work but also provide some direction to assess the use of political power or capital. Often a number of political environments exist within one organization. They are driven by the function of the unit, the managers and staff involved in the physical location, and many other factors. Each of these types of political environments may have both a positive and a negative effect on the organization as a whole. A leader's responsibility is to provide an ongoing assessment of power throughout the organization and evaluate its relative impact upon outcomes and morale. Table 41.4 outlines some possible leadership actions we might take based upon such an assessment.

REFLECTION Think of an organizational unit in which you have worked. Which metaphor would you use to characterize its political environment? Why? Do you see the metaphor from a positive or negative perspective? What did the leader(s) do to manage this environment? Was the outcome positive or negative?

TABLE 41.3 The Landscape of an Organizational Political Environment: A Metaphor

The Woods	**The High Ground**
Implicit norms, hidden assumptions, and unspoken routines comprise the woods Provides a structure for employees. A place where good ideas and necessary changes can get lost is reflective of the woods.	Formal authority is consistent with organizational systems; includes the rules, structures, policy guidelines, and procedures. Benefits of rules and procedures provide stability for the rocks and a check against groups within the organization moving away from stated goals. Overly bureaucratic rules and procedures and use of processes to challenge new ideas can prevent innovation and change.
The Weeds	**The Rocks**
Personal influence and informal networks govern the environment. Growth of natural relationship without any support (just like weeds) occurs. The weeds function without much need for direction and also form connections (a dense mat of weeds) through which little or nothing can grow. They may foster an opposition to needed change.	Formal sources of authority or interactions, especially when formal groups are "high status." This represents a stabilizing foundation, which may be helpful in a crisis. Rocks represent damaging sharp edges.

Jarrett M. The four types of organization politics. *Harv Bus Rev.* April 24, 2017. Available at: https://hbr.org/2017/04/the-4-types-of-organizational-politics.

STRATEGIES FOR ORGANIZATIONAL POLITICAL ACTION

As leaders, we must be prepared to recognize and adjust to the political norms where we work. Let's pretend that we are taking on a new leadership position. (This may have already happened or—who knows?—such an opportunity is right around the corner.) The first step we should take is to become familiar with the peculiarities of the specific organization through an assessment of the environment. How do you do this? Certainly, becoming familiar with the written documents regarding the mission, values, and processes of the area is initially important. Equally important is to introduce ourselves to our colleagues in the best possible light. Remember, we seem to get attached to our initial impression of people, and we find it very difficult to change our opinion of them, even when considerable evidence indicates the contrary.[6]

As new leaders, we should spend significant time in networking. Others will want to see and talk to us, so they can reduce the anxiety usually associated with the start of a new leader. In the initial discussions, we should actively work to reduce tension and to make others comfortable. We need to listen more than talk in these meetings. (That is why we all have two ears and only one mouth!) Listening deeply to others helps us to understand not only what they are saying but also what they are feeling. However, when we do talk, clear, straight-to-the-point communication, with a little humor thrown in, is always a plus.[7]

Developing relationships with our teams is, of course, the first priority. However, we also need to connect with others beyond the initial group. Don't forget to communicate with our bosses. Note: We are not bragging to communicate our activities, assessment, and plans moving forward—we are keeping them up-to-date.[7] One of us would readily admit that she had difficulty with this until she realized that her counterpart in another department took credit for the things that actually happened in nursing. After that, her report to her boss was longer because she wanted to be sure another group couldn't omit nurses from the reports of progress in the organization. Our bosses may also be anxious about how their "new hire" is working out. In addition, frequent communication can keep you on the right path. After all, we can't possibly learn everything we need to know about the organization during the interview process—or in the first months of a job. This ongoing interaction with others can give us additional information regarding the context in which we are working.

As we move through the first months of our jobs, we must treat everyone on our team equitably. We all have our favorite colleagues, but not showing preferential treatment will automatically level the political playing field. When one

TABLE 41.4 The Landscape Metaphor as a Framework for Political Action

Metaphor	Political Actions
Weeds	1. Get involved enough to understand the functioning of the networks or groups who form the weeds. 2. Include the network representatives in the planning of some aspect of the change. 3. Try to fill any vacancies in the network with people who are aligned with you and/or the change process. 4. Strengthen your relationship with other networks in the organization.
Rocks	1. Draw on the formal power structures, rather than fighting against them. 2. Redirect the energy of those who oppose the change through reasoned arguments or appealing to their interests.
The High Ground	1. Gather feedback from clients, customers, and other stakeholders and present the case for the change from this feedback. 2. Highlight, without blaming, how the current structure is preventing the organization from responding to the changing environment. 3. Emphasize that being risk averse is costly and may be riskier than trying something new. 4. Create a reward system for others who engage with the plan for change. 5. Set up a task force to examine the situation and to bridge silos to provide an opportunity outside of the typical organizational structure, which may provide an alternative source of power and support for change.
The Woods	1. Ask a variety of stakeholders about company functioning that is related to the change. 2. Establish benchmark information from surveys and specialist experts. 3. Use this information to bring implicit organizational routines and behaviors to the surface. Ask relevant groups to reflect on the extent to which the work they are focusing on will be most important in moving them forward.

Jarrett M. The four types of organization politics. *Harv Bus Rev.* April 24, 2017. Available at: https://hbr.org/2017/04/the-4-types-of-organizational-politics.

of us was in a leadership role where external socializing was common:

"I made a point to not socialize with any of my direct teams during work hours, except in groups. Even when one of my closest friends came to work in my area, we made a point to not spend a lot of time together during work hours. Because of our positions, we were often in meetings together; however, we tried to avoid the appearance of 'speaking in one voice.' (This process was helped by the fact that my friend and I had no difficulty disagreeing with each other—we did it all the time!)"

REFLECTION Reflect on what you just read in the previous section. Perhaps you have had the experience of being a new leader. Perhaps you can think of one of your colleagues who has been in a similar position. To what extent did the new leader follow the suggestions outlined earlier? What happened as a result? What did you learn from this reflection?

LL ALERT

- Don't limit networking to those above you or those who can improve your position in the organization.
- Don't worry about tension and discomfort in teams or meetings.
- Don't be afraid to assess and manage the political environment where you work.

SUMMARY

Politics are everywhere. Politics can be used to support the attainment of the organization's goals; however, political behavior, if used only for personal gain, can also be detrimental to the organization. Assessing on an ongoing basis the political climate of an organization is a critical competence of a leader. Using our values to guide us in making choices regarding political action is also vital to developing a leadership legacy. Used correctly, politics can make a positive difference in the outcomes of your organization and your career.

LL LINEUP

- Recognize that power has both positive and negative effects and assess the potential for both types of consequences before acting.
- Use organizational politics to meet the goals of the organization or unit.

REFLECTION What areas of organizational politics frighten you or make you reluctant to use it for good? What can you do about this? What skills do you hope to develop so that you can increase your competence in this area? If needed, how will you reframe involvement in politics to be a good thing?

42

Processes

All teams and organizations, regardless of their mission and/or structure, must use organizational processes to accomplish their identified goals. Our ability to develop a leadership trajectory requires that we know how to effectively use these processes to develop, implement, and/or evaluate the work for which we are responsible. Let's delve into the strategies to use processes to improve the outcomes of our work.

WHAT IS A PROCESS?

A process is a set of activities connected from a start to an end point. A process is similar to a procedure but is usually larger in scope. In fact, processes typically include procedures. Two types of processes are common: strategic and operational. Strategic processes happen periodically—for example, to guide the development of long-term goals. The operational processes involve regular everyday work. For example, most organizations have a set of operational processes that may include:

- Managerial
- Supply
- Production
- Marketing
- Sales and Delivery
- Research and Development
- Human Resources (hiring, evaluation, training)
- IT Development and Management
- Accounting

Using both types of processes effectively should be a core competency for nurse leaders. Depending on one's role in an organization, some of the processes are more critical than others. As an example of the use of a process, consider the orientation of new employees. A colleague of ours reported working in an education department of a medical center and hearing a number of concerns from nursing management that the initial orientation of new nursing staff was not effective. Specifically, new employees were not comfortable using the institution's policies related to interacting with the interprofessional team, dealing with patient privacy, and managing errors and missed care. Our colleague described the educational department's hesitation in addressing this concern. After all, talking about policies in a classroom is a recipe for participant boredom. However, our colleague realized that the organization was clear that the concerns had to be addressed. So, our colleague's approach to this concern illustrates the use of a process to identify an underlying problem and resolve it. The educational group developed questions that they felt they should ask various stakeholders to gain a deeper understanding of the problem. They also identified appropriate representatives of the stakeholders involved in the implementation of the policies who could shed light on the concerns expressed. The list of potential interviewees included:

- The relevant nurse managers
- The nursing directors' council
- Past and current orientees from nursing services
- A quality management representative, who dealt with issues of errors, including privacy violations and missed care
- The chief nursing officer and several of her teams
- The chief medical officer (CMO) and several physicians selected by the CMO
- The allied health council

Once the interviews were completed and the results analyzed, the group compared the feedback with their teaching-learning and evaluation plan for orientation sessions to determine whether they were capturing all the necessary content. They also considered *how* the material was being presented and evaluated to determine whether the presentation was sufficiently engaging for the orientees to remember what to do once they were on a unit. Determining whether the orientees knew where to get more information should it be needed as they began to practice without supervision was also important. Finally, the education group scheduled some follow-up evaluation activities after their new approach was implemented, so they could be sure that orientees' skills in these areas had improved.

This is an example of a process implemented in an organization in a relatively short period to resolve a problem. Similar and dramatically shorter processes were implemented in many hospitals to make them COVID ready. Let's now consider ways within an organization in which such a process can be implemented in a more formal way.

THE DEMING CYCLE (PDSA CYCLE)

Although many of us are familiar with the process known as the Plan, Do, Study, and Act (PDSA) cycle, we are always surprised to learn some leaders work in organizations that don't use some form of this cycle to solve problems. Implementing processes that focus on improving the way the team or organization works is an important part of the leader's role, regardless of the institution where they work. In the 1950s, a renowned statistician, W. Edward Deming, applied the scientific process to businesses processes to provide us with a simple way to evaluate complex organizations. The resulting process became known as the continuous quality improvement model, also referred to as the PDSA cycle; the Plan-Do-Study-Act; or the Deming cycle. This model represents a logical sequence of four repetitive steps that provide a framework for continuous improvement and learning. Table 42.1 outlines the steps in the PDSA cycle (https://www.isixsigma.com/dictionary/deming-cycle-pdca/).

The PDSA cycle emphasizes the following points. It must:

- Mirror the scientific process (formulating a hypothesis, collecting data, analyzing and interpreting the results, inferring the next steps to test the hypothesis).
- Begin with small-scale, iterative approaches to test interventions, allowing for flexibility to change based on the feedbacks.
- Predict the outcome, using what you know about the complex system with which you are dealing. This encourages an increasingly deep understanding of the system.
- Measure the resulting data over time to capture the inherent variability in complex organizations.
- Document the processes and findings to transfer the learning to other settings.[1]

REFLECTION Compare the process used by our colleague in the educational department described earlier with the PDSA cycle. In what ways was it similar? In what ways was it different? Would any differences affect the outcome?

PROCESSES IN HEALTH CARE

The health care industry, because of its complexity, is well known for the use of processes. This emphasis, in part, is likely driven by the work of Avedis Donabedian, who, in 1966, described a framework for assessing the quality of care in a variety of health care situations. He described the relationship among three concepts: structure, process, and outcome. In this model, *processes* are actions performed to improve patient health. *Structures* (also included in the Legacy *Leaders*-Ship Trajectory model) are defined as the

TABLE 42.1 Steps in the Plan, Do, Study, and Act (PDSA) Cycle

Steps	Definition	Effects
Plan	Plan ahead for change. Analyze and predict the result.	*Goal:* To understand what quality is in a particular context and what quality should be in this situation in the future. An attempt to improve outcomes and evaluate the extent to which leaders really understand the process.
Do	Execute the plan, taking small steps in controlled circumstances.	*Goal:* To test your proposed process. Start with small-scale implementation and evaluation. Use iterative changes during the process to test variables. Document every step. (Act as if this was a scientific experiment).
Study	Check and study the results.	*Goal:* To determine whether actual outcomes matched the prediction. In what way and why? How can the unexpected variables be tested? *These questions point out why Deming substituted Study for Check. He wanted to know "Why did it work?" rather than "Did it work?"*
Act	Take action to standardize or improve the process.	*Goal:* Implement recommended changes in a larger context. Track performance data over time, providing documentation to continue to improve. The Act step is also the first step of the next cycle.

Henshall A. How to use the Deming cycle for continuous quality improvement. December 1, 2017. Available at: https://www.process.st/deming-cycle/.

physical and organizational aspects of the care setting, such as facilities, equipment, personnel, operational, and financial. The *outcomes* to be improved include recovery, functional restoration, survival, and even patient satisfaction. According to Donabedian, evaluation of each of the three components of the framework is required to ensure quality care. For this reason, many health care organizations' quality plans identify criteria for evaluation in each component.[2] These same three concepts also apply to leadership processes.

PDSA CYCLE IN HEALTH CARE

The PDSA cycle has been applied in health care settings, as well as other types of businesses. For example, the Agency for Healthcare Research and Quality (AHRQ) Healthcare Innovative Exchange Center website (https://innovations.ahrq.gov/qualitytools/plan-do-study-act-pdsa-cycle) provides a succinct description of the PDSA cycle and gives examples of ways in which health care providers across the country are improving care through this approach.

The Institute of Healthcare Improvement (IHI), which focuses on improving health care through its Triple Aim framework (http://www.ihi.org/), builds upon the PDSA model through the Model for Improvement developed by Associates in Process Improvement (https://www.apiweb.org/index.php). The model addresses three questions: What are we trying to accomplish? How will we know a change is important? What change can we make that will result in improvement? Answers to this question lead to an emphasis on (1) improving the health of populations, (2) enhancing the experience for individuals, and (3) reducing the per capita cost of health care; in short, the Triple Aim Framework. This framework is then used to guide implementation of the PDSA cycle (Fig. 42.1).[3]

Since initiation of the Triple Aim Framework, a movement has grown to add an additional aim to this framework. For example, in 2014, Thomas Bodenheimer and Christine Sinsky[4] suggested that the consequence of the increased demands on health care providers have resulted in burnout. These high rates of burnout have many negative consequences for both patients and providers. Bodenheimer and Sinsky believe that improving the work lives of those who deliver care should serve as a fourth aim. For many organizations, this fourth aim is described as attaining joy in work.[5] The fourth aim is consistent with the years of work related to the establishment and evolution of the Magnet Recognition Program®.

Encouraging joy in work is not the only fourth aim to be posed. Derek Feeley[3] suggests that some organizations use pursuing health equity as the focus of the fourth aim, and the Military Health System has added readiness as their fourth aim. In an IHI blog, Feeley states that "IHI

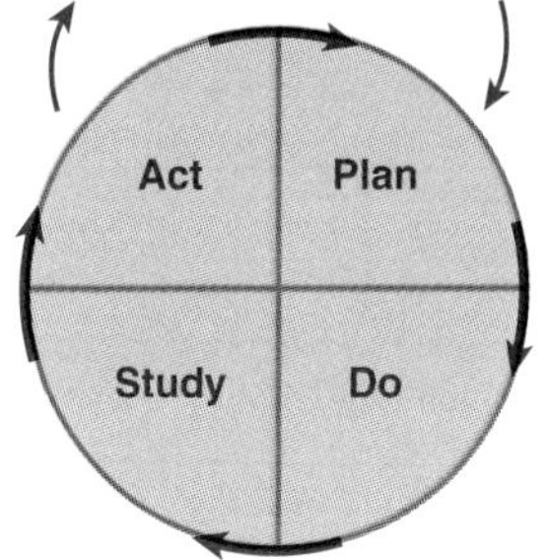

Fig. 42.1 The Institute of Healthcare Improvement Model by Associates in Process Improvement.

fully supports other organizations prioritizing these worthy efforts if a Quadruple Aim helps to deliver on the organizational strategy." However, he suggests four points to keep in mind when organizations do implement that fourth strategy. These include:

- Remember that the Triple Aim is about improving the lives of our patients; that focus should remain the highest priority.
- We haven't finished pursuing the original Triple aim; there is still work to be done.
- Don't lose focus on the optimal delivery of the Triple Aim.
- Measure what matters.[3]

REFLECTION What experience have you had with improvement processes in your work setting? Was the PDSA cycle used? Did you feel as if the process resulted in improvement in a particular context? What was the follow-up? What did you learn? Is there anything that you would change going forward?

DEVELOPING A NEW INITIATIVE

Nurse leaders are often responsible for leading the development of completely new initiatives, which require a special

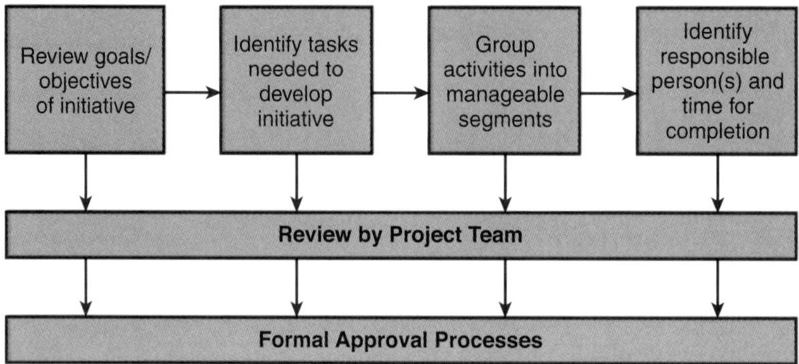

Fig. 42.2 Flowchart of the development of an organizational process

type of strategic process. Once the mission, goals, and objectives of the new initiative have been determined, the steps the developers take to make the new initiative a reality must be identified. The development team must list all the activities required to start the new initiative. This may include such items as mapping the services the initiative will provide, developing policies, hiring and training appropriate staff, marketing the product/service, determining needed physical space, and articulating coordination with other parts of the larger organization or service area. Grouping these activities into similar and manageable segments of work facilitates implementation. The team should also define the people responsible for each activity (or groups of activities) and the completion date(s) that should be expected. Usually, these are divided among the team, based on members' expertise. Throughout this process, the team leader(s) should seek approvals and/or permission from the appropriate groups within the organization and in the larger environment. Before each approval process, the responsible team should review the work to ensure congruence across the various components of the initiative. Following this type of process keeps the developmental team from missing important steps. Fig. 42.2 provides a schematic presentation or flowchart of this process.

WILL PROCESSES REDUCE MISSTEPS AND FAILURES?

Processes are designed to reduce the likelihood of missteps and failures as organizations take steps to achieve the mission or goal of the team or organization. There is no question that using a process plan to develop a new initiative, manage routine organizational activities, or improve the quality of a particular process is critical to assuring success. Does this mean that everything during the development process will go well? *Absolutely not!* Perhaps you have heard of the best laid plans…

Why is this so? Being involved in the implementation of processes involves not only the ability to think strategically and pay attention to detail, but also the ability to be flexible and problem-solve in the moment when things go sideways. All of us have had experience in using processes to plan activities, and one of us tells the story of starting a 50-bed psychiatric hospital:

"We followed a detailed planning process, and in general, all things went well. However effective the processes are planned and implemented, things can and will go wrong. The first week the hospital was open, something did, in fact, go wrong. Because the hospital was small, we contracted for laundry service from a full-service medical center close by. The hospital laundry staff was to deliver a certain quantity of linen on a scheduled basis. (Of course, we really didn't know how much linen we would need—after all, this was a psychiatric hospital where patients were up and about.) One night, a patient needed to have his bed changed during the night; unfortunately, no clean linen could be found in our hospital. A nurse who had played a critical role in the development of the hospital was on administrative call that night and received a frantic call from the nurse caring for the patient. What to do about getting more linen? The on-call administrative nurse asked her to call the on-call administrator of the medical center and arrange for one of the mental health techs to pick up some linen.

"As you might imagine, arranging such a linen pick-up at 2 AM was problematic. A number of phone calls with raised voices and frustrated staff—to say nothing of a patient who needed a dry bed—did nothing to resolve the problem until 8 AM the next morning at the usual delivery time. The person

who was most upset by the event was the administrative on-call nurse. (The nurse caring for the patient—and the patient—figured out how to use bedspreads to deal with the problem.) However, the nurse on administrative call sent in her resignation for her position the very next morning. Her rationale for the resignation was that a hospital should be able to count on fresh linen for patients at any time of the day or night.

"Of course, the nurse on administrative call was completely right: hospitals should always have fresh linens available. Certainly we had a glitch in our estimates, which meant our planning process was likely flawed. We redid the estimate of needed linen and tried to encourage the nurse to reconsider her resignation, referencing how helpful she had been in the opening of the hospital. Unfortunately, she said she couldn't work in a place that didn't have basic supplies in place. Upon reflection, I realized that this nurse, although competent and very helpful during the planning process, was not comfortable in situations where all of the processes were not established. Her inflexibility made working in a new facility a poor employment choice. As these things often do, the nurse went on to successful employment in a large, well-established hospital. And as we hired additional nurses, we made a point to emphasize the need for flexibility as we continued through our first 6 months of operation.

"This experience gave us some hints about revising our interview process. We recognized that our process needed to emphasize the 'soft skills' necessary to work in our environment. The Society for Human Resource Management (SHRM) notes that the hiring process includes (1) personnel requirements, (2) job posting, (3) interview process, (4) reference check, and (5) job offer (https://www.shrm.org/about-shrm/Pages/Membership.aspx). We determined that several of these areas in the hiring process were appropriate for emphasizing important soft skills. For example, flexibility was necessary to work in our new facility, and this characteristic was important to include in the job posting. Framing a question to assess the candidate's flexibility by a question such as 'Give an example of a time that you had to be flexible in your job duties' ensured that this characteristic is assessed in all of the job interviews. A similar question was included in the outline for checking references."

REFLECTION Consider your experience or the stories about shortages of vital equipment and supplies during the COVID-19 pandemic. What implications exist for the processes in your organization?

PREVENTING PROBLEMS THROUGH THE USE OF PROCESSES

An important use of processes is to prevent (or reduce) errors in implementation. As the example of the inadequate linen demonstrates, had the team crafted a process before the fact that addressed having an inadequate supply of any item in the off-hours, the "linen crisis" wouldn't have happened in the first place. (Hindsight is wonderful!) Once such a problem occurs, however, this experience allows us to consider what else could go wrong, to develop a process for staff to reach out to the administration for support, and to develop a process to address such situations.

ARE PROCESSES FOOL-PROOF?

Processes are meant to clarify actions in particular situations. Does this mean that there are never complications in implementation? Of course not. For example, those of us who have worked in a variety of organizations know that organizations often have different ways to manage a process. Most of us have had the experience where we implement a process we used in another institution, only to hear "We don't do that this way here." We have also heard new employees say, "The organization I worked at before didn't do it this way." These disagreements can be problematic, and we recommend several strategies to deal with these conflicts. First, seek to understand why the process has been set up in the way it has. There may be some unique organizational characteristics that require a particular approach. Second, go to the literature to see whether the evidence suggests a particular approach. Finally, keep an open mind—as the "linen crisis" illustrated, flexibility is an important trait.

The need for defined organizational processes to guide the activities of individuals who must work in concert to accomplish a goal is a key in a well-managed team or organization. As important as processes are to the work of an organization, as we have seen, things can go wrong. Each of the issues we encounter requires the expertise of flexible, patient, quick-thinking leaders—all skills that will facilitate the development of a Legacy *Leaders*-Ship Trajectory.

LL ALERT

- Don't expect the implementation of the process to go smoothly, with no "hiccups."
- Don't assume that all players are clear about their responsibilities.
- Don't forget to recognize that human emotions and behaviors can influence development and implementation.

SUMMARY

Organizational processes guide the accomplishment of organizational goals. Developing competence in leading these processes will provide individual leaders with a wide range of skills, including the ability to assess the needs of the organization and its many stakeholders, develop goals that meet the identified needs, organize a plan of action, evaluate results, deal with problems along the way, and use emotional intelligence to support others on the team throughout the process. As you plan ways to increase these types of skills, consider serving as a leader of a process improvement or new initiative team.

LL LINEUP

- Figure out which processes are "sacred," and deal with those very carefully.
- Acknowledge no process is perfect.

REFLECTION What specific skills do you think are critical for a nurse to effectively use a process as part of the leadership role? List as many as you can think of. Consider those skills that you feel you need to develop. What strategies will you use for development?

43

Relationships

How do things get done? Some people do everything themselves. Others tell people what to do. In reality, things get done through relationships. Relationships can be broadly defined as the way in which two concepts, objects or people, are connected.[1] Successful leaders understand about relationships and how to develop them. Interpersonal relationships are the glue that supports leaders to accomplish the vision and the goals they have established. Relationships are a part of the Environmental Triangle of the trajectory, because developing relationships is integral to developing a team. A team is essential to leading and leaving a legacy.

In one job experience, one of us was responsible for some 450 nurses and faculty:

"It seemed a bit overwhelming, and I questioned how I would come to know any of them. I decided to match this goal of learning to know people with one of my favorite things: teaching. I put all of them through a series of workshops focused on change, and we repeated the workshop with 50 to 60 staff in each one. My assistant (a non-nurse with a master's in business administration [MBA]) asked that one of the last workshops include Mike and Tom from maintenance. When asked, she said she wanted to develop a better relationship with them because we were in a building that was more than 100 years old. (I'm sure one of the elevators was original to the building.) After this outreach and the establishment of relationships over the 3 days of the workshop, we never waited 'days' for maintenance again. They liked us and from the workshop and had gotten to know many of us. We were no longer strangers asking for help; we were 'friends.' Things get done through relationships."

> **REFLECTION** Think of your best circle of friends. How did you connect with these people?

Interpersonal relationships constitute a close or strong association between two or more people. They usually grow gradually over time as people know one another better. Relationships are most often based on common beliefs and values, a common vision or goals, and common interests. These relationships are formed in the context of social, cultural, and other influences.

A GOOD RELATIONSHIP DEFINED

What constitutes a good relationship? Although trust is examined in detail in another chapter, we need to identify trust as the foundation of good relationships. Trust in your coworkers and colleagues forms a powerful bond to help in communication and effectively meeting the workplace goals. Trust creates openness and honesty with coworkers, and time is not wasted in guardedness and "watching your back." When trust is lacking, as Patrick Lencioni, author of the now classic *The Five Dysfunctions of a Team*, says, the team is dysfunctional.[2] The dysfunctional team spends its time figuring out who is trustworthy and how to protect themselves rather than being open and honest.

In addition, respect among leaders, coworkers, and peers is essential to working closely together in accomplishing goals. When team members are valued for their ideas and contributions, they often respond in the same manner. Developing solutions to problems based on joint creativity and insight produces outstanding results.

The following approaches contribute to creating meaningful relationships:

- Conscientiousness: Being conscientious about how we, as leaders, convey a message is taking responsibility for both our words and actions. This thought process extends to when we are feeling negatively or opposed to team members' ideas or suggestions, because the impact of negativity on the team is far reaching. Let's consider attitude. A negative attitude not only affects the atmosphere of the current discussion, it also affects the willingness of team members to disagree in the future. Even if leaders don't say anything, if they look upset, angry, or demonstrate negative physical gestures, the impact is the same. It prevents team members from voicing opposing views. We can see how being conscientious about positivity is important to the team.
- Opposing views: Opposition within the team is critical to sound decision-making, and strong leaders encourage

people to voice opposing views. Differing opinions allow leaders to examine issues from multiple perspectives and to consider these varying viewpoints before making decisions. The leader sets an environment that can encourage constructive opposition but does not include personal attacks that could damage relationships.

- Open communication: Honest and open communication is critical to building quality relationships. Effective communication is so important that a separate chapter is dedicated to the topic. With respect to relationships, the least desirable communication strategy is email and the most desirable is face to face. Remember to be open; clear; and congruent in word, tonality, body language, and facial expression.[3]

LEVELS OF RELATIONSHIPS

One way to think about relationships is to think about the people with whom you are very close compared with people who are only casual acquaintances. Multiple models exist about relationships, and the one that we use is based on work by Blaz Kos.[3] If we think about this in terms of circles, with you in the center, the other circles around you represent the level of relationships (Fig. 43.1):

- The Exchange Level: These are the people with whom you exchange services or create transactions, such as a stylist, a housekeeper, or your favorite bank teller. These are fairly casual relationships.
- The Participation Level: These are interactions with people from the nursing or the religious or similar communities that you see periodically and for which the interaction is focused on a specific activity or outcome. This level could include the Rotary Club, a climbing club, or a professional association. The purpose is more focused on the activity than on the relationship. Some work colleagues fall into this category.
- The Friendship Level: These are people who are close to you but you might not reveal intimate issues to them. They don't live with you, and they may not live in the same city, yet when you see them, the focus is on them rather than on the activity. These could be some important coworkers, people with whom you might share your vision or your dreams. You might share a "bad day" with friends who work closely with you.
- The Intimacy Level: These are the people who are the very closest to you and with whom you are the most open about your deepest thoughts and emotions—you trust them. You would be desolate without them. It is a relatively small group, perhaps five or six individuals, and some of them may be very close professional friends, a spouse, or a partner.

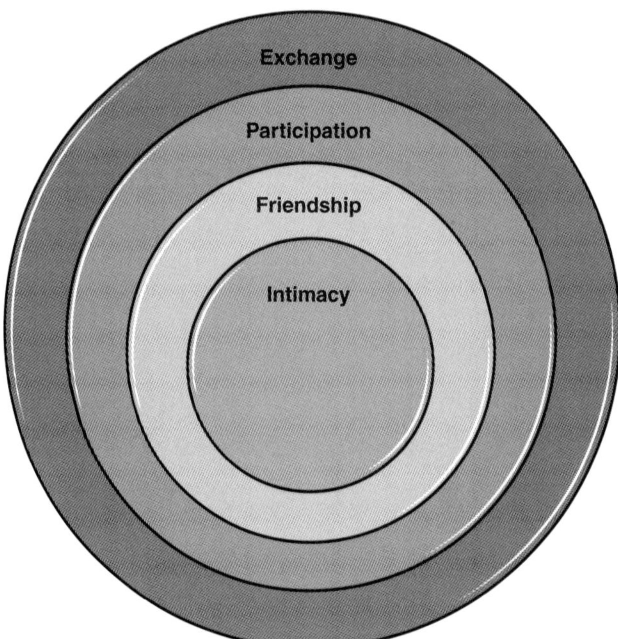

Fig. 43.1 Circle of relationships.

> **REFLECTION** Draw your own circles and identify the people you believe are in each. Do you want to increase the quantity or the quality of the people in the circles? Give some thought to how you connect to expand what you believe could be more meaningful.

THE FOUNDATION FOR DEVELOPING RELATIONSHIPS

Developing relationships is most often based on commonalties discovered between people. These commonalities can lead to a stronger connection and then to a deeper relationship. Among the first things to consider are beliefs and values.

Common Beliefs and Values

A belief is something one accepts as true or real; a firmly held opinion or conviction.[1] We have social, moral, intellectual, economic, and political beliefs. For example, some people have a social belief about waiting your turn in line and think about what happens when the belief is violated. Some people make comments about cutting in line and ask the person who cuts in to go to the end of the line.

Many of us have a belief about what constitutes respect for individuals. Entire patient care models are based on this respect, such as relationship-based care,[4] in which nurses have a respectful, trusting relationship with patients, families, peers, and other members of the health care team. And respect is demonstrated through how they interact with each other.

Values are essentially a belief about what is good, such as quality patient care, and what is bad, such as dishonesty. Values are abstract principles that serve to guide a person in life decision-making, including honesty, equality, harmony, order, wisdom, competitiveness, and the importance of hard work.

One aspect of relationships is that the people have common beliefs and values. Friends usually have a strong link regarding common beliefs and values, and a significant part of the relationship is based on these shared beliefs and values. In this respect they are alike or similar, and this serves as a foundation for the relationship.

Common Interests

Oftentimes, people develop relationships in part based on common interests. For example, two people could share a love of college football, they may have gone to the same school, and they follow the team and talk about football. For nurses, a common interest may be a specific clinical area.

"One of us has a best friend who was a master's-prepared nurse when I met her at a meeting of maternal-child nurses serving on a joint committee representing the American Nurses Association (ANA) and what was at the time the Nurses Association of the American College of Obstetrics and Gynecology (NAACOG; now the Association of Women's Health, Obstetric and Neonatal Nurses [AWHONN]).

"The goal was to establish joint guidelines for practice, and the group met multiple times in Kansas City. I discovered that we had common beliefs and values and common interests. We began to work together and wrote three graduate-level obstetric textbooks together. We had babies at nearly the same time, were inducted into the American Academy of Nursing the same year, and have remained friends over more than 40 years even though one of us lives in Minneapolis and the other lives in Denver. Distance does not affect the relationship. When we see each other (only a couple of times per year), we act as though we saw each other yesterday."

Common Vision or Goals

Vision is the ability to think about or plan the future with imagination and wisdom; it is the act of imagination, a mode of conceiving that can constitute unusual discernment or foresight.[5] People with a common vision share a dream and direction that other people want to follow. Leaders' visions go beyond written organizational mission statements and vision statements. The vision of leadership permeates the workplace and is manifested in the actions, beliefs, values, and goals of organizational leaders. In addition, the two nurses in the story also had a common vision—first the committee work and then the books, all of which were based on the vision of creating higher-quality care for mothers and infants.

Goals are the end or outcome toward which effort is directed; they are the object of a person's ambition; an aim or desired result. In education, goals are to be clearly defined and measurable. They allow the involved people to know when they have reached an outcome. Clearly, a common vision and goals are as much a basis for a relationship as are interests, values, and beliefs.

What Happens When No Common Goals, Values, and Interests Can Be Identified?

Relationships falter or don't form at all when no commonality exists between or among people. When conversations begin between people who don't know each other, they often begin with questions regarding where each person "came from" or where each went to school. The object in these questions is an attempt to find commonalities; to find likenesses to talk about.

One of the most difficult differences to bridge is education. Nurses are a confusing group to those external to the profession. We expect nurses prepared in an associate-degree program to build a professional relationship with physicians who have 8 to 10 years of postsecondary education and often come from very different backgrounds, beginning with the college attended (often a major academic center) compared with a community college. To bridge these differences, they might focus on the teamwork necessary for effective patient outcomes. The socioeconomic status is very different. A physician's income allows for living in a community that might differ greatly from that of where a nurse might live. An associate-degree nurse (ADN) may be the first person in the family to go to college. The physician may come from several generations of physicians or other highly educated family members such as lawyers or academicians. Two very different people may have to stretch to find any common ground. They frequently bridge these gaps by focusing on goals such as quality patient care.

Much has been reported about the millennial generation and how different they are from the baby boomers. Each grew up in a different situation in the world. For example, some baby boomers fought battles overseas in Vietnam. The millennial generation wasn't alive then. Yet they have local "battles" to endure. No baby boomer went to school through a security checkpoint or practiced terrorism alerts. Yet both generations care about other people. Getting to the level of conversation is the mutual challenge and goal. The latest generation likely would find stories about living without a smartphone barbaric.

STEPS IN BUILDING RELATIONSHIPS

Begin by creating the right positive mindset. This is crucial to career success. Positive relationships at work increase job satisfaction, and we feel more comfortable and less intimidated.[6] This mindset includes reaching out to peers and coworkers and asking them questions about themselves, about their jobs, and how they are progressing in their work. And *listening* when they reply. Remember most people like to talk about themselves and their lives. When reaching out to people to form relationships, focus on accepting people for who they are and to do so without judgment. For additional ideas about creating positive relationships in the workplace, see Table 43.1.

TABLE 43.1 Improving Work Relationships

Suggestions	Description
1. Share more of yourself at meetings.	Make yourself more approachable by sharing expertise, knowledge, and your personality. Prepare ahead for these meetings.
2. Speak positively about coworkers.	Say positive things about people in front of them and others: don't contribute to gossip.
3. Support another person's work.	Help colleagues meet their project goals.
4. Ask others to support your work.	Ask for help and bring others into your projects, which can support getting to know them better. You get more done.
5. Write thank-you notes.	Hand-write notes to people who are doing exemplary work, making positive contributions, and doing more than their job descriptions.
6. Ask questions.	Listen and let the other person share. Be interested and then share something about yourself.
7. Initiate subsequent interactions.	Get to know each other better, through phone, email, and in-person conversations.
8. Attend activities outside of work.	Go to lunch or do something in the evenings or on weekends.
9. Share information.	Discuss topics that might vary depending on what you have in common or what you each want to learn. The topic can be work related or a hobby or other interests.
10. Introduce yourself at social events.	Interact with people at these events, where people are more likely to let down their guard. Relate to them on a personal level.

Adapted from Garfinkle J. Building positive relationships at work. Available at: https://garfinkleexecutivecoaching.com/articles/build-positive-work-relationships/building-positive-relationships-at-work.

Collect information about people and make every effort to remember their names and information. Discover hobbies they enjoy, the activities of their children, and the vacations they take. Attempt to see if you have friends or acquaintances in common. You might be surprised how many people you know in common. Find out what interests and values you may have in common. Assume that others also want to form connections.

Demonstrate knowledge, caring, and thoughtfulness. Ask a person to coffee. Discover what they did on the weekend. Ask for some help with thinking through a problem, and express value for their thinking. Create unexpected acts of kindness. This might be a handwritten thank-you note, or it could be sending someone an article that reflects what you know about their interests.

One of us was in a senior position in an academic medical center:

"I had been hired to address specific issues in maternal-child services. However, the chief pediatrician had a strong supportive relationship with my predecessor and was not pleased to have a person come into the role whose main clinical expertise was in obstetrics. It was clear I had to determine how to build a relationship with this individual other than pediatrics. I worked very hard at reaching out and at one point discovered that the pediatrician loved to sail. He had a very impressive sailboat and spent most summer weekends on the boat. From that point on, I sent him everything I found about sailing—articles, special books, and pictures. I worked very hard with the pediatric staff and implemented programs and initiatives to improve care. It was important to have the right positive mindset, to collect helpful information about him, and to go out of my way to establish acts of thoughtfulness. After about 6 months, he began to soften and believe I might not be so bad after all. We grew to be colleagues. It was well worth the time and energy put into building the relationship."

OBSTACLES TO BUILDING GOOD RELATIONSHIPS

Barriers to creating strong positive relationships are many.[6] However, some examples to emphasize what doesn't work in creating effective work relationships include the following:

- Moralizing—which can be construed as commenting on issues of right and wrong, typically with an unfounded air of superiority or from an overly critical point of view. Such comments or observations tend to shut down communication and harm relationships.
- Arguing—expressing diverging or opposite views in a heated or angry way. Anger enflames others and makes them defensive or fearful.
- Excessive storytelling—dominating the conversation in a self-centered way is distracting and creates an atmosphere of polite nonlistening. This does little to create a positive relationship.
- Preaching—telling the other person what they should do in certain situations, which could also be viewed as lecturing.
- Blocking communication—interrupting the conversation with your story or advice so that it stops or prevents the other person from talking.
- Talking too much—dominating the conversation.

These are only five examples of how to obstruct the creation of positive relationships. We all likely have many more. It is valuable to remember the times when we have been in a conversation with someone in which we wanted only to leave or disengage from the individual. These experiences serve as a reminder of what not to do.

LL ALERT

- Don't moralize, argue, or preach.
- Don't interrupt.

SUMMARY

We've discussed the importance of relationships in getting things done. Understanding what constitutes a good relationship and the common values, beliefs, interests, vision, and goals can lead to important and valued relationships. Not all relationships are the same and varying levels of relationships exist in all our lives. Some people create obstacles to developing relationships that are problematic, and it would be helpful to have a dialogue with individuals that demonstrate behaviors impeding the building of effective relationships.

LL LINEUP

- Be in relationships with others: it's how to lead a legacy.
- Create relationships of varying intensities to create diverse views and resources.

REFLECTION Think about the last time you were introduced to a new person, one you haven't met before. What happened? How did the conversation go? Were you uncomfortable? Did you connect or did you "write the person off"? What were the factors in the interaction that influenced you? What did you learn? Reflect on these questions and discover if there are aspects of the interaction that you would do differently.

44

Strategy

What is strategy? One definition describes a high-level plan to achieve one or more goals under conditions of uncertainty.[1] Strategy definitions are frequently tied to warfare, which includes several subsets of skills such as tactics, logistics, equipment, and training.[2] One example would be the famous General George Patton from WWII. A classic movie, *Patton*, was produced focusing on his life during the war. In the North African campaign, he replaced an American general who had been soundly defeated by German General Erwin Rommel. Patton proceeded to develop a plan in which he completely routed the Germans. In the film, he stands on a hill with his field glasses, overlooking the battle field with the retreating Germans, and says, "Rommel, you magnificent bastard, I read your book!!" It is a classic scene in which we see strategy laid out. Patton not only knew about tank warfare, he had studied his enemy, read Rommel's writings on tank warfare, and devised strategies to counter him. This is how strategy is enacted.

STRATEGY, IMPLEMENTATION, AND EXECUTION

Meaningful distinctions exist among strategy, implementation, and execution. To be a strategy wonk like Ken Favaro, we have to appreciate the differences; they are valuable to our discussion.[3] Favaro thinks of strategy in two parts: corporate strategy and business unit strategy. A corporate strategy is composed of three basic choices:

- What are the capabilities that distinguish this company or business?
- What is the comparative advantage of the business in adding value to patients or businesses?
- What businesses should this organization be in?

The responses to these questions drive the functions, the daily work of the staff, and how they measure success. They are great questions we each should ask ourselves.

For the business unit or area, another three key decisions must be addressed. They are:

- Who are the customers or patients that define our target market?
- How do we differentiate our products and services with these clients and patients through identification of a value proposition?
- What are the capabilities that make our services better than others attempting to deliver on that same value proposition?[3]

REFLECTION Think about these questions and how they relate to services you provide.

Implementation relates to the decisions and activities required to accomplish the strategies for both corporate and business unit/area. When the corporation has the capabilities, the advantages, the portfolio, and the skills needed and desired and the business unit/area has the patients, value proposition, and skills necessary, its strategy is also complete. However, specific strategies are rarely fully implemented due to the rapid change of the environment. Before full implementation, the situation has usually changed. Consequently, strategy is continually evolving or being adapted to remain relevant. Thus a gap nearly always exists between the strategy and where the business unit/area is. Closing this gap is implementation. We could also think of this as rapid-cycle improvement.

Execution is defined as the decisions and activities required to evolve the implemented strategy into a business success. For example, when a nurse-sensitive indicator is significantly improved due to the problem-solving and improved patient service related to the indicator, this is excellence in execution.

These three concepts (strategy, implementation, and execution) serve as the determinant of the organization's results or outcomes. However, when the strategy is poor, the implementation is also poor. And the execution is unsuccessful when the strategy and implementation are wanting. Neither does a great strategy ensure great implementation and execution. When all are successful, the nurse-sensitive indicator now exceeds the national benchmark.

STRUGGLING WITH STRATEGY

Leaders might struggle with strategy. They know strategies are important in aligning decision-making in their operations, but crafting strategy is not easy, and leaders can become embroiled in the process.[3] Confusion can exist about what a business strategy is and is not. Watkins defines business strategy as a set of guiding principles that can engender a desired pattern of decision-making within the organization.[3] Business strategy is about "how" people in the organization make decisions and allocate resources toward the identified goals. In reality, the specific strategy provides a roadmap that defines what actions should be taken in given circumstances. The clarity of these rules and principles supports workers in prioritizing to reach the identified goals.

Strategy is the "how" of resource allocation to accomplish the mission. Michael Watkins compares this to the "what," or the desired mission of the organization; the "whom," or the value network of people who will collaborate in the effort; and the "why," or the vision and incentives that motivate the people to reach the goals. Watkins further implies that it is not possible to develop strategy before addressing the mission and goals. Furthermore, strategy cannot be developed in isolation from a thorough understanding of the partners involved. When considering all four of these elements (how, what, whom, why) in an appropriate sequence, the development of an effective strategy can be demystified.

This thought process can be helpful in clarifying for nurse leaders the rationale for devoting time to considering strategy. For example, when we decide to pursue Magnet® designation or redesignation, we must think carefully about the "how," the strategy of working toward the goal, including such aspects as enrolling the members of the C-Suite, especially the financial members. "How" do we build a case for the advantages of being designated a Magnet® organization, not just for nursing but for the entire facility. "How" would we create or describe our model of nursing care? How would we address all aspects of the Magnet® guidelines? What has to be accomplished to address each Magnet® Source Of Evidence (SOE), and who is involved in each aspect? How do we select the best possible Magnet® coordinator? How do we support this person to help identify subgroups to work on various aspects? What resources, workshops, knowledge, and information could support the Magnet® coordinator and other team members? How do we strategize these aspects? Questions such as these support the development of a "Magnet® Strategy" and increase the possibility of a successful effort.

"It was not surprising that two major hospitals in the city decided to apply for the Magent® designation at about the same time. Competition exists everywhere, including in health care and nursing. I was called in by one of the organizations to review their application, which had been returned without a recommendation, for a site visit. After reading the hundreds of pages, it became clear. The strategy for seeking Magnet® status was evident. The key people in the organization, including the chief executive and financial officers and physicians, were on board with securing the designation, and the chief nursing officer was highly committed. What was missing was the detail for how to execute that high-level view into the unit-area operations. Sources of evidence were present; however, from the document, I couldn't trace a theme across the various units and services. Unlike some organizations that give up, the people in this one did not and later submitted a noteworthy document."

A BUSINESS PERSPECTIVE

According to *Harvard Business Review*, strategic thinking is about analyzing opportunities and problems from a broad perspective or point of view and analyzing and understanding the impact our actions could have on the future of our organizations at all levels.[4] When thinking strategically, we rise above the day-to-day operations and consider the larger environment. What is going on around our business? What is happening with competitors? What is happening in the general field of health care? Asking questions and challenging assumptions are critical. Have we gathered the complex data related to our operation? Can we interpret what we find and use any insights we have acquired to select a course of action?

> **REFLECTION** What changes has your organization made as a result of the coronavirus pandemic? How will you assure yourself and others you are prepared for a similar event in the future? Please consider both the positive and negative experiences people in health care have had.

Leaders at most levels of the organization need to think strategically. If we are leading a team, we need to think strategically and to support the team to think strategically. What prevents leaders from thinking strategically? Of course, one of the major aspects of a failure to think strategically is that we do not have the time or cannot make the time to think strategically, either in team activities or in our daily activities. In addition, research has shown that less than 20% of employees understand the organization's purpose and objectives and less than 25% of employees believe that their activities and job descriptions are linked to any

TABLE 44.1 Attributes of Strategic Thinkers

Attributes	Descriptions
Curiosity	Take a genuine interest in what happens in your area, organization, industry, and the broader business environment.
Consistency	Be persistant in pursuing and meeting goals and objectives.
Agility	Acquire the ability to adapt activities and shift to new ideas when new information suggests the importance of doing so.
Focus on the future	Consider impending short-term changes on a consistent basis. Watch for both opportunities and threats looming in the future.
Understand the world outside of your business	Identify trends and patterns in the industry outside and be willing to have discussions with people outside of your organization.
Openness	Be welcoming to new ideas from peers, employees, and partners such as physicians, patients and families, and industry vendors.
A broader perspective	Strive to increase your knowledge and experience so you can see connections across unrelated fields of knowledge.
Questioning	Ask yourself if you should be doing what you're doing. Are you focused on the right things? Are there things you should stop doing? Change your approach? How are you creating value?

Adapted from *HBR Guide to Thinking Strategically*. Boston, MA: Harvard Business Review Press; 2019.

overall organizational strategy.[5] This indicates a significant divide between what employees do every day and the overarching organizational goals and objectives. A conscious effort to think strategically requires asking great questions, evaluating the pros and cons of potential decisions, being able to let go of old ideas and projects, and even being able to reject exciting ideas that do not fit with the overall priorities. Leaders who are successful in becoming strategic thinkers demonstrate certain personal traits, behaviors, and attitudes that support strategic thinking, including curiosity, consistency, agility, a focus on the future, an understanding of the world outside of our business, openness, a broader perspective, and a questioning attitude. Further discussion of these attributes can be found in Table 44.1.

DEVELOPING STRATEGIC THINKING

The work required to develop strategic thinking skills is methodical and demanding. We must be exposed to strategic roles in the organization and be curious while synthesizing a broad range of information. In addition, we must be able to use our experiences in wide-ranging activities to learn to connect the dots of various unique and unusual patterns. These activities begin with a solid foundation and knowledge regarding what is happening in health care generally. We also must increase our knowledge by reading widely, including such journals and magazines as *Modern Healthcare*, *Harvard Business Review*, and futuristic journals such as *The Futurist*. The goal is to learn more about what happens in the world at large, beyond our day-to-day work. This can lead to a better understanding of trends both in health care and across the business world.

REFLECTION Think about how the information might affect health care and your organization. Plan to attend at least two to four national or international conferences, which could be meetings such as the annual meeting of the American Organization for Nursing Leadership (AONL) or a business leadership conference. Such activities serve to update information you will need to think more creatively and strategically. What do you need to learn? How will such meetings contribute to your knowledge base to be a better leader?

Finding time to think, plan, and read—to stay current—is not easy. Structuring these activities in our calendar often works well. Block 30 minutes a couple of times per week just to think about information and issues outside your organization. Block reading time. It isn't necessary to read every article in a journal, just to know what's there and which information would benefit you at this point in time. Block national meetings and treat them as time to reconnect with colleagues and learn about some of the latest developments. It requires discipline to not be sidetracked from these important activities by daily work and crises. Make learning a priority for your work life. Learning supports us to think differently about issues and problems.

TABLE 44.2 **Seven Steps for Making Better Decisions**

Decision-Making Step	Discussion
Identify five preexisting organizational goals that will be affected by this decision.	Focus on what is important. Avoid making up reasons for decisions after the fact.
Identify three to five reasonable options.	Expand your choices to improve your decision-making even though it may be difficult to look for options.
Identify the most important information that is missing.	Identify what we don't need among the excessive amount of information we are exposed to every day. Ruling out unnecessary data can be critical to the decision.
One year from today, what will be the impact of this decision?	Describe in a story the expected outcome of your choice. This can stimulate similar stories that can broaden our perspectives.
Involve a team of stakeholders, recipients of your services.	Reduce your bias and increase buy-in from stakeholders through considering many perspectives.
Document what was decided and why. What was the level of team support?	Establish a basis for measuring outcomes and written comments by effective documentation. This can increase the commitment of the team.
Schedule a follow-up debrief several months into the decision.	Check in on the decision at an appropriate later date. This allows for an evaluation of the decision and the outcomes and supports the learning if it isn't working as anticipated.

Adapted from Larson E. Seven steps for making faster, better decisions. In: *HRA Guide to Thinking Strategically.* Boston, MA: Harvard Business Review Press.

ALIGNED DECISION-MAKING

Decisions that all levels of leaders make must be aligned with the overall organizational strategies and with what applies to the area over which the leader has responsibility. Be more strategic in decisions we make—even the small decisions. They need to align with each level of decision-making and strategy. How do we as leaders and our team members learn to make decisions that are in accord with the corresponding strategies? For one thing, we use evidence in our decision-making, and even more importantly, we can institute a process related to decision-making. A step-by-step process can be used to support leaders in making decsions using this process. It's a great list, but it is only effective if we use it (see Table 44.2).

ZOOM IN AND ZOOM OUT

Rosabeth Moss Kanter, a famous management theorist at Harvard, describes the importance of being able to focus on both detail and the 30,000-foot level.[6] She describes leaders who in crisis are frozen in the "zoom in" phase, that translates to all the detail around specific issues. She uses the BP oil spill in the Gulf of Mexico as an example. The BP chief executive officer (CEO) could only focus on the details and blaming others rather than being able to also see the big picture of what the disaster meant to the public and the industries that were so profoundly affected by the spill. Zooming in brings important details into tight focus. Although lacking context, opportunities can be compelling when focusing on the details. The picture emerges. Zooming in allows for a closer look at the contributing details, which can be critical for problem-solving.

However, when zooming out, we lose detail in deference to seeing the big picture and understanding issues from a totally different perspective. When we zoom out, we can map the whole territory or see the patterns. The important thing for leaders is that their zoom button doesn't get stuck in one position, but remains flexible so that we can see close up for the necessary detail and further away for the broader perspective or big picture. Another way to think about zoom in and zoom out is that some people cannot see the forest for the trees. And some leaders are focused on the bug sitting on the bark of the tree and have no idea they are in a forest. This is another way to think about zooming in (on the bug) and zooming out to see the huge beautiful forest and the important countryside that includes the forest. The important learning is to refrain from choosing one perspective over another and instead appreciate a continuum of perspectives. And to be able to both zoom in and zoom out.

LL ALERT

- Don't make snap decisions and judgments that are likely to result in negative outcomes.
- Don't avoid thinking about corporate strategy, even if you aren't directly involved in its development.

SUMMARY

In thinking about a goal, we must consider how it aligns with the overall goals and objectives of our organizations. Considering the problems and opportunities for our area of responsibilities from a broad perspective allows us to see the whole picture. We need to consider the competitors—what is the situation like in our communities? Considering advantages and disadvantages of our "plan" helps us create better plans.

LL LINEUP

- Be clear about strategy and zoom in and out to maintain perspective.
- Remember strategy is the how of resource allocation.

REFLECTION As a leader, what was the last carefully evaluated decision you made? How did you go about making the decision? Was it a gut-level decision? Or was it carefully considered? Who else was involved? Who did you discuss it with? What was the outcome of that decision? What did you learn that would be useful to future decision-making?

45

Structure

When one of us was a young faculty member, she heard a colleague present the results of his dissertation:

"The question addressed by the research was 'How does the work environment affect the nurse's job performance?' Until that time, it had never occurred to me that the environment of an organization had any impact on the individual's work. I thought that you went to work, did your best, and your success was dependent on your efforts. That meant that you could succeed anywhere. (Well, I was really young!) Although the specifics of the presentation are lost to history, I walked away with the realization that the work environment can have a huge impact on the productivity of us all."

ORGANIZATIONAL STRUCTURE

The structure of an organization is the grouping of people to accomplish the work of the organization, outlining the typical lines of authority, communications, and rights and duties of the organization. The structure determines how the roles, power, and responsibilities are assigned, controlled, and coordinated and ways that information flows among the different levels of management. It also establishes relationships among a business's managers and workers. The choice of the structure of the organization depends upon the organization's objectives and strategies. In a centralized structure, the top layer of management has most of the decision-making power, with tight control over departments and divisions in a centralized structure. In a more decentralized structure, the decision-making power is more widely distributed, and departments, divisions, and groups may have different levels of independence.[1]

> **REFLECTION** What sort of structure is present in the organization where you work? What effect does this have on the decision-making in your own job function?

IMPACT OF STRUCTURE

The organizational structure of any work group plays a huge role in the motivation, behavior, and productivity of the participants. Functional, team-based, divisional, and matrix structures represent the most common organizational approaches. Table 45.1 outlines the definitions of these structure forms and the potential implications. This table demonstrates that choice(s) of the type of structure designed for an organization requires thoughtful consideration of the goals of the organization, because structure does matter.

Safi Bahcall, a theoretical physicist turned business entrepreneur, in the book, *Loonshots: How to Nurture the Crazy Ideas That Win Wars, Cure Diseases, and Transform Industries*, notes that structure is as critical as the culture of an organization. He applies the work of science policy adviser Vannevar Bush's WWII-era theories on how to encourage radical breakthroughs or innovation. In the same way that a small change in temperature can transform rigid ice into flowing water, the work of organizations can be altered based on rather small structural changes.[2]

"A colleague of ours describes the effect of a change in a component of the organizational structure of a facility where she worked. For years, the staff of the quality department collected relevant data from the service lines, analyzed the results, and reported this information to the executive council, without sharing it with the concerned staff. If changes were needed, the appropriate executive would ask for responses from the service lines. As you can image, this set up a feeling of 'us' against 'them,' which made it difficult for line staff to accept responsibility for any changes that needed to be made. To improve the situation, the structure was changed to integrate a quality manager into each of the service line teams. Those persons coordinated the quality management process in the service area by collecting data and working with their teams to determine priorities for change. Our colleague was

TABLE 45.1 Effects of Organizational Structures

Type of Structure	Definition	Potential Effects
Functional ("Mechanistic")	Top-down power hierarchy, with decision-making authority pushed up as high as is practically possible. Many rules for a predictable order. Workers grouped according to function; results in narrow, standardized jobs.	Goal: efficiency from the point of view of the top of the hierarchy. Individual creativity and initiative limited. Results: insular behavior among groups.
Team-based	Fluid teams resulting in decentralized authority. Uses fluid employee teams to take charge of company goals and projects. Decentralized authority to push down to employees.	Employees respond = initiative, creativity, and enthusiasm. Team capabilities support effective communication, problem-solving, and diversity. Result: employee behavior exhibits initiative, creativity, and enthusiasm.
Divisional	Groups dedicated to a single concern (e.g., medical-surgical division within a health care system; college within a university). Typically found in large organizations.	Decentralizes power; focuses attention on issues specific to smaller groups. Creates redundancy (e.g., every division has to have its own equipment). Leads to insular behavior among groups.
Matrix	Combines a permanent functional organization with divisional structures that pull employees from across functional areas to work in teams on divisional projects.	Increases the flexibility within groups by using the team-based structure, while maintaining the efficiency of the functional approach. Built-in potential for conflict between divisional and functional managers, resulting from territorial and competitive behavior.

surprised by how this (relatively) small structure change positively influenced staff engagement in this process."

As the previous story implies, the structure of the organization can affect two important components of the processes critical to the employees' motivation and ultimately their productivity: the placement of authority and the way in which communication flows. When close supervision from above is needed and that need is driven by, for example, safety concerns, the behavior of the manager and the processes of communication and supervision must be well defined for everyone involved. When creativity to allow employees to innovate is called for, less supervision is needed. Employees expected to be creative must be allowed to consider "wild and crazy" options, make mistakes, and profit from those. In this approach, the communication systems must also be defined, but the path to communication may be quite different. If our organizational structures are not set up properly, information may not travel where it is needed. For example, if middle management teams do not have effective channels of communication with the executive team (and vice versa), important organizational information could take days before it reaches the appropriate or entire staff.[3]

ORGANIZATIONAL STRUCTURE AND MOTIVATION

Effective corporate organizations have clear reporting lines. This means if people have an idea, challenge, issue, or problem, they know exactly who to talk to. When companies do not have a strong organizational structure, opportunities and complaints can both be lost. To avoid this, building strong communication channels into their organizational structure can ensure that employees know they have both the opportunity to share ideas and the chance to discuss problems. This also creates a culture where everyone is accountable for success and error. The more accountable everyone is, the more likely we are to work toward success.

For an organization to be fully successful, the majority of people at all levels must be highly motivated. Sherman suggests that motivation can be stimulated by the presence of two components within an environment, including confidence in the organization and shared goals. Let's take a look at these factors more closely.[4]

Confidence

The organizational structure that makes people feel secure in their jobs allows them to turn their attention to their work, thus encouraging them to do the best job possible. This security may involve hiring from within when possible and promoting effective employees. Simon Sinek makes this same point in his Ted Talk presentation.[5] A good leader has many things to attend to, and one of them is to make staff feel safe.

> **REFLECTION** Consider what percentage of positions in your organization are filled from within. Unless the percentage is great, what could you do to increase that percentage?

Shared Goals

Employees are more motivated when they share the goals of the organization. The organizational structure that facilitates transparency of actions throughout the organization is more likely to encourage employee motivation. This type of transparency is best ensured by an effective communication process throughout the organization. This open communication encourages employees to consider how they can contribute to established goals.[4]

EFFECT OF MOTIVATION

Some years ago, one of us was part of an organization that was undergoing multiple management reorganizations in response to the changing market:

"The new president and his executive council made some swift decisions that were important to achieve new goals that had been set for the organization. In all this rapid change, the upper administration decided to eliminate the component for which I was responsible. The plan was for me to continue my work, but with a slightly different goal and scope. There was one problem, however. The person on the executive council responsible for the change in direction didn't tell me or my team and allowed the announcement of that change, as well as a number of other new initiatives, to be disclosed to the entire workforce, without my team being forewarned.

"You can imagine the result of this move on the subsequent motivation of this team."

> **REFLECTION** Have you ever been involved in a situation where the organization (and its structure) failed you and/or your team? What happened, and how did it affect the team members? If you had been in a leadership role, what would you have done?

ASSESSING THE ORGANIZATIONAL STRUCTURE

If the organization's structure has such an impact on our work environment, isn't it important that we assess the structure anytime that we join an organization? Here are some questions that you might ask when considering a move to a new position:

1. What is the organizational structure of the organization?
2. Are the company's management and decision-making practices centralized or decentralized?
3. What is the company's policy regarding hiring from within the organization for other jobs?
4. How many of the executives have risen from a lower position within this organization?
5. What type of succession does your company have for employees who demonstrate promise and aptitude?
6. Outside of my team (group), which parts of the organization, will I work with most closely?
7. What types of employee development opportunities are available?

The answers that an organization's representative may give to these questions must, of course, be taken in context. However, some answers that potentially raise a red flag might include:

Question: Are the company's management and decision-making practices centralized or decentralized? *Answer:* Most decisions regarding goals, strategy, tactics, hiring and firing, and resource allocation are made by the executive team.

Question: What is the company's policy regarding hiring from within for other jobs? *Answer:* We sometimes hire internal candidates for middle-management positions, but rarely for executive positions.

Question: How many of the executives have risen from a lower position within this organization? *Answer:* None.

LL ALERT

- Don't underestimate the power of structure.
- Don't assume that the "org chart" is an accurate reflection of how things really work.

- Don't accept a new position with the idea that you will change the structure unless you truly have the authority to do such.
- Don't allow surprises to go unchallenged.

SUMMARY

Organizational structure is not just some drawing that is put in the organization's management documents. As we have seen, the organizational structure matters to the employees at all levels. The structure influences the rights and responsibilities of the organization and its employees, goals and strategies used, communication among all groups of stakeholders, defined decision-making process, the accountability of all parties, and many other factors that influence the motivation and productivity of all involved with the organization. It is important to consider these factors when accepting a position or when circumstances change within the organization, since Legacy *Leaders*-Ship is influenced by the environment in which we work. Finding an environment (or more than one over the course of our careers) in which we can flourish is a critical step in developing our Legacy *Leaders*-Ship Trajectory.

LL LINEUP

- Be certain nursing is positionally appropriate within the organization.
- When productivity is low, consider whether the structure is a contributing factor.

REFLECTION In what ways does your organization influence your Legacy *Leaders*-Ship? What does this mean for your immediate future? Are there steps you should take to maximize your legacy?

46

Exiting

Most of us leave positions in the course of our professional lives, and ultimately, many will retire from professional roles completely. A number of reasons explain why we leave a position. On occasion, we leave because although we love the organization and our position, we have an opportunity for growth in a new position that is absent in our current situation. Sometimes we leave because the environment has changed and the "fit" between the job and our skill set no longer meets our needs or that of the organization. And sometimes our spouse moves and so do we. Finally, at some point, we may decide to retire completely from our professional lives. The plans we make for these transitions, as well as their implementation, can affect the development of our careers and the satisfaction we feel at its end.

> **REFLECTION** You may have already had the opportunity to exit a position. What were the reasons that you left? What did you do to prepare for leaving? What were your feelings regarding the change? What strategies did you use to deal with the feelings? What lessons did you learn from making this transition?

THE CONCEPT OF EXITING

The Free Dictionary defines exiting as the act of going away or out.[1] In the context of the Legacy *Leaders*-Ship Trajectory model, exiting also refers to leaving a team or organization, often for another position, thus transferring our energy and commitment to a new situation. The exiting may or may not be by our own choice. In either circumstance, the way we exit will influence our lives and/or subsequent careers in a variety of ways. Learning effective strategies to exit can pay multiple benefits over the course of our leadership trajectory.

LEAVING A POSITION WE LOVE

We are very lucky if we love the work we do, the people with whom we work, and the environment in which we spend a great deal of the time. In a situation where we feel so positive, we tend to identify strongly with our work in that setting. So when we leave that position, we feel a significant loss, even if it is our choice to move on.

Several strategies will help us leave *well* the job we love. It is natural and appropriate to mourn the loss of the job. However, even as we have been able to commit to this job, we must also be able to commit to moving on. We should take time to say goodbye to those with whom we worked and recognize the contributions that they have made to our career. We should pay attention to those people with whom we will continue to associate. In many cases, associates that we value will continue to be a part of our circle of contacts beyond the current position. Despite leaving this position, we are keeping what we learned during our tenure—and will be able to build upon this knowledge and skills for the rest of our careers.[2] Deep reflection on all aspects of exiting helps us identify the lessons learned.

LEAVING UNDER CONFLICT

Leaving a position under conflict may include being terminated for cause or for reasons that are unrelated to performance, such as when personnel are "downsized" for financial or reorganizational purposes. Even when the termination (or resignation under negative circumstances) is not a reflection of our performance, these situations not only generate sadness that we would feel anytime we are leaving a job but also shock, anger, regret, guilt, worry, and fear of the future. Despite the feelings generated when we first hear that we have been terminated for any reason, we should avoid broadcasting the news until we have had time to process the loss and develop a message of the events for professional contacts. Sharing our feelings only with family or close friends with whom we have a personal, trusting relationship is also a smart idea.[3]

Particularly in a "downsizing" situation when a lapse of time before the termination date is prolonged, others may be asked to assist with transition of work duties. Although often difficult, being helpful in this transition will typically work to the benefit of the employee who is leaving. At the very least, others in the organization may see the cooperation as a reason for future recommendations.

Throughout the transition, the terminated employee must not criticize the supervisor or other leadership members or blame colleagues for factors that resulted in the termination. Despite the temptation to justify our own behaviors or attack those who may have had an impact on the loss of our job, it is best to remain positive. Former colleagues at all levels may have the opportunity to provide feedback for background checks by future employers. It is to everyone's best interest that our leave-taking be as positive as possible.[3]

REFLECTION Have you ever been terminated or "downsized"? How did this make you feel? How did you cope with these feelings as you moved toward another position or role? If you have never had this experience, have you observed the responses of others who have? What did you learn from these observations?

A STORY OF BEING "DOWNSIZED"

A few years ago, one of us was an administrator for a mental health service as part of a large health system.

"I was hired to lead a reorganization of the service in response to the increasing level of managed care as a reimbursement strategy of psychiatric/substance abuse service by many insurance companies. The goal of the reorganization was to streamline care delivery and reduce the cost of care. Over a 2-year period, a new approach was developed and implemented, meeting the goal of cost reduction without negative impact on patient outcomes. However, the change had its detractors among powerful stakeholders. Because the larger organization was continuing to downsize administrators and other employees across the health system, those who were not happy with the changes in mental health lobbied for the service to be moved to another component of the organization. As a result, I was also 'downsized.'

Although being downsized or terminated is a traumatic situation, regardless of the circumstances, fortunately, I had a great support system and the opportunity to participate in a career transition service. The worst thing that ever happened professionally turned into a great opportunity. My subsequent job changed my career trajectory and set the stage for the rest of my career. Out of termination came opportunity. And, as I always say, I may have lost this particular job, but the experience I gained has paid dividends throughout my career."

RETIREMENT

As we age, society expects us to retire. For some of us, this is a desired state; for others, perhaps it is a more difficult decision. A qualitative study of academic physicians who were anticipating retirement gives us an example of views about looming retirement. One of the quotes from the respondents summed up this group's concerns about retirement:

What is your value as a person when you're finished? What are the things that make you happy; make you feel fulfilled? What are the activities that will fill the void?[4]

The consensus of the respondents in this study was retirement is a transition. Respondents didn't anticipate an abrupt end to their careers in academic medicine, but rather a scaling back of work duties, a gradual career transition into a state of less demanding paid work. They described the need to strategically manage the challenge of retirement. This includes managing the time frame leading up to retirement, developing new objectives, and reprioritizing their goals. The perceptions of these individuals regarding retirement were consistent with psychological theory that indicates individuals with strong work identities may have difficulty with the transition to retirement.[4]

Of course, many people look forward to retirement and make the transition with a minimum amount of stress. One of us was recently at her 50-year anniversary of college graduation.

"It was interesting to talk to those nurses who were present. Some in this group were working full-time, some were working part-time, and some were gratefully enjoying their lives without being employed. As one of the 'job-free' nurses said, 'I am so busy I don't know when I would have time for a job.' Perhaps our expectations are the key to a happy retirement—whatever that looks like to us."[5]

Others choose to deal with retirement by reformatting it into "preferment." When leaving a leadership position, these individuals focus on what they prefer to do, which could look like dedicating more time to grandchildren, writing, gardening, or traveling to places they have longed to see or focusing on one aspect of nursing that was always the most appealing work. Maybe they can even complete their "bucket list" of adventures. Preferment also translates into avoiding those activities that were most aggravating, such as daily commutes or dealing with impossibly difficult people. This kind of reframing of the process supports a positive outlook about retirement.

Steps for Retirement Planning

To combat the potential stress of retirement and manage our expectations about this period, the Council on Disability suggests steps that potential or actual retirees can use in this transition:

- Give yourself time to adapt to the process.
- Craft a mission statement: What will be your focus during retirement? List the things that you want to achieve and the things you would regret not doing before.
- Assess your resources, including asking yourself, "Can I change my situation or my perception of the situation if I want to?"
- Maintain connections and friendships.
- Exercise and otherwise manage your health.
- Ask for help from wise friends or a professional in evaluating your options.[6]

PREPARATION FOR EXITING

Regardless of why we might exit a job or a career, we need to prepare for the transition. Certainly, part of that transition may include financial planning and appropriate concern for our current and future health. Equally important is the psychological preparation for making the transition. Three emotional fears affect us as we exit a job, role, or career: loss of professional status (related to self-image), fear of change, and concern over how to spend free time. Answering the following questions can help us analyze our readiness to exit from a particular job.

1. ***Do you enjoy your job? Does it provide a sense of meaning to your life?***
   If you have the option to stay and the answer to these questions is yes, perhaps you should stay, unless you can replace that sense of meaning with some other passion. If you do not have the option to stay, identifying areas of passion is important so that you can determine other activities or positions that engender those feelings.
2. ***Is your job so stressful that you are considering retirement or changing jobs?***
   Analyze the components of your job stimulating this stress. Consider whether retirement or a change in job or career trajectory is the answer.
3. ***Does your job provide the major social interactions and connections in your life? Do you have hobbies or interests about which you are excited? How can you replace these activities and social interactions if you exit from your current job?***
   Consider what activities and people will fill up your time. Even if you continue to work at your current job or another one, recognizing that having activities that connect you to others not associated with your job or career provides you with options to broaden your horizons. This may even be a meaningful nonworker role. However, exiting requires you to replace that self-identify with new descriptors. Try on new descriptions of your potential based upon what you hope for in the future.
4. ***Have you considered possible conflicts that might arise after the exit? How will you manage this potential?***
   Your family or other support system may have ideas about how you spend your time that conflict with your own dreams and aspirations for the transition—and perhaps later. How will you handle this?[7]

REFLECTION Imagine that you are considering retirement. (This is a good exercise, even if you believe you have several years to work before you move toward retirement.) How would you answer the questions posed earlier? Based on the answers you have today, what strengths do you have to support moving through the transition of retirement? What feelings or actions should you change now to make the transition more positive later?

EVIDENCE ON SUCCESSFUL LEADERSHIP TRANSITIONS

Particularly when the leader is retiring, opportunities exist for the outgoing leader to serve as a resource to guide the new leader in building relationships with key stakeholders, understanding the cultural norms and agendas, and navigating the political nuances of the organization. Marla Weston, previously the chief executive officer (CEO) of the American Nurses Association (ANA), wrote of her work in supporting the interim ANA CEO and then the new ANA CEO via a leadership handoff.[8] She provides guidance for both the incoming and outgoing leader, which is synthesized in Table 46.1.

MULTIGENERATIONAL LEADERSHIP

The wave of complete or partial retirement of the baby boomers has begun. However, for a variety of reasons, older workers are staying in the workforce. As a result, having a boss (or leader) who is younger than some of the

TABLE 46.1 Guidance for Leadership Transition

Guidance for Incoming Leaders	Guidance for Outgoing Leaders
Rely on the depth of experience of the outgoing leader, particularly when they are giving historical context and advising you of potential landmines, pitfalls, or roadblocks.	Inform generously—don't hold back; instead alert the new leader to opportunities and challenges they haven't yet recognized.
Confidently "own" your roles and decisions.	Coach—support the new leader's own competence by enhancing his or her thinking and encouraging action.
Be open to new ways of responding.	Speak up to avoid mistakes.
Be bold (not rash) in action. Combine detached objectivity and willingness to make change with an "insider's" understanding of the environment.	Encourage a fresh perspective. Help the new leader change the status quo and reexamine priorities.
Share honestly, including your struggles.	Establish trust through confidentialities. Stay out of the limelight. Redirect when others ask your opinions. Introduce new leaders to critical stakeholders and supporters.

Adapted from weston m. leadership transitions: ensuring success. *nurse leader.* 2018;16:304-7.

employees is no longer uncommon. How does this work? In the blog, Knowledge @ Wharton, Chip Conley, a former hotelier who now works at Airbnb as head of global hospitality and strategy, where the CEO is two decades younger, addresses this situation. Conley promotes the notion of an "intergenerational potluck" in today's workplace where "everyone brings something to the table."[9]

Conley notes that because of our dependency on digital intelligence in today's organizations, those who hold powerful positions are frequently 10 years younger than similar leaders 20 years ago. In addition, we are living on average 10 years longer than before, creating a new 20-year gap for people in mid-life and beyond. He suggests, however, that the "modern elder" can bring wisdom to the table through emotional intelligence, leadership skills, and strategic thinking. The wisdom of the modern elder is derived from being able to see patterns faster than the younger employee, because they have seen a lot of patterns, as well as the implications of them.[9] In short, each group has competencies and each requires the expertise of the other to address the current complex world. Using both types of skills, they can manage the complexity of the current work environment.

Given that intergenerational workforces are becoming the norm, leaders must provide an environment in which all generations can work effectively. Common leader behaviors that can disrupt a team or organization's work include:

- Demonstrating a lack of respect for or being critical of another generation's competencies.
- Belittling experiences from the past or the current environment.
- Refusing to learn new skills.
- Being unwilling to ask for help in an area in which you are not comfortable.
- Saying, "This hasn't worked in the past, so it can't work now."

The intergenerational differences don't necessarily lead to exiting. Failure to adapt, however, can.

LL ALERT

- Don't micromanage what you see as your legacy from afar.
- Don't keep critical information from your successor.
- Don't fall behind in critical skills if you wish to continue to work.
- Don't ignore signs that you might be terminated or downsized (especially during a time of major transitions) if you wish to remain in charge of yourself.

SUMMARY

Exiting positions or work roles is inevitable through a lifetime of work. Using the strategies that support our transitions can enhance our leadership trajectory and our enjoyment of the time we spend in our professional lives. The Legacy *Leaders*-Ship Trajectory model provides us all with a process to develop a reputation of leadership that reflects the best of who we are. We must implement strategies required for lifelong learning, including self-assessing, reflecting, and framing; influencing; advocating; coaching; mentoring; visioning; and searching for wisdom in a manner that demonstrates character, commitment, connectedness, compassion, and confidence. We can then look back upon our professional lives with satisfaction. We will recognize our mistakes and failures as an integral part of our journey and celebrate our successes, finding closure to this role.

The Legacy *Leaders*-Ship Trajectory model is designed to help us take what we might think of as our ordinary talents and foster them in a way that allows us to engage in creating some incredible and sustainable work that benefits employees and patients alike. The model outlines a plan for our leadership development over a lifetime by recognizing that leading is a journey for which the destination is our legacy. Our professional lives involve many destinations, which require us to exit a job or a role to take on a new journey to a different destination.

LL LINEUP

- Always be prepared to "move on."
- Leaving is your last opportunity to make a good impression and facilitate a legacy.

REFLECTION Use the Legacy Leaders-Ship Trajectory model to review your progress toward wisdom and a legacy at this point in your career. Which personal characteristics do you possess? Which characteristics do you see as weaknesses? What might you do in the next 6 months to strengthen your personal characteristics? Assess the environment characteristics. Are there areas here that could affect your leadership growth? How comfortable are you in enacting the steps toward your legacy? This assessment will provide you with a roadmap for continued growth. Continue this assessment every so often during your leadership journey as a strategy to stay on track.

CONCLUSION

This is the end of the book but not the end of your journey. As Dietrich Bonhoeffer said, "There is meaning in every journey that is unknown to the traveler."[1] We discover things about ourselves as we move through life, and we can either capitalize on that information or ignore it. We are really confident that you got the message about reflecting on who you are and who you are becoming. Leadership is all about creating conditions, relationships, and outcomes, even when you are not in an official position to do so. Leadership is your super power that allows you to influence and inspire others to action.

As you read the book, you may have had thoughts of personal values we didn't mention, other key concepts that would be essential for you personally, and environmental elements important to you in your development as a leader. If you did, good for you! If you did not, know that we provided you with a place to start and afterward, with more reflection and learning, you, too, can identify your additional thoughts about what else you want or need to know.

Experience is a rich resource we often don't consider in an active manner. One of the strategies we used in this book that we hope you will carry forward in your day-to-day lives is the idea of reflection—and actually recording what you are thinking. When you do this, you have to think clearly about your experience. Then, later, when you review your old entries, you can find personal growth, which is a great reinforcer for the effort you invest in your self-learning.

Because leadership is a journey and learning is never-ending, you know you are not done. You may be done reading the book, but you are not done learning about leadership and how leaders create legacies. We are confident you got the big point: you have to be part of a team of leaders committed to the same mission if you want an idea to live on past your physical presence. Your opportunity lies within yourself to identify what your next steps are so that you can be your best in contributing to the profession of nursing and the people we serve.

This is now your opportunity to take on some wonderfully wild idea about what you need to know and tell someone you have to do it because it is a requirement for reading the book! (If you want to send us those ideas, we'd love to read them! The email address is TheLeadershipTrajectory@gmail.com.) Too often we read a book, mark it off our to-do list, and move on to the next thing. We all do it, in part because we are so busy and in part because sometimes we just want to hear or see what the answer is and move on. Yet each chapter has had one or more reflections. Now you can have a BIG REFLECTION: Living your life as a leader leading to a legacy.

REFLECTION What did the book help you understand about what you need to do next in learning leadership? What did you feel most insecure with? What did you feel most comfortable with? How will you use this knowledge? What wonderfully wild idea do you want to explore? Please, grab that opportunity now and do something with it.

Earlier in the book, we told you that the literature and our Circle of Advisors offered many words that would be important for us to consider and that we condensed those words down to a manageable number. We presented the content, chapter by chapter, without integrating the concepts because each relates to the other and has a different meaning when combined with different elements. For example, go back and pull random chapter titles and think what is possible when two or three personal elements are combined together and then what those might mean when combined with two or three of the environmental elements. The message of the book is this: leadership is about potential and how you combine what happens to you with key concepts about being a leader. This message shapes you and sets a course for your leadership journey. Our task was to provide a basic core for your consideration. Your task is to enhance that core so that it is meaningful to you, and your other task is to be sure you have a cadre of people you call leaders going on the journey with you so that you create a leadership legacy—something that lives on after you leave your position or the organization or the profession.

Your journey may have taken new twists—we hope so, because they are enriching. Your journey probably had highs and lows, and we hope you have learned to "hold the ship steady" through those turbulent waters. We also know that if you are engaged in the meaning of the Legacy *Leaders*-Ship Trajectory model, you can help create something of great meaning for your colleagues and the people we all serve. (Yes, we said that a few paragraphs earlier. It is a point worth repeating.)

One last thing: if you chose to develop your own trajectory from Fig. 2.2, we hope you will snap a photo of it and email us with your ideas. We know leadership is individual, and we would love to know your perspective. Happy journey!

REFLECTION What is your leadership trajectory story? Who comprises your *Leaders*-ship team?

REFERENCES

Preface

1. @AdamMGrant A. Good leadership books (a) introduce original ideas, (b) back them with evidence & experience, (c) make them engaging. December 27, 2018. Available at: https://twitter.com/AdamMGrant/status/1078275853153374208. Accessed December 30, 2018.
2. Cook T. Commencement address. Stanford, CA: Stanford University; June 16, 2019. Available at: https://news.stanford.edu/2019/06/16/remarks-tim-cook-2019-stanford-commencement.

Chapter 1: Leading to Legacies

1. Goodwin DK. Leadership in turbulent times. New York: Simon & Schuster; 2018.
2. Bissell CT. Risk more than others think is safe. Care more than others think is wise.Dream more than others think is practical. Expect more than others think is possible. Goodreads. Available at: https://www.goodreads.com/quotes/247659-risk-more-than-others-think-is-safe-care-more-than. Accessed December 30, 2018.
3. Tribute to Herb Kelleher. Dallas Morning News. January 6, 2019. Available at: https://www.dallasnews.com/business/southwest-airlines/2019/01/03/southwest-airlines-legendary-co-founder-herb-kelleher-dies-87.
4. Berger J. Invisible influence: the hidden forces that shape behavior. New York: Simon & Schuster; 2016.
5. Sinek S. Start with why: how great leaders inspire everyone to take action. New York: Penguin Books; 2009.
6. Maxwell J. Great leaders never walk alone. Nordic Business Report. December 16, 2015. Available at: https://www.nbforum.com/nbreport/john-c-maxwell-great-leaders-never-walk-alone/. Accessed December 30 2018.
7. Fernandez-Araoz C, Roscoe AY, Aramaki K. Turning potential into success: the missing link in leadership development. *Harv Bus Rev*. 2017:86-93.
8. Gratton L. The challenge of scaling soft skills. MIT Sloan. August 6, 2018. Available at: https://sloanreview.mit.edu/article/the-challenge-of-scaling-soft-skills/. Accessed December 30, 2018.
9. McClure M, Poulin M, Sovie M, Wandelt M. Attraction and retention of professional nurses. Washington, DC: American Academy of Nursing; 1983.
10. Institute for Healthcare Improvement. The quadruple aim. September 4, 2017. Accessed December 30, 2018. Available at: http://lippincottsolutions.lww.com/blog.entry.html/2017/09/05/moving_from_triplet-uouA.html.
11. Watson J. Caring science theory. Watson Caring Scinece Institute. Accessed December 30, 2018. Available at: https://www.watsoncaringscience.org/jean-bio/caring-science-theory/.
12. Miranda L-M. Hamilton. Available at: https://hamiltonmusical.com/new-york/.
13. Boothe A, Yoder-Wise P, Gilder R. Follow the leader: changing the game of hierarchy in health care. *Nurs Adm Q*. 2019;43:76-83.
14. Tagliareni SJ, Brewington JG. Roving leadership: breaking through the boundaries. Philadelphia, PA: Wolters Kluwer; 2018.
15. Cialdini R. Influence: science and practice. 5th ed. New York: William Morrow; 2008.

Chapter 2: Legacy *Leaders*-Ship: The Model

1. US Bureau of Labor Statistics. Employment by major industry sector. Available at: https://www.bls.gov/emp/ep_table_201.htm.
2. Thompson D. Health care just became the U.S.'s largest employer. January 9, 2018. Available at: https://www.theatlantic.com/business/archive/2018/01/health-care-america-jobs/550079/.
3. Sinek S. Start with why: how great leaders inspire everyone to take action. London: Penguin Books, LTD; 2011.
4. International Labour Organization. Inception report for the global commission on the future of work. Geneva: International Labour Organization; 2017.
5. International Labour Organization and Gallup. Towards a better future for women and work: voices of women and men. 2017. Available at: http://www.ilo.org/wcmsp5/groups/public/-dgreports-dcomm-publ/documents/publication/wcms_546256.pdf.
6. Wright LM, Bell JM. Beliefs and illness: a model for healing. Calgary, Alberta, Canada: 4th Floor Press; 2009.
7. Oxford Dictionary. Model. Available at: www.Oxforddictionaries.com. Accessed December 30, 2018.
8. Miranda L-M. Hamilton. Available at: https://hamiltonmusical.com/new-york/.
9. Batcheller J, Yoder-Wise P. Creating insight when the literature is absent: the circle of advisors. *Nurs Adm Q*. 2011;35, 4:338-43.
10. Cain LB, Cronin SN, Nelson D, Meredith DA, Newman KP, Rudolf S. A tool to identify key behaviors and attributes of high-performing nurses. *J Nurs Adm*. 2018;48:197-202.
11. Hughes V. Standout nurse leaders…what's in the research? *Nurs Manag*. 2017;48:16-24.
12. Kouzes JM, Posner BZ. Learning leadership: the five fundamentals of becoming an exemplary leader. San Francisco: Wiley; 2016.
13. Kowalski KE, Yoder-Wise P. Five Cs of leadership. *Nurse Leader*. 2003;1:26-31.
14. Henderson J. Closing keynote. Presented at: American Organization of Nurse Executives Conference; Indianapolis, IN; April 15, 2018.

15. Institute of Medicine. The future of nursing: leading change, advancing health. Washington, DC: The National Academies Press; 2011.
16. Tye J, Dent B. Building a culture of ownership in healthcare: the invisible architecture of core values, attitude, and self-empowerment. Indianapolis, IN: Sigma Theta Tau International; 2017. p 205.

Chapter 3: The Profession and Values

1. Van Gogh V. Available at: https://www.goodreads.com/quotes/620676-your-profession-is-not-what-brings-home-your-weekly-paycheck.
2. Gallup Poll. 2018. Available at: https://news.gallup.com/poll/1654/Honesty-Ethics-Professions.aspx.
3. The DAISY Foundation. Available at: https://www.daisyfoundation.org/.
4. Hayes S. 10 signs you know what matters. *Psychology Today.* 2018;53-59, 90.
5. Miles JM, Scott ES. A new leadership development model for nursing education. *J Prof Nurs.* 2019;35:5-11.
6. Gardner JW. *On leadership*. New York: Free Press; 1990.
7. Kowalski K, Yoder-Wise PS. The five "Cs" of leadership. *Nurse Leader.* 2003;1:26-31.
8. Lencioni P. The five dysfunctions of a team. San Francisco: Jossey-Bass; 2002.
9. Brown B. Rising strong: the reckoning, the rumble, the resolution. New York: Random House; 2015.
10. Groysberg B, Lee J, Price J, Cheng JYJ. The leader's guide to corporate culture: how to manage the eight critical elements of organizational life. *Harv Bus Rev.* 2018:44-52.
11. Rath T. Strengths finder 2.0. New York: Galllup Press; 2007.
12. Cuddy A. Presence: bringing your boldest self to your biggest challenges. New York: Back Bay Books; 2015.
13. Kowalski P. Building effective teams. In: Yoder-Wise PS, editor. Beyond leading and managing in nursing. 7th ed. St Louis: Elsevier; 2006. p. 355.
14. Maxwell J. Today's word: commitment. 2019. Available at: https://johnmaxwellteam.com/commitment/.
15. Lindsay D. An interview with Hennings C. A force of character. *J Character Leaders Dev Fall.* 2018;5,1:20-26.
16. Maxwell J. Your success stops where your character stops. You can never rise above the limitations of your character. Goodreads. Available at: https://www.goodreads.com/quotes/205069-your-success-stops-where-your-character-stops-you-can-never. Accessed December 30, 2018.
17. Johnson S. Farsighted: how we make decisions that matter the most. New York: Riverhead Books; 2018.

Chapter 4: Lifelong Learning

1. Institute of Medicine. The future of nursing: leading change, advancing health. Washington, DC: The National Academies Press; 2011.
2. Bleich MR. Our GOLDEN Anniversary: guiding, orienting, leading, developing, educating, nurturing. *J Contin Educ Nurs.* 2019;50:383-4.
3. Coleman J. Make learning a lifelong habit. 2017. Available at: https://hbr.org/2017/01/make-learning-a-lifelong-habit?autocomplete=true.
4. O'Donnell JT. #1 Career skill everyone needs to succeed. 2019. Available at: https://www.workitdaily.com/career-skill-everyone-needs/.
5. Brassey J, van Dam N, Coates K. Seven essential elements of a life-long learning mind-set. 2019. Available at: https://www.mckinsey.com/business-functions/organization/our-insights/seven-essential-elements-of-a-lifelong-learning-mind-set?cid=other-eml-alt-mip-mck&hlkid=6f43374516d344afb1465e60d533e628&hctky=2599421&hdpid=4a586936-e25d-452d-83b4-969eb0daa091.
6. Staats BR. Never stop learning: stay relevant, reinvent yourself, and thrive. Boston: Harvard Business Review Press; 2018. p 5.
7. Maxwell J. Today's word: value. The John Maxwell Team. Available at: https://johnmaxwellteam.com/value/. Accessed March 10, 2019.
8. Tegmark M. Life 3.0: being human in the age of artificial intelligence. New York: Alfred A. Knopf; 2017.
9. Ancona D, Gregersen H. The power of leaders who focus on solving problems. April 16, 2018. Available at: https://hbr.org/2018/04/the-power-of-leaders-who-focus-on-solving-problems.
10. Selingo J. The third education revolution. 2018. Available at: https://www.theatlantic.com/education/archive/2018/03/the-third-education-revolution/556091/.
11. Rogers EM. Diffusion of innovations. 3rd ed. New York: Free Press of Glencoe; 1983.
12. Gino F, Staats B. Why organizations don't learn. *Harv Bus Rev.* 2015:110-8.
13. Kouzes JM, Posner BZ. Learning leadership: the five fundamentals of becoming an exemplary leader. San Francisco: Wiley; 2016.
14. Finkelstein S. The best leaders are great teachers. *Harv Bus Rev.* 2018:142-5.
15. Moldoveanu M, Narayandas D. The future of leadership development. *Harv Bus Rev.* 2019:41-8.
16. Ivy S. Georgia Tech envisions 'deliberate innovation, lifetime education' in new report. April 25, 2018. Available at: News.gatech.edu.
17. Staats BR. Never stop learning: stay relevant, reinvent yourself, and thrive. Boston: Harvard Review Press; 2018.
18. Merriam-Webster. Available at: https://www.merriam-webster.com/dictionary/failure.
19. Nightingale F. Notes on nursing. Digital Library, University of Pennsylvania. 1859. Available at: https://search.yahoo.com/yhs/search;_ylt=AwrC3Os2vDhdrigA5gQPxQt.;_ylc=X1MDMjExNDcwMDU1OQRfcgMyBGZyA3locy1wdHktcHR5X21hcHMEZ3ByaWQDcTU5dVFhcjJUZnU3WXdTbDFDdG9CQQRuX3JzbHQDMARuX3N1Z2cDMARvcmlnaW4Dc2VhcmNoLnlhaG9vLmNvbQRwb3MDMARwcXN0cgMEcHFzdHJsAzAEcXN0cmwDNzIEcXVlcnkDbmlnaHRpbmdhbGUlMjBuZXZlciUyMGNvbnNpZGVyJTIwb3Vyc2VsdmVzJTIwZmluaXNoZWQlMjBhcyUyMG51cnNlcyUyME5vdGVzJTIwb24lMjBOdXJzaW5nBHRfc3RtcAMxNT

YzOTk5MzA3?p=nightingale+never+consider+ourselves+finished+as+nurses+Notes+on+Nursing&fr2=sb-top&hspart=pty&hsimp=yhs-pty_maps¶m1=20190427¶m2=cf04d7b8-b426-4cb2-aa20-f17bb9607297¶m3=maps_%7EUS%7Eappfocus1¶m4=d-ccc6-lp0-cp_1588105121-bb9%7EFirefox%7Enightingale+never+consider+ourselves+finished+as+nurses+how+to+improve%7ED41D8CD98F00B204E9800998ECF8427E&type=1588105121. Accessed March 10, 2019.

Chapter 5: Purpose

1. Sinek S, Mead D, Docker P. Find your why: a practical guide for discovering purpose for you and your team. New York: Portfolio/Penguin; 2017.
2. Groysberg B, Lee J, Price J, Cheng, JYJ. The leader's guide to corporate culture: how to manage the eight critical elements of organizational life. *Harv Bus Rev.* 2018:44-52.
3. Alimujiang A, Wiensch A, Boss J, et al. Association between life purpose and mortality among US adults older than 50 years. *JAMA Network Open.* 2019;2:e194270.
4. Hayes SC. 10 signs you know what matters. *Psychology Today.* 2018;53-9, 90.
5. McRaven WH. Make your bed: little things that can change your life…and maybe the world. New York, NY: Grand Central Publishing; 2017.
6. Hedges K. The power of presence: unlock your potential to influence and engage others. New York: AMACOM; 2012.
7. Brown B. Rising strong: how the ability to reset transforms the way we live, love, parent and lead. New York: Random House; 2017.
8. Duckworth A. Grit: the power of passion and perseverance. New York: Scribner; 2016.
9. Tye J, Dent B. Building a culture of ownership in healthcare: the invisible architecture of core values, attitude, and self-empowerment. Indianapolis, IN: Sigma Theta Tau International; 2020.
10. Csikszentmihalyi M. Creativity: the psychology of discovery and invention. New York: Harper Perennial; 2013.
11. Burke D, Flanagan J, Ditomassi M, Hickey PA. Characteristics of nurse directors that contribute to registered nurse satisfaction. *J Nurs Adm.* 2017;47:219-25.
12. Hinds PS, Britton DR, Coleman L, et al. Creating a career legacy map to help assure meaningful work in nursing. *Nurs Outlook.* 2015;63:211-8.
13. Quinn RE, Thakor AV. Creating a purpose-driven organization. Harv Bus Rev 2018:78-85.
14. Pink D. Drive: the surprising truth about what motivates us. New York: Riverhead; 2009.

Chapter 6: Self-Assessing

1. Kouzes JM, Posner BZ. Learning leadership: the five fundamentals of becoming an exemplary leader. San Francisco: Wiley; 2016.
2. Pink D. Drive: the surprising truth about what motivates us. New York: Riverhead; 2009.
3. Ashkenas R, Manville B. The fundamentals of leadership still haven't changed. 2018. Available at: https://hbr.org/2018/11/the-fundamentals-of-leadership-still-havent-changed.
4. Keltner D. Managing yourself: don't let power corrupt you. *Harv Bus Rev.* 2016:112-5.
5. *Langford J, Clance PR.* The impostor phenomenon: recent research findings regarding dynamics, personality and family patterns and their implications for treatment. Psychotherapy *1993;30:495-501.*
6. Clance P. Clance IP Scale. Pauline Rose Clance. Available at: https://paulineroseclance.com/pdf/IPTestandscoring.pdf. Accessed March 20, 2019.
7. Kruger J, Dunning D. Unskilled and unaware of it: how difficulties in recognizing one's own incompetence lead to inflated self-assessments. J Pers Soc Psychol 1999;77:1121-34.

Chapter 7: Reflecting

1. Watkins A. Reflective practice as a tool for growth. Ausmed. 2018. Available at: https://www.ausmed.com/cpd/articles/reflective-practice. Accessed January 28, 2019.
2. Kouzes JM, Posner BZ. Learning leadership: five fundamentals of becoming an exemplary leader. San Francisco: Wiley & Sons; 2016.
3. Beard A. Life's work: an interview with Deepak Chopra. Harv Bus Rev 2018:160.
4. Argyris C, Schön DA. Organizational learning: a theory of action perspective. Addison-Wesley OD series. 1. Reading, MA: Addison-Wesley; 1996.
5. Johns C. Becoming a reflective practitioner. 5th ed. Hoboken, NJ: John Wiley & Sons; 2017.
6. Hendricks J, Mooney D, Berry C. A practical strategy approach to use of reflective practice in critical care nursing. Intensive *Crit Care Nurs.* 1996;12:97-101.
7. Sherman R. Reflecting on your leadership practice. *Nurse Leader.* 2018;16:278-9.
8. Porter J. Why you should make time for self-reflection, (even if you hate doing it). March 21, 2017. Available at: https://hbr.org/2017/03/why-you-should-make-time-for-self-reflection-even-if-you-hate-doing-it. Accessed January 28, 2019.
9. Routledge C. Keeping a reflective diary & reflective questions. Available at: https://cw.routledge.com/textbooks/9780415537902/data/learning/8_Reflection%20in%20Practice.pdf. Accessed January 28, 2019.
10. Kramer H. How self-reflection can make you a better leader. 2016. Available at: https://insight.kellogg.northwestern.edu/article/how-self-reflection-can-make-you-a-better-leader. Accessed August 27, 2019.
11. Drucker Institute. High time for think time. February 16, 2011. Available at: http://www.druckerinstitute.com/2011/02/high-time-for-think-time/. Accessed January 28, 2019.

12. Sherman R. Reflecting on your leadership practice. *Nurse Leader.* 2018;16:278-9.
13. Center for Creative Leadership. How journaling can improve your resiliency. Available at: https://www.ccl.org/multimedia/podcast/reflection-for-resilience-2/. Accessed January 28, 2019
14. McClure P. Reflection on practice. Making practice-based learning work. Available at: https://cw.routledge.com/textbooks/9780415537902/data/learning/8_Reflection%20in%20Practice.pdf. Accessed January 28, 2019.

Chapter 8: Framing

1. Goffman E. Frame analysis: an essay on the organization of experience. Boston: Northeastern University Press; 1974.
2. Grant AM, Hofmann DA. It's not all about me: motivating hand hygiene among health care professionals by focusing on patients. *Psychol Sci.* 2011;22:1494-9.
3. Yoder-Wise PS. The power of yet. *Nurs Educ Perspect.* 2019;49:315.
4. Cialdini R. Principles of persuasion. Influence at work. 2020. Available at: https://www.influenceatwork.com/principles-of-persuasion/. Accessed March 22, 2020.
5. Cialdini R. The power of persuasion. Stanford Executive Briefings. Availabel at: https://searchworks.stanford.edu/view/10008836. Accessed March 22, 2020.

Chapter 9: Influencing

1. Merriam-Webster. Definition of "influence." Available at: https://www.merriam-webster.com/dictionary/influence.
2. Merriam-Webster. Definition of "inspiration." Available at: https://www.merriam-webster.com/dictionary/inspiration.
3. Cialdini R. Influence: science and practice. Boston: Allyn and Bacon; 2001.
4. Shillam CR, Adams JM, Bryant DC, Deupree JP, Miyamoto S, Gregas M. Development of the Leadership Influence Self-Assessment (LISA ©) instrument. Nursing Outlook 2017;66:130-7.
5. Cialdini R. Pre-suasion: a revolutionary way to influence and persuade. New York: Simon & Schuster; 2016.

Chapter 10: Advocating

1. Joint Commission. Speak up initiatives. 2018. Available at: https://www.bing.com/search?q=speak+up+campaign&form=EDGSPH&mkt=en-us&httpsmsn=1&plvar=0&refig=d0e59a36ec714aba9bcc363dfee579bb&sp=4&qs=AS&pq=speak+up&sk=EP1AS2&sc=8-8&cvid=d0e59a36ec714aba9bcc363dfee579bb&cc=US&setlang=en-US. Accessed March, 2019.
2. American Nurses Association. Code of ethics for nurses. Available at: https://www.nursingworld.org/practice-policy/nursing-excellence/ethics/code-of-ethics-for-nurses/. Accessed July 27, 2019.
3. The Commonwealth Fund, New York Times, & Harvard T.H. Chan School of Public Health. 2019. *Americans' values and beliefs about national health insurance reform.* Available at: https://cdn1.sph.harvard.edu/wp-content/uploads/sites/94/2019/10/CMWF-NYT-Harvard_Final-Report_Oct2019.pdf.
4. Trivers RL, Newton HP. The crash of flight 90: doomed by self-deception? *Science Digest.* 1982:66–7, 111.
5. Pierce BR. Speaking up: it requires leadership maturity. *Nurse Leader.* 2016:413-8.
6. Maxfield J, Grenny R, McMillan KP, Switzler A. Silence kills: the seven crucial conversations for healthcare. VitalSmarts. 2005. Available at: https://www.aacn.org/nursing-excellence/healthy-work-environments/~/media/aacn-website/nursing-excellence/healthy-work-environment/silencekills.pdf?la=en.
7. Maxfield D, Grenny J, Lavendaro R, Groah L. The silent treatment: why safety tools and checklists aren't enough to save lives. 2011.
8. Clark CM. Seeking civility. *Am Nurse Today.* 2014;9:18-46.
9. American Organization of Nurse Executives. For the role of the nurse executive in patient safety. AONE Guiding Principles. 2007. Available at: http://www.aone.org/resources/role-nurse-executive-patient-safety.pdf.
10. Daum K. 5 Reasons you should speak up (even when you think you shouldn't). 2014. Available at: https://www.inc.com/kevin-daum/5-reasons-you-should-speak-up-even-when-you-think-you-shouldnt.html.
11. American Nurses Association. Speak to be heard: effective nurse advocacy. 2012. Available at: https://www.americannursetoday.com/speak-to-be-heard-effective-nurse-advocacy/.
12. Winkler County. Texas criminal case against nurses. Available at: www.texasnurses.org.
13. Tomajan K. Advocating for nurses and nursing. *Online J Issues Nurs.* 2012;17. Available at: http://ojin.nursingworld.org/MainMenuCategories/ANAMarketplace/ANAPeriodicals/OJIN/TableofContents/Vol-17-2012/No1-Jan-2012/Advocating-for-Nurses.html#Skills.
14. Buerhaus P. Nurse practitioners: a solution to America's primary care crisis. American Enterprise Institute. 2018. Available at: http://www.aei.org/wp-content/uploads/2018/09/Nurse-practitioners.pdf. Accessed July 27, 2019.
15. Johnson I. A rural "grow your own" strategy building providers from the local workforce. *Nurs Admin Q.* 2017;41:346-52.

Chapter 11: Coaching

1. Weintraub JR, Hunt JM. 4 Reasons mangers should spend more time on coaching. 2015. Available at: https:/hbt.org/2015/05/4reasons-managers-should-spend-more-time-on-coaching#.
2. Reckmeyer M, Robison J. Strengths based parenting: developing your children's innate talents. New York: Gallup Press; 2016.
3. International Coach Federation (ICF). Available at: https://coachfederation.org/.

4. Kimsey-House H, Kimsey-House K, Sandahl P, Whitworth L. Co-active coaching: changing business transforming lives—the proven framework for transformative conversations at work and in life. 4th ed. Boston: Nicholas Brealey Publishing; 2018.
5. Berger W. A more beautiful question: the power of inquiry to spark breakthrough ideas. New York: Bloomsbury; 2014.
6. Stone D, Heen S. Thanks for the feedback: the science and art of receiving feedback well. New York: Penguin Books; 2015.
7. Yoder-Wise P. Kowalski K. Beyond leading and managing: administration for the future. St Louis: Elsevier; 2006.

Chapter 12: Mentoring

1. Maxwell JC. Mentoring 101: what every leader needs to know. Los Angeles: Harper Collins in association with Yates and Yates; 2008.
2. Reh FJ. A guide to understanding the role of a mentor. 2019. Available at: https://www.management-mentors.com/resources/coaching-mentoring-differences.
3. Quintana A. Unpublished data collected for HRSA Diversity project. Denver, CO: Colorado Center for Nursing Excellence; 2017.
4. Sawatzky JA, Enns CL. A mentoring needs assessment: validating mentorship in nursing education. J Prof Nurs 2009;25:145-50.
5. Slimmer L. A teaching mentorship program to facilitate excellence in teaching and learning. J Prof Nurs 2011;28:182-5.
6. Zachary L. The mentor's guide: facilitating effective learning relationships. 2nd ed. San Francisco: John Wiley & Sons; 2012.
7. Ontario Nurses' Association. The ONA mentor toolkit. 2013. Available at: https://www.ona.org/wp-content/uploads/ona_thementortoolkit_201303.pdf
8. Buckingham M, Goodall A. The feedback fallacy. *Harv Bus Rev.* 2019:92-101.
9. McBride AB, Campbell J, Woods NF, Manson SM. Building a mentoring network. *Nurs Outlook.* 2017;65:305-14.
10. Kouzes JM, Posner BZ. Learning leadership: the five fundamentals of becoming an exemplary leader. San Francisco: Wiley; 2016.

Chapter 13: Visioning

1. Kennedy JF. Speech at Rice University, Houston, TX. September 12, 1962. Available at: https://er.jsc.nasa.gov/seh/ricetalk.htm.
2. Bennis W. Leadership is the capacity to translate vision into reality. Available at: https://www.brainyquote.com/quotes/warren_bennis_121713. Accessed July 27, 2019.
3. Bates Communication. How leaders develop and communicate a vision. 2010. Available at: https://www.bates-communications.com/articles-and-newsletters/articles-and-newsletters/bid/57961/How-Leaders-Develop-and-Communicate-a-Vision.
4. Kotter J. How to create a powerful vision for change. 2011. Available at: https://www.forbes.com/sites/johnkotter/2011/06/07/how-to-create-a-powerful-vision-for-change/#41be684951fc.
5. Goodnow C. 4 Ways to develop and communicate your vision. 2018. Available at: https://www.bates-communications.com/bates-blog/how-to-develop-and-communicate-your-vision. Accessed July 26, 2019.
6. Stoner JL. The key to visions that work. 2014. Available at: https://www.seapointcenter/vision-statements/.

Chapter 14: Wisdom

1. Robert Wood Johnson Foundation. Wisdom at work. The importance of the older and experienced nurse in the workplace. Princeton, NJ: Robert Wood Johnson Foundation; 2006.
2. Conley C. Wisdom at work: the making of a modern elder. New York: Crown Publishing; 2018.
3. Bodenheimer T, Sinsky C. From triple to quadruple aim: care of the patient requires care of the provider. *Ann Fam Med.* 2014;12:573-6.
4. McClure M, Poulin M, Sovie M, Wandelt M. Attraction and retention of professional nurses. Washington, DC: American Academy of Nursing; 1983.
5. Dictionary.com. Definition of "wisdom." Available at: https://www.dictionary.com/browse/wisdom.
6. Matney SA, Avant K, Staggers N. Toward an understanding of wisdom in nursing. Online J Issues Nurs 2016;21. Available at: http://ojin.nursingworld.org/MainMenuCategories/ANAMarketplace/ANAPeriodicals/OJIN/TableofContents/Vol-21-2016/No1-Jan-2016/Articles-Previous-Topics/Wisdom-in-Nursing.html.
7. Brown SC. Learning across the campus: How college facilitates the development of wisdom. *J Coll Stud Dev.* 2004;45:134-48.
8. Ulrich B, Barden C, Cassidy L, Varn-Davis N. Critical Care Nurse Work Environments 2018: findings and implications. *Crit Care Nurse.* 2019;39:67-84.
9. Thielking M. Time's Up tackles gender bias and harassment in health care. Sci Am March 1, 2019. Available at: https://www.scientificamerican.com/article/times-up-tackles-gender-bias-and-harassment-in-health-care/.
10. Time's Up. Times Up Foundation. Available at: https://www.timesuphealthcare.org. Accessed March 22, 2020.
11. National Health Care Retention & RN Staffing Report. 2018. Available at: https://nsinursingsolutions.com/Documents/Library/NSI_National_Health_Care_Retention_Report.pdf Accessed March 22, 2020.
12. Kouzes JM, Posner BZ. Learning leadership: the five fundamentals of becoming an exemplary leader. San Francisco: Wiley; 2016.
13. Batcheller J, Yoder-Wise PS. Creating insight when the literature is absent: the circle of advisors. *Nurs Adm Q.* 2011;35:338-43.

14. Torbert WR, Cook-Greuter S. Action inquiry: the secret of timely and transforming leadership. San Francisco: Berrett-Koehler; 2004.
15. Rooke D, Torbert WR. 7 Transformations of leadership. *Harv Bus Rev.* 2005;83:66-76.

Chapter 15: Accountability

1. Battié R, Steelman VM. Accountability in nursing practice: why it is important for patient safety. *AORN J.* 2014;100: 537-41.
2. Rache M. Accountability: a concept worth revisiting. Am Nurse Today. March 2012. Available at: https://www.americannursetoday.com/accountability-a-concept-worth-revisiting/. Accessed July 27, 2019.
3. Latimore-Volkmann L. A no-nonsense coach, Vic Fangio promises no "death by inches" for this Broncos team. Available at: Milehighreport.com. Accessed January 12, 2019.
4. Sherman R. Promoting professional accountability and ownership: nursing leaders set the tone for a culture of professional responsibility. *Am Nurse Today.* 2019;14:24-6.
5. American Nurses Association. Code of ethics for nurses with interpretive statements. Silver Springs, MD: American Nurses Association; 2015.
6. Skousen T. Choose Accountability. 2016. Available at: https://www.partnersinleadership.com/insights-publications/responsibility-vs-accountability/. Accessed March 7, 2019.
7. Surbhi S. Difference between responsibility and accountability. 2016. Available at: https://keydifferences.com/difference-between-responsibility-and-accountability.html. Accessed March 7, 2109.
8. Partners in Leadership. Landmark workplace study reveals "crisis of accountability. 2014 Available at: https://www.partnersinleadership.com/news/press-releases/landmark-workplace-study-reveals-crisis-of-accountability/.

Chapter 16: Agility

1. Bourton S, Lavoie J, Vogel T. Leading with inner agility. McKinsey & Company. 2018. Available at: https://www.mckinsey.com/business-functions/organization/our-insights/leading-with-inner-agility.
2. Brown B. Rising strong: the reckoning, the rumble, the resolution. New York: Random House; 2015.
3. David S. Connecting organizational and individual values. March 12, 2019.
4. David S, Congleton C. Emotional agility. 2013. Available at: https://hbr.org/2013/11/emotional-agility?autocomplete=true.
5. Institute for Healthcare Improvement. Available at: http://www.ihi.org/resources/Pages/HowtoImprove/ScienceofImprovementTestingChanges.aspx.
6. Schwaber K, Sutherland J. The scrum guide. 2017. Available at: https://www.scrumguides.org/docs/scrumguide/v2017/2017-Scrum-Guide-US.pdf#zoom=100.
7. Coleman J. The best strategic leaders balance agility and consistency. January 4, 2017. Available at: https://hbr.org/2017/01/the-best-strategic-leaders-balance-agility-and-consistency?autocomplete=true.
8. Rigby DK, Sutherland J, Noble A. Agile at scale: how to go from a few teams to hundreds. *Harv Bus Rev.* 2018:88-96.
9. Trepanier S, Nordgren M. Improvisation for leadership development. *J Contin Educ Nurs.* 2017;48:151-3.

Chapter 17: Attitudes

1. Merriam-Webster. Definitions. https://www.merriam-webster.com/dictionary/attitude.
2. Swindoll C. Attitude. 2015. Available at: https://insight.org/resources/daily-devotional/individual/the-value-of-a-positive-attitude. Accessed February 2, 2010
3. Bradberry T. Here's why your attitude is more important than your intelligence. 2017. Available at: https://www.weforum.org/agenda/2017/08/heres-why-your-attitude-is-more-important-than-your-intelligence. Accessed February 1, 2019.
4. Darlington N. Life isn't about what happens to you, it's about how you react to it. 2018. Available at: www.lifehack.org/446739/life-isnt-about-what-happens-to-you-its-about-how-you-react-to-it. Accessed July 29, 2019
5. Tully S, Tao H. Work-related stress and positive thinking among acute care nurses: a cross-sectional survey. *Am J Nurs.* 2019;119: 24-31.
6. Cherry K. Attitudes and behavior in psychology. 2018. Available at: http://www.verywellmind.com/attitudes-how-they-form-change-shape-behavior-2795897. Accessed February 3, 2010.
7. Dweck C. Mindset: the new psychology of success. 2nd ed. New York: Ballentine Books; 2016.
8. Duckworth A. Grit: the power of passion and perseverance. New York: Simon and Schuster; 2016.
9. Steinberg T. "Positive reframing" as optimistic thinking. 2012. Psychology Today blogs. Available at: https://www.psychologytoday.com/us/blog/in-the-face-adversity/201209/positive-reframing-optimistic-thinking. Accessed February 10, 2019.
10. McGauran D. 7 Cognitive behavioral techniques to help reframe your thinking. 2016. https://www.activebeat.com/your-health/7-cognitive-behavioral-techniques-to-help-reframe-your-thinking/?streamview=all. Accessed February 10, 2019.
11. Scott E. 4 steps to shift perspective and change everything: how to reframe situations so they create less stress. 2018. Available at: https://www.verywellmind.com/cognitive-reframing-for-stress-management-3144872. Accessed February 10, 2019.
12. Clear J. The Akrasia effect: why we don't follow through on what we set out to do and what to do about it. 2018. Available at: https://www.bing.com/search?q=The+Akrasia+Effect%3A+Why+We+Don%E2%80%99t+Follow+Through+on+What+We+Set+Out+to+Do+and+What+to+Do+About+It.

+&form=EDNTHT&mkt=en-us&httpsmsn=1&plvar=0&refig=ee39cc52b0894bf9cc34d7e2e6a5fcb1&sp=-1&pq=&sc=8-0&qs=n&sk=&cvid=ee39cc52b0894bf9cc34d7e2e6a5fcb. Accessed February 10, 2019.
13. Pressfield S. The war of art: break through the blocks and win your inner creative battles. New York: Black Irish Entertainment; 2012.
14. Clear J. Procrastination: a scientific guide on how to stop procrastinating. 2018. Available at: https://jamesclear.com/procrastination. Accessed February 10, 2019.

Chapter 18: Authenticity

1. George B, Sims P, McLean A, Mayer D. Discovering your authentic leadership: why self-awareness is so critical. Authentic leadership. Emotional intelligence. *Harv Bus Rev.* 2018:1-39.
2. George B, Sims P. True north: discover your authentic leadership. San Francisco: John Wiley and Sons; 2007.
3. Avolio BJ, Gardner WL. Authentic leadership development: getting to the root of positive forms of leadership. *Leadersh Q.* 2005;16:315-38.
4. Ibarra H. The authenticity paradox. Authentic leadership. Emotional intelligence. Harv Bus Rev 2015:39-71.
5. Goffee R, Jones G. Managing authenticity: the paradox of great leadership. *Harv Bus Rev.* 2005.
6. Seppala E. What bosses gain by being vulnerable: the psychology of human connection. Authentic leadership. Emotional intelligence. *Harv Bus Rev.* 2018:71-86.
7. Brown B. Dare to lead. Brave work. Tough conversations. Whole hearts. New York: Random House; 2018.
8. American Nurses Association. Healthy work environment. 2020. Available at: https://www.nursingworld.org/practice-policy/work-environment/. Accessed, 2020.
9. American Association of Critical Care Nurses. Building a healthy work environment. 2019. Available at: https://www.aacn.org/nursing-excellence/nurse-stories/building-a-healthy-work-environment
10. Wong CA, Laschinger H, Cummings GG. Authentic Leadership and nurses' voice behavior and perception of care quality. *J Nurs Manag.* 2010;18:889-900.
11. Giallonardo L, Wong C, Iwasiw C. Authentic leadership of preceptors: predictor of new graduate nurses' work engagement and job satisfaction. *J Nurs Manag.* 2010;18:993-1003.
12. Laschinger HK, Borgogni L, Consiglio C, Read E. The effects of authentic leadership, six areas of worklife, and occupational coping self-efficacy on new graduate nurses' burnout and mental health: a cross-sectional study. *Int J Nurs Stud.* 2015;52:1080-9.

Chapter 19: Capacity

1. Merriam-Webster. Definition of "capacity." Available at: https://www.merriam-webster.com/dictionary/capacity.
2. Bennis WG, Thomas R. Crucibles of leadership. HBR's 10 must reads. Boston: Harvard Business Review Press; 2018. p 9-24.
3. Boss J. How to build your leadership capacity. Forbes.com. 2017. Available at: https://www.forbes.com/sites/jeffboss/2017/09/08/how-to-build-your-leadership-capacity/#6185ae716496.
4. Gilkey R, Kilts C. Cognitive fitness. On mental toughness. HBR's 10 must reads. Boston: Harvard Business Review Press; 2018. p 37-52.
5. Hogg B. Building leadership capacity. White paper. Bill Hogg and Associates. 2019. Available at: https://www.billhogg.ca/white-paper-building-leadership-capacity/.
6. Dotiwala F, Unni N. Developing leadership capabilities. McKinsey and Company. 2013. Available at: https://www.mckinsey.com/business-functions/operations/our-insights/developing-leadership-capabilities.

Chapter 20: Courage

1. Hamric A, Arras J, Mohrmann M. Must we be courageous? *Hastings Center Rev.* 2015:33-40.
2. Sportsman S, Converse C. Courageous leadership. Collaborative Momentum Consulting. 2018. Available at: www.collaborativemomentum.com/courageousleadership/.
3. Tardanico S. Ten traits of courageous leaders. Forbes. January 15, 2013. Available at: https://www.forbes.com/sites/susantardanico/2013/01/15/10-traits-of-courageous-leaders/#22612c74fc0d. Accessed January 2019.
4. Muehlbauer P. Have the moral courage to do the right thing. Straight talk. *ONS Connect.* 2014;29:39.
5. Didert J. Cultivating everyday courage. *Harv Bus Rev.* 2018: 128-35.
6. Sack K. Sheriff charged in the Texas whistle-blowing care. 2011. New York Times. Available at: https://www.nytimes.com/2011/01/15/us/15nurses.html.
7. Maxwell D, Grenny J, McMillan R, Patterson K, Switzler A. Silence kills: the seven crucial conversations for health care. Agency for Healthcare Research and Quality, PSNeT: Patient Safety Network. 2005. Available at: https:psnet.ahrq.gov/resources/1149.
8. Okuyama A, Wagner C, Bijnen B. Speaking up for patient safety by hospital-based health care professionals: a literature review. *BMC Health Serv Res.* 2014;14:61.
9. Morrow KJ, Gustavson AM, Jones J. Speaking up behaviors (safety voices): a metasynthesis of qualitative research studies. *Int J Nurs Stud.* 2016;64:42-51.

Chapter 21: Creativity

1. Alda A. Creativity quotes. Available at: https://daringtolivefully.com/creativity-quotes. Accessed March 25, 2019
2. Dragoon J. What is creativity's value—in marketing, in business? Forbes. October 4, 2010. Available at: https://www.forbes.com/2010/10/04/facebook-zuckerberg-twitter-wendy-kopp-creativity-advertising-cmo-network.html#73c07d2b8007. Accessed March 22, 2019.

3. Burrus D. Creativity and innovation: your keys to a successful organization. 2017. Available at: https://www.huffingtonpost.com/daniel-burrus/creativity-and-innovation_b_4149993.html. Accessed March 24, 2019
4. Johnson I. A rural "grow your own" strategy; building providers from the local workforce. Nurs Adm Q 2017;41:346-52.
5. Christensen C. The innovator's dilemma: when new technologies cause great firms to fail. Boston: Harvard Business Review; 2016.
6. Christensen C, Grossman J, Hwang J. The innovator's prescription: a disruptive solution to healthcare. New York: McGraw-Hill; 2009.
7. Weberg D, Davidson S. Leadership for evidence-based innovation in nursing and health professions. 2nd Ed. Burlington, MA: Jones and Bartlett Learning; 2019.
8. Sokolova S. The importance of creativity and innovation in business. Available at: https://www.linkedin.com/pulse/importance-creativity-innovation-business-siyana-sokolova. Accessed March 23, 2019.
9. McCaffrey T. Brainswarming: because brainstorming doesn't work. 2014. Available at: https://www.bing.com/videos/search?q=brainswarming+video&view=detail&mid=4085C5AFC6C7304B99C84085C5AFC6C7304B99C8&FORM=VIRE.
10. Maney K. Shelter from the storm: why brainswarming is the future of collaboration. 2013.
11. Vozza S. Forget brainstorming, try brainswarming instead. Available at: https://www.entrepreneur.com/author/stephanie-vozza. Accessed March 23, 2019.
12. Adams C. What is brainswarming and how does it compare to brainstorming? Available at: https://www.modernanalyst.com/Careers/InterviewQuestions/tabid/128/ID/3483/What-is-Brainswarming-and-how-does-it-compare-to-Brainstorming.aspx. Accessed March 25, 2019.

Chapter 22: Integrity

1. Lewis C. Integrity quote. Available at: https://www.goalcast.com/2018/03/26/15-c-s-lewis-quotes/c-s-lewis-quote1/.
2. Merriam-Webster. Definition of "integrity." Available at: https://www.merriam-webster.com/dictionary/integrity.
3. Cambridge Dictionary. Definition of "integrity." Available at: https://dictionary.cambridge.org/dictionary/english/integrity. Accessed May 29, 2020.
4. Sternberg L. What is the relationship between courage and integrity? 2016. Available at: https://leadershiplaboratory.wordpress.com/2016/06/04/what-is-the-relationship-between-courage-and-integrity/.
5. Ruiz D. Quotes. Available at: https://www.brainyquote.com/quotes/don_miguel_ruiz_182401?src=t_integrity.
6. Eisenhower D. Integrity quote. Available at: https://www.brainyquote.com/quotes/dwight_d_eisenhower_109026?src=t_integrity.
7. Heathfield S. Did you bring your ethics to work today? 2018. Available at: https://www.thebalancecareers.com/did-you-bring-your-ethics-to-work-today-1917741.
8. Sherwood M. 6 Ways to rebuild integrity. Available at: https://fmidr.com/integrity/.

Chapter 23: Intelligence

1. Merriam-Webster. Definitions. Available at: https://meriam-webster.com/.
2. Psychology Today. Emotional intelligence. Available at: https://www.psychologytoday.com/us/basics/emotional-intelligence. Accessed May 29, 2020.
3. Psychology Today. Intelligence: IQ giftedness. Available at: https://www.psychologytoday.com/us/basics/intelligence. Accessed April 26, 2019.
4. Psychology Today. No, your IQ is not constant: implications are profound. 2018. Available at: https://www.psychologytoday.com/us/blog/memory-medic/201805/no-your-iq-is-not-constant. Accessed April 26, 2019.
5. Gardner H. Frames of mind: the theory of multiple intelligences. New York: Basic Books; 1983.
6. Thatchenkery T, Metzker C. Appreciative intelligence: seeing the mighty oak in the acorn. 2006.
7. Kowalski KE. On call staffing. *Am J Nurs.* 1973;73:10.
8. Kowalski KE, Bowes WA. Parental response to the loss of a stillborn infant. *Contemp Obstet Gynecol.* 1976;8:53-7.
9. Goleman D. Emotional intelligence: why it can matter more than IQ. New York: Bantam Dell; 1995.
10. Bariso J. 13 Signs of high EI. Available at: https://www.inc.com/justin-bariso/13-things-emotionally-intelligent-people-do.html.
11. Ruiz DM. The four agreements. San Rafael, CA: Amber-Allen Publishing; 1997.
12. Herman A. Visual intelligence: sharpen your perception, change your life. New York: Houghton, Mifflin Harcourt Publishing Company; 2016.
13. BBC News. "Infomania: worse than marijuana. 2005. Available at: http://news.bbc.co.uk/2/hi/uk/4471607.stm. Accessed March 25, 2020.
14. Herman A. Distractions are making us dumber. Available at: http://www.visualintelligencebook.com/blog/distractions. Accessed May 2, 2019.

Chapter 24: Mindfulness

1. Kleiner A, Schwartz J, Thomson J. The wise advocate: the inner voice of strategic leadership. New York: Columbia University Press; 2019.
2. Dye CF, Garman AN. Exceptional leadership: 16 critical competencies for healthcare executives. 2nd ed. Chicago: Health Administration Press; 2015.
3. Smith JA, Suttie J, Jazaieri H, Newman KM. The state of mindfulness science. Greater Good Magazine. December 5, 2017. Available at: https://greatergood.berkeley.edu/article/item/the_state_of_mindfulness_science.
4. Storoni M. This 2-minute breathing exercise can help you make better decisions, according to a new study. 2019. Available at: https://www.inc.com/mithu-storoni/this-2-minute-breathing-exercise-can-help-you-make-better-decisions-according-to-a-new-study.html.

5. Powell A. Researchers study how it seems to change the brain in depressed patients. Harvard Gazette. April 9, 2018. Available at: https://news.harvard.edu/gazette/story/2018/04/harvard-researchers-study-how-mindfulness-may-change-the-brain-in-depressed-patients/.
6. Van Dam NT, van Vugt MK, Vago DR, et al. Mind the hype: a critical evaluation and prescriptive agenda for research on mindfulness and meditation. *Perspect Psychol Sci.* 2017;13:36-61.
7. Powell A. When science meets mindfulness. April 9, 2018. Available at: https://news.harvard.edu/gazette/story/2018/04/harvard-researchers-study-how-mindfulness-may-change-the-brain-in-depressed-patients/.

Chapter 25: Presence

1. Burke D, Flanagan J, Ditomassi M, Hickey PA. Characteristics of nurse directors that contribute to registered nurse satisfaction. *J Nurs Adm.* 2017;47:219-25.
2. Hewlett SA. Executive presence: the missing link between merit and success. New York: HarperCollins; 2014.
3. Hedges K. The power of presence: unlock your potential to influence and engage others. New York: AMACOM; 2012.
4. Kouzes JM, Posner BZ. The leadership challenge: how to make extraordinary things happen in organizations. 5th ed. San Francisco: Jossey-Bass; 2012.
5. Maxwell on presence.The John Maxwell Team. Presence. Available at: https://johnmaxwellteam.com/2019-presence. Accessed March 22, 2020.
6. Heath K, Flynn J, Holt MD. Women, find your voice. *Harv Bus Rev.* 2014:118-21.
7. Huang K, Yeomans M, Brooks AW, Minson J, Gino F. It doesn't hurt to ask: question-asking increases liking. *J Pers Soc Psychol.* 2017;113:430-52.
8. Shellenbarger S. How to look smarter. January 13, 2015. Available at: https://www.wsj.com/articles/how-to-look-smarter-1421189631.
9. Chib VS, Adachi R, O'Doherty JP. Neural substrates of social facilitation effects on incentive-based performance. *Soc Cogn Affect Neurosci.* 2018;13:391-403.
10. Yoder-Wise PS, Benton KK. The essence of presence and how it enhances a leader's value. *Nurse Leader.* 2017;15:174-8.
11. Cuddy A. Presence: bringing your boldest self to your biggest challenges. New York: Little, Brown & Co; 2015.

Chapter 26: Resilience

1. Human Performance Institute. Available at: https://www.jnj.com/tag/human-performance-institute. Accessed March 8, 2019
2. Kester K, Wei H. Building nurse resilience. *Nurs Manage.* 2018;49:42-5.
3. Grant A. Oval office lessons. FastCompany 2018:30-2.
4. Brigham T, Barden C, Dopp AL, et al. A journey to construct an all-encompassing conceptual model of factors affecting clinician well-being and resilience. NAM Perspectives. Washington, DC: National Academy of Medicine; 2018. Available at: https://nam.edu/journey-construct-encompassing-conceptual-model-factors-affecting-clinician-well-resilience/. Accessed March 8, 2019.
5. Steege LM, Pinekenstein BJ, Arensault Knudsen E, Rainbow JG. Exploring nurse leader fatigue: a mixed methods study. J Nurs Manage 2017;25:276-86.
6. Prestia AS. Transformational resiliency. *Nurse Leader.* 2016:354-7.
7. Rodin J. The resiliency dividend. New York: Public Affairs; 2014.
8. Brown B. Rising strong. New York: Spiegel & Grau; 2015.
9. Carpio RC, Castro LP, Huerto HM, Highfield MEF, Mendelson S. Exploring resilience at work among first-line nurse managers. *J Nurs Admin.* 2018;48:481-5.
10. Bernard N. Resilience and professional job: a toolkit for nurse leaders. *Nurse Leader.* 2019:43-8.
11. Press Ganey. Burnout and resilience: a framework for data analysis and a positive path forward. 2018. Available at: https://www.pressganey.com/resources/white-papers/burnout-and-resilience-a-framework-for-data-analysis. Accessed December 26, 2018.
12. Valcour M. Managing yourself: beating burnout. *Harv Bus Rev.* 2016:98-101.
13. Sandberg S, Grant A. Resilience. Available at: https://hbr.org/ideacast/2017/04/sheryl-sandberg-and-adam-grant-on-resilience.html. Accessed May 15, 2019.
14. Ignatius A. Above all, acknowledge the pain. *Harv Bus Rev.* 2017:142-7.
15. Gill R, Orgad S. The amazing bounce-backable woman: resilience and the psychological turn in neoliberalism. *Sociol Res Online.* 2018;23:477-96.

Chapter 27: Risking

1. Oxford English Dictionary. Definition of "risk." Available at: https://en.oxforddictionaries.com/definition/risk.
2. Goodreads. Available at: https://www.goodreads.com/quotes/9819-only-those-who-will-risk-going-too-far-can-possibly.
3. Piscione DB. (2014) The risk factor: the seven characteristics of bold risk-takers. December22, 2014. Available at: https://www.linkedin.com/pulse/7-characteristics-bold-risk-takers-deborah-perry-piscione.
4. Griffin J. To have a great career, be a risk taker. Available at: https://www.forbes.com/sites/jillgriffin/2018/04/27/to-have-a-great-career-be-a-risk-taker/#34f1243574a2.
5. Nieboer J. Group member characteristics and risk-taking by consensus. *J Behav Exp Econ.* 2015;57:81-8.
6. Tersigni A. Breaking bias: gender equity is imperative in health care. Modern Healthcare. 2019. Available at: https://www.modernhealthcare.com/opinion-editorial/breaking-bias-gender-equity-imperative-healthcare. Accessed March 2020.

7. Tull M. How taking risks evokes leadership success. December 6, 2017. Available at: https://www.huffingtonpost.com/megan-tull/how-taking-risks-evokes-l_b_10843744.html. Accessed February 2019.
8. Crenshaw J, Yoder-Wise P. Creating an environment for innovation: the risk-taking leadership competency. *Nurse Leader.* 2013:24-7.

Chapter 28: Spirituality

1. University of Minnesota. Taking charge of your health and wellbeing. What is spirituality? Available at: https://www.takingcharge.csh.umn.edu/what-spirituality.
2. Puchalski C. What is spirituality? Available at: https://www.takingcharge.csh.umn.edu/what-spirituali. Accessed March 2020.
3. Recomparison.com. Religion vs. spirituality. Available at: http://recomparison.com/comparisons/101393/religion-vs-spirituality/.
4. Anonymous. 12 Symptoms of spiritual awakening. Available at: https://www.bing.com/images/search?q=12+symptoms+of+spiritual+awakening&qpvt=12+symptoms+of+spiritual+awakening&FORM=IGRE.
5. Merton T. Quotes. Available at: https://www.azquotes.com/author/10004-Thomas_Merton.
6. University of Minnesota. Interview with Matthieu Ricard. Available at: https://www.takingcharge.csh.umn.edu/interview-matthieu-ricard.
7. Krentzman A. Why is spirituality important? Available at: https://www.takingcharge.csh.umn.edu/enhance-your-wellbeing/purpose/spirituality/why-spirituality-important.
8. Greater Good in Action at Berkeley. Nine steps to forgiveness. Available at: https://ggia.berkeley.edu/practice/nine_steps_to_forgiveness.
9. Thoresen C, Luskin F. The Stanford forgiveness project. Available at: http://www.hawaiiforgivenessproject.org/Stanford.htm.
10. Brussat F, Brussat M. What is spirituality? Available at: https://www.spiritualityandpractice.com/about/what-is-spirituality.

Chapter 29: Timing

1. Merriam-Webster. Definition of "timing." Available at: https://www.merriam-webster.com/dictionary/timing.
2. Kingston MB. Voice of the president: career transitions. *Voice Nurs Leader.* 2019;17:1
3. Botelho EL, Powell KR, Kincaid S, Wang G. What sets successful CEOs apart. *Harv Bus Rev.* 2017:70-7.
4. Nightingale F. Notes on nursing, what it is and what it is not. New York: D. Appleton and Company; 1860.
5. Pink DH. When: the scientific secrets of perfect timing. New York: Riverhead Books; 2018.

Chapter 30: Truthfulness

1. Silva L. Honesty. The real benefits of honesty in the workplace. Unconventional wisdom/influential minds. 2017. Available at: https://www.influencive.com/real-benefits-honesty-workplace/.
2. Firestone L. Five ways to build trust and honesty in your relationships. Psychology Today June 29, 2015. Available at: https://www.psychologytoday.com/us/blog/compassion-matters/201506/5-ways-build-trust-and-honesty-in-your-relationship.
3. Schnackenberg AK, Tomlinson EC. Organizational transparency: a new perspective on managing trust in organization-stakeholder relations. *J Manag.* 2016;42:1784-810.
4. Arruda W. Five ways to identify a company with a culture of transparency. Forbes Blog. March 11. 2018. Available at: https://www.forbes.com/sites/williamarruda/2018/03/11/five-ways-to-identify-a-company-with-a-culture-of-transparency/#60a9fad64804.
5. Richman J. Five examples of companies succeeding through transparency. Entrepreneur Blog. May 27, 2016. Available at: https://www.entrepreneur.com/article/274636.
6. Wille A. Transparency and business: four critical things business owners need to know. Klipfolio. 2017. Available at: https://www.klipfolio.com/blog/transparency-and-business.
7. SkillsYouNeed. Develop the skills you need for life. Skills for life. 2019. Available at: https://www.skillsyouneed.com/.
8. Universal Class. The role of truthfulness in collaboration. Available at: https://www.universalclass.com/articles/business/the-role-of-truthfulness-in-collaboration.htm.

Chapter 31: Trust

1. Reich RB. The common good. Toronto, Ontario, Canada: Knopf; 2018.
2. Moore M. Trust: essential to healthy work environments. RNL: Reflections on Nursing Leadership. Sigma 2019. Available at: https://www.reflectionsonnursingleadership.org/features/more-features/trust-essential-to-healthy-work-environments.
3. Fisher AS, Neesha Hathy, EVP at Charles Schwab, on why you should stretch yourself even if you don't feel it. ThriveGlobal. 2019. Available at: https://thriveglobal.com/stories/neesha-hathi-evp-at-charles-schwab-on-why-you-should-stretch-yourself-even-if-you-dont-always-feel-it/
4. Lexico. Definition of "trust." Available at: en.oxforddictionaries.com/definition/trust.
5. Zak P. Neuro-science of Trust. Harv Bus Rev 2017:83-90. Available at: https://hbr.org/2017/01/the-neuroscience-of-trust.
6. Braun S, Peus C, Weisweiler S, Frey D. Transformational leadership, job satisfaction, and team performance: a multilevel mediation model of trust. *The Leaders Q.* 2013;24:270-83.
7. Mo S, Shi J. Linking ethical leadership to employee burnout, workplace deviance and performance testing the mediating roles of trust in leader and surface acting. *J Bus Ethics.* 2017;144:293-303.

8. Xiong K, Lin W, Li JC, Wang L. Employee trust in supervisors and affective commitment: the moderating role of authentic leadership. *Psychol Rep.* 2016;118:829-48.
9. Covey S. How the best leaders build trust. Leadership Now Blog 2019. Available at: https://www.leadershipnow.com/CoveyOnTrust.html.
10. Horsager D. You can't be a great leader without trust—here's how to build it. Forbes Leadership Forum. October 2012. Available at: forbes.com/sites/forbesleadershipforum/2012/10/24/you-cant-be-a-great-leader-without-trust-heres-how-you-build-it/#58b7a21f4ef7..
11. Berman J. The three essential Warren Buffet quotes to live by. Forbes Blog. April 24, 2014. Available at: https://www.forbes.com/sites/jamesberman/2014/04/20/the-three-essential-warren-buffett-quotes-to-live-by/#376bdf536543.
12. Grossman D. Six actionable steps to building trust with employees. September 14, 2016. Available at: http://www.yourthoughtpartner.com/blog/bid/59619/leaders-follow-these-6-steps-to-build-trust-with-employees-improve-how-you-re-perceived.
13. Schawbol D. Joel Peterson: how to build a high trust organization. Forbes Blog. August 3, 2016. Available at: https://www.forbes.com/sites/danschawbel/2016/08/03/joel-peterson-how-to-build-a-high-trust-organization/#790036011346.
14. Zenger J, Tolkman J. How leaders build trust. Adapted from "Three elements of trust." Harvard Business Review Blog. June 26, 2019. Available at: https://hbr.org/tip/2019/06/how-leaders-build-trust. Accessed March 2020.

Chapter 32: Vulnerability

1. Brown B. Dare to lead: brave work, tough conversations, whole hearts. New York: Random House; 2018.
2. Brown B. Vulnerability. 2010. Available at: https://www.youtube.com/watch?v=iCvmsMzlF7o.
3. Swoboda K. The benefits of practicing vulnerability in the office. Entrepreneur. 2014. Available at: https://www.entrepreneur.com/article/239424.
4. Stempniak M. Nurse leaders must "take off their armor," be vulnerable to succeed. 2017. Available at: https://www.hhnmag.com/articles/8193-nurse-leaders-must-take-off-their-armor-be-vulnerable-to-thrive.
5. Williams D. The importance of being courageously vulnerable at work. Forbes. 2018. Available at: https://www.forbes.com/sites/davidkwilliams/2013/07/18/the-best-leaders-are-vulnerable/#5927c2723c1d.
6. Seppala E. What bosses gain by being vulnerable. *Harv Bus Rev.* 2014. Available at: https://hbr.org/2014/12/what-bosses-gain-by-being-vulnerable.

Chapter 33: Alliances

1. Grant A. WorkLife podcast. Worklife. 2018. Available at: https://www.ted.com/podcasts/worklife. Accessed March 22, 2020.
2. Straw J, Scullard M, Kukkonen S, Davis B. The work of leaders: how vison, alignment and execution will change the way you lead. San Francisco: Wiley; 2013.
3. Hackman R. Leading teams: setting the stage for great performances. Boston: Harvard Business School Publishing Corporation; 2002.
4. Leavitt M, McKeown R. Finding allies, building alliances: 8 elements that bring—and keep—people together. San Francisco: Jossey-Bass; 2013.
5. Brenan M. Nurses again outpace other professions for honesty, ethics. 2018. Available at: https://news.gallup.com/poll/245597/nurses-again-outpace-professions-honesty-ethics.aspx.

Chapter 34: Communication

1. Merriam-Webster. Definitions. https://www.merriam-webster.com/
2. American Organization of Nurse Executives. AONE Nurse Executive Competencies. Chicago, IL: American Organization of Nurse Executives; 2015.
3. Bellundi N. Mehrabian's 7-38-55 rule of personal communication. 2008. Available at: http://www.rightattitudes.com/2008/10/04/7-38-55-rule-personal-communication/.
4. Crane TG. The heart of coaching: using transformational coaching to create a high-performance culture. San Diego, CA: FTA Press; 1999.
5. The Entrepreneur Success Institute. Build attitude ahead of aptitude. 2013. Available at: http://theentrepreneursuccessinstitute.com/build-attitude-ahead-of-aptitude/. Accessed June 14, 2020.
6. Murphy M. Saying the word "you" is a good way to start fights and make people mad. Forbes. Oct 1, 2017.
7. Greenleaf Counseling. Communication filters. 2018. Available at: http://greenleafcounseling.org/communication-filters/.
8. Doyle A. Learn about active listening skills with examples. 2018. Available at: https://www.thebalancecareers.com/active-listening-skills-with-examples-2059684.
9. Zenger J, Folkman J. What great listeners actually do. *Harv Bus Rev.* 2016. Available at: https://hbr.org/2016/07/what-great-listeners-actually-do.

Chapter 35: Contribution

1. Potter TM. In two words, what do nurses contribute to healing? Reflections on nursing leadership. Sigma. 2016. Available at: https://www.reflectionsonnursingleadership.org/features/more-features/Vol42_4_in-two-words-what-do-nurses-contribute-to-healing.
2. Rosa B. What nurses really contribute to health care: part 1 of an education do-over. HuffPost Contributor Platform. 2016. Available at: https://www.huffpost.com/entry/what-nurses-really-contribute-to-health-care_n_9550926.
3. Aiken L, Clarke S, Sloan D, Sochaski J, Silber J. Hospital nurse staffing and patient mortality, nurse burnout, and job dissatisfaction. *JAMA.* 2002;288:1987-93.

4. Avalere Health. Optimal nurse staffing to improve quality of care. American Nurses Association. 2015. Available at: https://www.semanticscholar.org/paper/Nurse-staffing-and-patient-outcomes-in-critical-%3A-A-Sevransky/a5569d733f6171c770043f9e53504e99be7362f4.
5. Robert Wood Johnson Foundation. Nurses take on new and expanded roles in health care. Patient centered care: RWJF Collection. January 20, 2015. Available at: https://www.rwjf.org/en/library/articles-and-news/2015/01/nurses-take-on-new-and-expanded-roles-in-health-care.html.

Chapter 36: Culture

1. Schein P. Organizational culture and leadership. 5th ed. Hoboken, NJ: Wiley; 2017
2. AMN Healthcare. Nurse executive survey: clinical leadership trends & strategies. 2017. Available at: htts://www.amnhealthcare.com/industry-research/survey/nurseexecutive-survey/. Accessed March 25, 2019.
3. Groysberg B, Lee J, Price J, Cheng Y. The leader's guide to corporate culture: how to manage the eight critical elements of organizational life. *Harv Bus Rev.* 2018:49.
4. Gothamculture. What is organizational culture? Available at: https://gothamculture.com/what-is-organizational-culture-definition/. Accessed March 29, 2019
5. Pisano G. The hard truth about innovative cultures. *Harv Bus Rev.* 2019:62-71.
6. Gino F. Case study: can you fix a toxic culture without firing people? *Harv Bus Rev.* 2018.
7. Carucci R. 3 Ways senior leaders create a toxic culture. *Harv Bus Rev.* 2018.
8. Tye J, Dent B. Building a culture of ownership in healthcare: the invisible architecture of core values, attitude and self-empowerment. Indianapolis, IN: Sigma Theta Tau International; 2017.
9. Duckworth A. Grit: the power of passion and perseverance. New York: Simon and Schuster; 2016.
10. Lee TH, Duckworth AL. Organizational grit. *Harv Bus Rev.* 2018.

Chapter 37: Engagement

1. Harter J. Employee engagement on the rise in the US. August 28, 2018. Available at: https://news.gallup.com/poll/241649/employee-engagement-rise.aspx. Accessed April 2020.
2. Kahn WA. Psychological conditions of personal engagement and disengagement at work. *Acad Manage J.* 1990;33:692-724.
3. Roth T. Create a culture of high energy and commitment: the four levels of leadership. Engagement starts with your leaders. Wilson Learning Worldwide. 2016. Available at: https://www.wilsonlearning.com/wlw/articles/l/engagement-leaders.
4. CustomInsight. What causes employee disengagement? Employment Engagement Survey. 2019. Available at: https://www.custominsight.com/employee-engagement-survey/research-employee-disengagement.asp.
5. Markos S, Sridevi MS. Employee engagement: the key to improving performance. *Int J Bus Manage.* 2010;5:89-96.
6. Tims M, Bakker AB, Xanthopoulou D. Do transformational leaders enhance their followers' daily work engagement? *Leadership Q.* 2011;22:121-31.
7. Seaton H. Leadership and employee engagement: 5 startegies to engage employees in 2018. 2018. Available at: https://www.flashpointleadership.com/blog/leadership_and_emplyee_engagement.
8. Gruman J, Saks A. Performance management and employee engagement. *Human Resource Management Review.* 2011; 21:123-36.
9. Carasco-Saul M, Kim W, Kim T. (2014) Leadership & employment engagement: Proposing research Agendas through a review of the literature. *Human Resource Development Review.* 2014;14:38-63.
10. Moore K, Ciampi V. Leadership engagement always trumps employee engagement. Forbes 2016. Available at: https://www.forbes.com/sites/karlmoore/2016/08/31/leadership-engagement-always-trumps-employee-engagement/#4ca614e14944.

Chapter 38: Governance

1. Mitchell R. The crucial difference between governance and management. Indiana Philanthropy Alliance. 2011. Available at: https://www.inphilanthropy.org/sites/default/files/resources/Crucial%20Difference%20Between%20Governance%20%26%20Management-AKT%20LLP-2011.pdf.
2. Noble A. Behind all good leadership is good governance. World Economic Forum. 2012. Available at: https://www.weforum.org/agenda/2012/06/behind-all-good-leadership-is-good-governance/.
3. Bajic E. Why companies need to build more diverse boards. Available at: https://www.forbes.com/sites/elenabajic/2015/08/11/why-companies-need-to-build-more-diverse-boards/#3d544863662c. Accessed April 23, 2020.
4. Schoning M, Noble A, Heinecke A, Archleitner A, Mayer J. The governance of social enterprises: managing your organization for success. Schwab Foundation for Social Entrepreneurship. World Economics Form. 2012. Available at: http://www3.weforum.org/docs/WEF_Governance_Social_Enterprises_2106_light.pdf.
5. Health Care Trustees of New York State. Boardroom basics: what every health care trustee needs to know. 2008. Available at: http://htnys.org/governance/docs/boardroom_basics.pdf.
6. Gaunci G, Mederios N. Shared governance that works. Minneapolis, MN: Creative Health Care Management; 2018.
7. Olson G. Exactly what is "shared governance"? Chronicle of Higher Education. June 23, 2009. Available at: https://www.chronicle.com/article/Exactly-What-Is-Shared/47065.

Chapter 39: Inclusion

1. Liswood L. The loudest duck: moving beyond diversity while embracing differences to achieve success at work. Hoboken, NJ: Wiley; 2011.
2. Holmes K. Mismatch: how inclusion shapes design. Cambridge, MA: The MIT Press; 2018.

3. Heath T. Perspective: Lisa Wardell walked into a meeting with 14 white, male bankers—and she ran the room. March 22, 2019. Available at: https://www.washingtonpost.com/business/economy/a-black-woman-walks-into-a-meeting-with-14-white-male-bankers--and-runs-the-room/2019/03/22/53b04ff4-4bf4-11e9-93d0-64dbcf38ba41_story.html. Accessed March 22, 2019
4. Duhigg C. What Google learned from its quest to build the perfect team. The New York Times. Available at: https://www.nytimes.com/2016/02/28/magazine/what-google-learned-from-its-quest-to-build-the-perfect-team.html. Accessed February 25, 2016.
5. Lencioni P. The five dysfunctions of a team: a leadership fable. San Francisco, CA: Jossey-Bass; 2002.
6. Eberhardt JL. Biased: uncovering the hidden prejudice that shapes what we see, think, and do. New York: Viking; 2019.
7. Kanigel R. The diversity style guide. Hoboken, NJ: Wiley; 2019.
8. Wharton. Diversity isn't enough: cultivating a sense of belonging at work. 2019. Available at: http://knowledge.wharton.upenn.edu/article/belonging-at-work/.
9. Gostick A, Elton C. The best team wins: the new science of high performance. New York: Simon & Schuster; 2018. p 5.
10. Bourke J, Espedido A. Why inclusive leaders are good for organizations, and how to become one. 2019. Available at: https://hbr.org/2019/03/why-inclusive-leaders-are-good-for-organizations-and-how-to-become-one?utm_medium=email&utm_source=newsletter_weekly&utm_campaign=insider_activesubs&utm_content=signinnudge&referral=03551.

Chapter 40: Innovation

1. Idea to value. Available at: https://www.ideatovalue.com/inno/nickskillicorn/2016/03/innovation-15-experts-share-innovation-definition/#anal. Accessed July 28, 2019.
2. Crenshaw JT, Yoder-Wise PS. Creating an environment for innovation: the risk-taking leadership competency. *Nurse Leader.* 2013;11:24-7.
3. Anthony SD. Build an innovation engine in 90 days. *Harv Bus Rev.* 2014;60-8.
4. Hill LA, Brandeau G, Truelove E, Lineback K. Collective genius. *Harv Bus Rev.* 2014:94-102.
5. Yoder-Wise PS. Creating wise forecasts for nursing: the Wise Forecast Model©. *J Continuing Educ Nurs.* 2011;42:387.
6. Sawhney M, Khosla S. Managing yourself: where to look for insight. *Harv Bus Rev.* 2014:126-9.
7. Ancona D, Gregersen H. The power of leaders who focus on solving problems. 2018. Available at: https://hbr.org/2018/04/the-power-of-leaders-who-focus-on-solving-problems. Accessed March 19, 2019.
8. Innovation Resource Consulting group. Available at: https://www.innovationresource.com/innovation-skills/.
9. Bahcall S. Loonshots. New York: St. Martin's Press; 2019.
10. Bahcall S. The innovation equation: the most important variables are structural, not cultural. *Harv Bus Rev.* 2019: 74-81.
11. Kim SJ, Park M. Leadership, knowledge sharing, and creativity: the key factors in nurses' innovative behaviors. *J Nurs Adm.* 2015;45:615-21.
12. Pisano G. The hard truth about innovative cultures. *Harv Bus Rev.* 2019:62-71.
13. Stilgenbauer DJ, Fitzpatrick JJ. Levels of innovativeness among nurse leaders in acute care hospitals. *J Nurs Adm.* 2019;49:150-5.

Chapter 41: Politics

1. Jarrett M. The four types of organization politics. Harvard Business Review. April 24, 2017. Available at: https://hbr.org/2017/04/the-4-types-of-organizational-politics.
2. Wroblewski M. The impact of power and politics in organizational productivity. November 14, 2018. Available at: https://smallbusiness.chron.com/impact-power-politics-organizational-productivity-35942.html.
3. French JRP Jr, Raven B. The bases of social power. In: Cartwright D, editor. Studies in social power. Ann Arbor (MI): Institute for Social Research; 1959.
4. Quimby M. Using your power for good. The Strategic Thinker. 2019. Available at: https://thesystemsthinker.com/organizational-politics-using-your-power-for-good/.
5. Prestia A, Sherman R, Demezier C. Chief Nursing Officers' experiences with moral distress. *J Nurs Adm.* 2017;7:101-7.
6. Jones B. First impressions. Psychology Today. 2019. Available at: https://www.psychologytoday.com/us/basics/first-impressions.
7. Gleeson P. Power, influence & politics in the workplace. February 4, 2019. Available at: https://smallbusiness.chron.com/impact-power-politics-organizational-productivity-35942.html.

Chapter 42: Processes

1. Henshall A. How to use the Deming cycle for continuous quality improvement. December 1, 2017. Available at: https://www.process.st/deming-cycle/.
2. McDonald KM, Sundaram V, Bravata D, et al. Care coordination (Vo. 7) closing the quality gap: a critical analysis of quality improvement strategies. Technical Reviews, no. 9.7, report no. 04(07)-0051-7, June 2007. Available at: https://www.ncbi.nlm.nih.gov/books/NBK44008/.
3. Feeley D. The triple aim or the quadruple aim. Institute for Healthcare Improvement Blog. November 28, 2017. Available at: http://www.ihi.org/communities/blogs/the-triple-aim-or-the-quadruple-aim-four-points-to-help-set-your-strategy.
4. Bodenheimer T, Sinsky C. From triple to quadruple aim: care of the patient requires care of the provider. *Ann Fam Med.* 2014;12:573-6.
5. Gergen Barnett KA. In pursuit of the fourth aim in health care: the joy of practice. *Med Clin North Am.* 2017;10:1031-40.

Chapter 43: Relationships

1. Merriam-Webster. Definition of "relationship." Available at: https://www.merriam-webster.com/.
2. Lencioni P. The five dysfunctions of a team: a leadership fable. San Francisco: Jossey Bass; 2002.
3. Kos B. Relationship circles—the most important diagram of your life. 2018. Available at: https://agileleanlife.com/relationship-ircles/. Accessed August 27, 2018.
4. Manthy M. Relationship-based care: a model for transforming practice. Minneapolis, MN: Creative Health Care Management; 2004.
5. Sias PM. Organizing relationships: tradition and emerging perspectives on workplace relationships. Thousand Oaks, CA: SAGE Publications; 2009.
6. Garfinkle J. Building positive relationships at work. 2018. Available at: https://garfinkleexecutivecoaching.com/articles/build-positive-work-relationships/building-positive-relationships-at-work.

Chapter 44: Strategy

1. SHRM. Understanding organization structure. Society of Human Resources Management Blog. Available at: https://www.shrm.org/resourcesandtools/tools-and-samples/toolkits/pages/understandingorganizationalstructures.aspx. Accessed April 2020.
2. Cambridge Dictionary. Definition of "strategy." Available at: https://dictionary.cambridge.org/dictionary/english/strategy. Accessed May 30, 2020.
3. Watkins MD. Demystifying strategy: the what, who, how, and why. Harvard Business Review. 2007. Available at: https://hbr.org/2007/09/demystifying-strategy-the-what. Accessed March 2007.
4. Harvard Business Review. HBR guide to thinking strategically. Boston: Harvard Business Review Press; 2019.
5. Schiemann W. Aligning performance management with organizational strategy, values and goals. In: Smither J, Manuel L, editors. Performance management: putting research into action. San Francisco: Josey-Boss; 2009.
6. Kanter R. Managing yourself: zoom in, zoom out. Harvard Business Review. 2011. Available at: https://hbr.org/2011/03/managing-yourself-zoom-in-zoom-out.

Chapter 45: Structure

1. Johnson S. The effects of organizational structure on behavior. Houston Chronical Blog. 2019. Available at: https://smallbusiness.chron.com/effects-organizational-structure-behavior-65759.html.
2. Bahcall S. Loonshots: how to nurture the crazy ideas that win wars, cur diseases, and transform industries. New York: St. Martin's Press/ Macmillan Press; 2019.
3. Root GN. The impact of organizational structure on productivity. Houston Chronical blog. 2019. Available at: http://smallbuisness.chron.com/impact-organization-structure-productivity-21902.htm.
4. Sherman F. The effects of an organizational structure on employee motivation. May 29, 2019. Bizfluent Blog. Available at: https://bizfluent.com/list-7486634-effects-organizational-structure-employee-motivation.html Accessed April 2020.
5. Sinek S. Why good leaders make you feel safe. Available at: https://www.ted.com/talks/simon_sinek_why_good_leaders_make_you_feel_safe.

Chapter 46: Exiting

1. Petriglieri G. How to leave a job we love. Harvard Business Review. November 15, 2018. Available at: https://hbr.org/2018/11/how-to-leave-a-job-you-love.
2. Doyle A. Top ten things not to say or do if you are fired. Career Advisor. The Balance Careers. January 6, 2019. Available at: https://www.thebalancecareers.com/top-things-not-to-say-or-do-if-you-re-fired-2063942.
3. Silver M, Pang NC, Williams SA. "Why give up something that works so well?" Retirement expectations among academic physicians. *Educ Gerontol.* 2015;41:333-47.
4. Potocnink K, Tordera N. The influence of the early retirement process on satisfaction with early retirement and psychological wellbeing. *Int J Aging Hum Dev.* 2010;70:251-73.
5. The Council for Disability. The emotional stages of retirement. Council for Disability Blog. May 23, 2016. Available at: https://blog.disabilitycanhappen.org/the-emotional-stages-of-retirement/.
6. Riggion R. Are you psychologically ready to retire? Four critical questions you need to ask yourself before making this decision. Psychology Today. January 9, 2015. Available at: https://www.psychologytoday.com/us/blog/cutting-edge-leadership/201501/are-you-psychologically-ready-retire.
7. Jayson S. Are you afraid to retire: recognize the emotional fear factors to make the leap. AARP. October 31, 2017. Available at: https://www.aarp.org/retirement/planning-for-retirement/info-2017/.
8. Weston M. Leadership transitions: ensuring success. *Nurse Lead.* 2018;16:304-7.
9. Conley C. Wisdom at work: why the modern elder is relevant. Knowledge @ Wharton. http://knowledge.wharton.upenn.edu/article/wisdom-workplace-modern-elder-relevant.

Conclusion

1. A-Z Quotes. Available at: https://www.azquotes.com/quote/365726. Accessed April 18, 2020.

INDEX

Page numbers followed by "*f*" indicate figures, "*t*" indicate tables.